AF291430

ADVANCED METHODS IN BIOMEDICAL SIGNAL PROCESSING AND ANALYSIS

ADVANCED METHODS IN BIOMEDICAL SIGNAL PROCESSING AND ANALYSIS

Edited by

KUNAL PAL

SAMIT ARI

ARINDAM BIT

SAUGAT BHATTACHARYYA

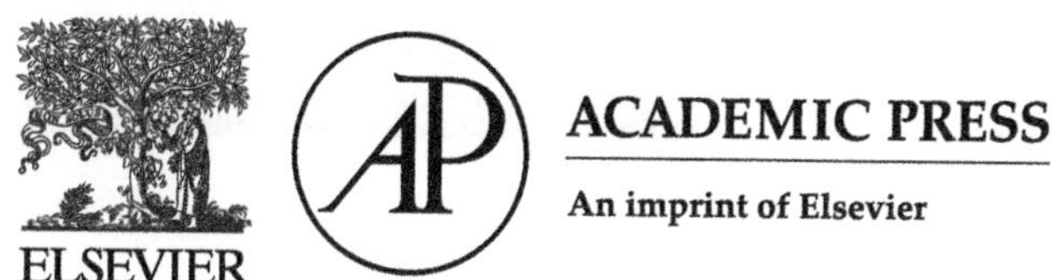

ACADEMIC PRESS

An imprint of Elsevier

Academic Press is an imprint of Elsevier
125 London Wall, London EC2Y 5AS, United Kingdom
525 B Street, Suite 1650, San Diego, CA 92101, United States
50 Hampshire Street, 5th Floor, Cambridge, MA 02139, United States
The Boulevard, Langford Lane, Kidlington, Oxford OX5 1GB, United Kingdom

Copyright © 2023 Elsevier Inc. All rights reserved.

No part of this publication may be reproduced or transmitted in any form or by any means, electronic or mechanical, including photocopying, recording, or any information storage and retrieval system, without permission in writing from the publisher. Details on how to seek permission, further information about the Publisher's permissions policies and our arrangements with organizations such as the Copyright Clearance Center and the Copyright Licensing Agency, can be found at our website: www.elsevier.com/permissions.

This book and the individual contributions contained in it are protected under copyright by the Publisher (other than as may be noted herein).

Notices
Knowledge and best practice in this field are constantly changing. As new research and experience broaden our understanding, changes in research methods, professional practices, or medical treatment may become necessary.

Practitioners and researchers must always rely on their own experience and knowledge in evaluating and using any information, methods, compounds, or experiments described herein. In using such information or methods they should be mindful of their own safety and the safety of others, including parties for whom they have a professional responsibility.

To the fullest extent of the law, neither the Publisher nor the authors, contributors, or editors, assume any liability for any injury and/or damage to persons or property as a matter of products liability, negligence or otherwise, or from any use or operation of any methods, products, instructions, or ideas contained in the material herein.

ISBN 978-0-323-85955-4

For information on all Academic Press publications
visit our website at https://www.elsevier.com/books-and-journals

Publisher: Mara Conner
Acquisitions Editor: Tim Pitts
Editorial Project Manager: Fernanda A. Oliveira
Production Project Manager: Kamesh Ramajogi
Cover Designer: Miles Hitchen

Typeset by STRAIVE, India

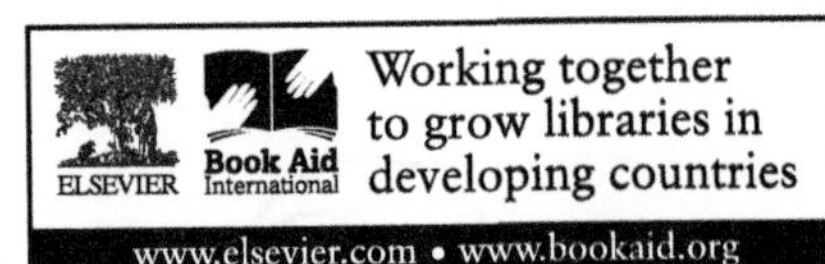

Contents

Chavali Ravikanth, Bikash K. Pradhan, Deepti Bharti, Angana Sarkar, Ananya Barui, Preetam Sarkar, Satyapriya Mohanty, and Kunal Pal

Contributors

Jaya Prakash Allam Department of Electronics and Communication Engineering, National Institute of Technology Rourkela, Rourkela, Odisha, India

Arfat Anis Department of Chemical Engineering, King Saud University, Riyadh, Saudi Arabia

Samit Ari Department of Electronics and Communication Engineering, National Institute of Technology Rourkela, Rourkela, Odisha, India

B. Arya Bio-signals and Medical Instrumentation Laboratory, Department of Biotechnology and Medical Engineering, National Institute of Technology Rourkela, Odisha, India

Indranil Banerjee Department of Bioscience and Bioengineering, Indian Institute of Technology, Jodhpur, India

Ananya Barui Center of Healthcare Science and Technology, Indian Institute of Engineering Science and Technology, Shibpur, India

Deepti Bharti Department of Biotechnology and Medical Engineering, National Institute of Technology, Rourkela, India

Saugat Bhattacharyya Ulster University, Londonderry, United Kingdom

M. Boreyko Glushkov Institute for Cybernetics of National Academy of Science of Ukraine, Kyiv, Ukraine

Pranjali Borkar Molecular Medicine Laboratory, Department of Microbiology, AIIMS, Bhopal, India

I. Chaikovsky Glushkov Institute for Cybernetics of National Academy of Science of Ukraine, Kyiv, Ukraine

Sumit Chakravarty Department of Electrical Engineering, Kennesaw State University, Marietta, GA, United States

Rashmi Chowdhary Department of Biochemistry, AIIMS, Bhopal, India

B. Dhananjay Bio-signals and Medical Instrumentation Laboratory, Department of Biotechnology and Medical Engineering, National Institute of Technology Rourkela, Odisha, India

Zahra Emrani Medical Image and Signal Processing Research Center, Isfahan University of Medical Sciences, Isfahan, Iran

Mahnaz Etehadtavakol Department of Medical Physics, School of Medicine; Poursina Hakim Digestive Diseases Research Center, Isfahan University of Medical Sciences, Isfahan, Iran

Yu. Frolov Glushkov Institute for Cybernetics of National Academy of Science of Ukraine, Kyiv, Ukraine

A. Kazmirchuk National Military Medical Clinical Center "GVKG", Kyiv, Ukraine

Chen Liu Sun Yat-Sen University, Guangzhou, China

Manoja K. Majhi Department of Biotechnology and Medical Engineering, National Institute of Technology, Rourkela, India

Anvita Gupta Malhotra Molecular Medicine Laboratory, Department of Microbiology, AIIMS, Bhopal, India

Satyapriya Mohanty Department of Cardiothoracic and Vascular Surgery, All India Institute of Medical Sciences (AIIMS), Bhubaneswar, India

Suraj K. Nayak Department of Biotechnology and Medical Engineering, National Institute of Technology, Rourkela, India

I. Nedayvoda Glushkov Institute for Cybernetics of National Academy of Science of Ukraine, Kyiv, Ukraine

E.Y.K. Ng School of Mechanical and Aerospace Engineering, College of Engineering, Nanyang Technological University, Singapore, Singapore

Kunal Pal Department of Biotechnology and Medical Engineering, National Institute of Technology, Rourkela, India

Anton Popov Electronic Engineering Department, Igor Sikorsky Kyiv Polytechnic Institute, Kyiv, Ukraine

Bikash K. Pradhan Department of Biotechnology and Medical Engineering, National Institute of Technology, Rourkela, India

M. Primin Glushkov Institute for Cybernetics of National Academy of Science of Ukraine, Kyiv, Ukraine

Saeed Mian Qaisar Electrical and Computer Engineering Department; Communication and Signal Processing Lab, Energy and Technology Research Center, Effat University, Jeddah, Saudi Arabia

Chavali Ravikanth Department of Biotechnology and Medical Engineering, National Institute of Technology, Rourkela, India

Haider Raza University of Essex, Colchester, United Kingdom

Deepak K. Sahu Department of Biotechnology and Medical Engineering, National Institute of Technology, Rourkela, India

Saunak Samantray Department of ETC, IIIT Bhubaneswar, Odisha, India

Angana Sarkar Department of Biotechnology and Medical Engineering, National Institute of Technology, Rourkela, India

Preetam Sarkar Department of Biotechnology and Medical Engineering, National Institute of Technology, Rourkela, India

Sarman Singh Molecular Medicine Laboratory, Department of Microbiology, AIIMS, Bhopal, India

J. Sivaraman Bio-signals and Medical Instrumentation Laboratory, Department of Biotechnology and Medical Engineering, National Institute of Technology Rourkela, Odisha, India

N. Prasanna Venkatesh Bio-signals and Medical Instrumentation Laboratory, Department of Biotechnology and Medical Engineering, National Institute of Technology Rourkela, Odisha, India

Slawomir Wilczynski Department of Basic Biomedical Sciences, Medical University of Silesia, Katowice, Poland

Feature engineering methods

Anton Popov

Electronic Engineering Department, Igor Sikorsky Kyiv Polytechnic Institute, Kyiv, Ukraine

1. Machine learning projects development standards and feature engineering

Feature Engineering is a set of actions devoted to preparation of the raw data collected from the objects under investigation to the use by algorithms of automated analysis. The steps in feature engineering are the following:

1. *Exploratory data analysis and data preprocessing*— understanding the quality and quantity of the input data and preparing it for further use.
2. *Feature extraction*—converting the available data into descriptive features.
3. *Feature reduction* by either selection of useful features or reducing the dimensionality of the feature vector to keep only the valuable features for further use.

Projects related to machine learning are being developed according to common practices which are formalized in a form of standards and frameworks. One of the most popular one is called CRISP-DM [1]: cross-industry standard process in data mining. It was developed in 1997, and since then it has a wide application in many domains where machine learning is used in data analysis for real applications. The CRISP-DM workflow is presented in Fig. 1.

The process of machine learning model development starts with understanding the business domain and formulating the problem which should be solved. This problem is associated with data and ultimately should be solved using the data available. Then starts the first stage of the Feature Engineering process: Data Understanding and exploration. After the characteristics of data are available and it is clear what it is possible to do with them, engineers start preparing the data for training the models. In terms of

Advanced Methods in Biomedical Signal Processing and Analysis. https://doi.org/10.1016/B978-0-323-85955-4.00004-1
Copyright © 2023 Elsevier Inc. All rights reserved.

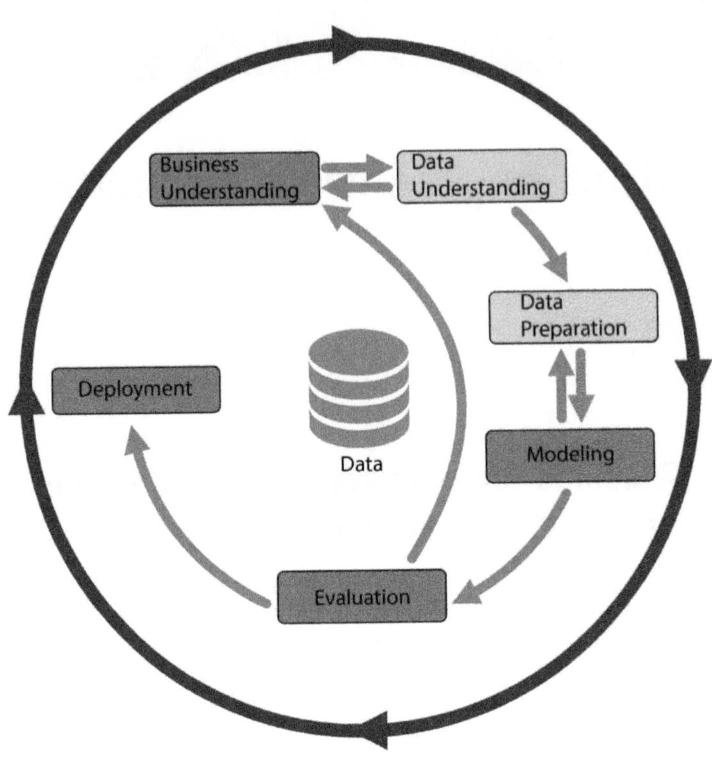

Fig. 1 CRISP-DM process diagram. Stages of feature engineering highlighted in *green* (gray in the print version). (For interpretation of the references to color in this figure legend, the reader is referred to the web version of this article.)

Feature Engineering, the stages of data processing, feature extraction and feature reduction are implemented and they constitute the Data Preparation stage. Then the features are ready for model training and evaluation of their performance. This CRISP-DM stage either finishes the process, if business goals are achieved, or it requires another iteration of requirements clarification from the business perspective, and then walking through the data preparation, feature extraction and reduction, model training and evaluation. So, feature engineering is embedded in the standard process of machine learning models development, and distributed across its two stages: Data Understanding and Data Preparation.

Same is valid for other existing data science project development frameworks, such as KDD and SEMMA [2]—every project has the stages related to data exploration, extraction and preparation of features.

2. Exploratory data analysis

Every investigation of either a single patient visiting the doctor, or a large cohort of multicentral clinical studies starts from collecting a lot of raw data from participating subjects. This data is collected in different forms, such as text, electrophysiological measurements, introscopy results, etc., and is devoted to the aim of supporting the clinical decision [3]. Before supplying the collected data into the automated decision support system based on machine learning, one needs to assure the quality and operability of this data. This is done at the first stage of Feature Engineering: Exploratory Data Analysis (EDA) [4,5]. EDA is aimed at helping the research engineer to look at the data and improve it, before making any assumption about the object or process under investigation.

EDA is a set of actions for the first analysis of collected data, summarization of its characteristics and getting insights of the required preparation of the data for further use in machine learning algorithms. The aim of EDA is the understanding the data and planning of its preparation for further use. To that aim, the research engineer should first understand what types of data are available, what is their quality, and how to improve it. During EDA the research engineer understands the variables which are available, cleans the dataset to get rid of the possible noise and artifacts or unnecessary variables, and analyses the relationships between the variables. Also, the understanding of the amount of data is gained during EDA, and the strategy and limitations of the model training is supplemented with the knowledge of the data available.

2.1 Types of input data

Everything we know about the object or process under analysis, should be turned into data. Data is the representation of our object of interest, and it is used for formalizing our knowledge about it. Depending on which characteristics of the object are of interest, the corresponding types of data should be extracted. Then we need to transform them into features for further processing. Also, sometimes we want to convert one type of data to another, which better fits to extracting features and doing machine learning.

Classification of data types can be implemented in many ways [6]. For the tasks of feature engineering it is useful to define the data types based on the types of mathematical operations which one can apply to the data. For example, for such information as gender, tumor location, eye color, or type of disease, only the comparison operation is allowed (equal/nonequal), and it is not possible to define which value is larger or smaller. This type of data is called *nominal*.

If we have a stage of disease (I, II, and III), pain level (no pain, mild, moderate, severe), etc., they could be arranged in some natural order. With such data, not only equality can be defined, but also we can tell which is larger or lower; this is *ordinal* data type. Finally, we can have *numerical* data, which can take any value, either continuous (e.g., weight and high of the subject, dimensions of the region in the CT image, blood pressure, etc.) or discrete (days of treatment duration, age, number of subjects in a group).

Separate types of numerical data are the signals of different types. First, these could be time series, which is the ordered sequence of values obtained in the result of measuring some process. The example is the electrocardiogram (ECG) recording—the result of the measurement of voltage difference on the body emerged due to the electrical activity of the heart. ECG is the samples of digitized values of this voltage recorded with a certain time interval. Second type of numerical signals are images, which are two-dimensional data recorded from the area of the object. The example is an X-ray image—the distribution of the intensity of the X-rays passed through the patient's body. This image can be continuous (when present on the special film), or discrete (when measured in a digital form with the matrix of X-ray detectors).

Another special type of the data is text, e.g., description of the patient state in the electronic records. This can be used for automated extraction of the meaningful information which is not presented with standard nominal or ordinal data, but rather is explained in various words by many authors. To process the text, operations such as stemming, lemmatization, and tokenization are applied first, and then the words are encoded to numerically represent text.

In biomedical applications, all types of data are used and are represented in various formats [7], and often the machine learning algorithms need to use the data of different types and even modalities. For example, logistic regression can use continuous data about heart rate and ECG time-magnitude characteristics as input, and the class of severity (ordinal values) as output. Or deep neural networks can use time series of the measurement of vital signs and accelerometry data from wearable device in addition to the age of a subject and time of the day, to define the level of fatigue. Despite the various nature of data and different types, often the data values are converted and coded into numerical values for more convenient representation in machine learning models. But the researcher should be careful in interpreting these values. For example, if we code the eye color $1=$ "brown," $2=$ "blue," $3=$ "gray," the numerical values 1, 2, 3 do not have any mathematical meaning. We cannot say that $3>2$, because nominal values are not subject to more or less operations. Also, when extracting the statistical features from the nominal data, only the *mode* value (most probable value) can be defined, but not mean value.

2.2 Data preparation and preprocessing

Before describing the methods of EDA, lets introduce some important definitions. First, we will call a *variable* the quantitative or qualitative property which we measure. For example, age, eye color, type of diabetes, blood sugar level, systolic and diastolic pressure, are all the variables of different types which we can obtain during measurements. Each variable when we measure it takes a state, which we will call the *value*. So when we do the experiments and collect the data, we will measure values of the variables from every subject. Finally, we will call an *observation* (or the data point, data sample, data instance) the set of values of different variables measured for each particular subject. The observation is the instance of the dataset. It will contain the set of the values, each describing the variables collected for each subject.

2.2.1 Missing values treatment

When looking at the data, most obvious problem is when some values of variables are missed. These data points could be not recorded because of failures or experiment design, unspecified, or unknown. The treatment of these missing values depends on the knowledge of the experiment design [8]. Knowing the reasons of the missing data to appear in the dataset can help in decision about the treating the data: how the data was obtained, what is the characteristics of the source? Are there any patterns or regularities in missing data, which can be used as an additional feature of the data source? Finally, can we rely on the dataset with such amount of missing values. Valid question to ask in exploring the data set with missing data, are whether the occurrence of missing values in one variable depends on the other variables, or it is random. Studying the distribution of the missing data occurrences together with other information about the object or process under analysis can give useful insights [9–11].

There are two approaches in treatment the missing values: one can either *drop* the corresponding observations completely from the dataset, or *impute* the missing values somehow. Also, depending on the amount of the missing data and the potential impact on the analysis results, one can decide to postpone the analysis until more data is collected.

Removing samples with missing values. In case we found that the occurrence of missing data is random, and its fraction is small, it is safe to just remove the samples containing missing values in one variable from the dataset.

Encoding as "missing." If we suspect that missing *categorical* values occurred not in a complete random manner, and there might be useful to know that particular value is not available, it is possible to introduce new category in the variable (missing), and use it in further analysis.

Imputation. In case we would like to have some values instead of missing values of the variables, we can impute it [12]. The simplest approach is to substitute the missing values with the mean or median of the nonmissing values. For categorical variables, one can impute the most common category instead of missing one, or chose one of the category from the available categories by sampling procedure.

Predicting missing values. If we see that the missing values occurred not in random manner, but their behavior may be explained by other variables, the strategy could be to calculate the missing values in one variable from the values of other variables with the prediction model. If relations between variables exists, the prediction can provide reliable estimates of the missing values to impute in the dataset [13]. The simple approach could be using the regression models for numerical variables, or logistic regression for categorical variables.

2.2.2 Encoding the categorical variables

If dataset contains categorical variables, their values should be converted into numerical values during preprocessing [14,15].

The simplest case is binary categorical values which can be encoded either as 0 or 1 (e.g., "healthy"/"disease") or -1 and 1.

For categorical variables taking more than two possible values, we have two cases: ordinal and nominal.

In case of ordinal categorical variable, e.g., having some state of a subject coded with the letters A to D, we have ranked values. So we can just encode each value with the *integer number*, from 1 to 4 in our example.

In case on nominal categorical values, they do not have any quantitative relations between each other, so if we encode them with the sequence of number, that might cause the unwanted fictional ordinal relationship. To avoid this, the *one-hot-encoding* procedure is used [16].

First, one need to calculate the number N of the unique values of nominal variable. In the previous case, (letters from A to D), there are four values. Then, each instance of the variable for each subject will be encoded as a vector with dimension 4. Each coordinate of the vector is binary (0 or 1), and will encode the corresponding value:

$$
\begin{aligned}
A &: \quad [1 \quad 0 \quad 0 \quad 0] \\
B &: \quad [0 \quad 1 \quad 0 \quad 0] \\
C &: \quad [0 \quad 0 \quad 1 \quad 0] \\
D &: \quad [0 \quad 0 \quad 0 \quad 1]
\end{aligned}
$$

In that way, the nominal categorical variable with four values (A, B, C, or D) is encoded as the sparse vector with mostly zeroes, and 1 in one coordinate.

2.2.3   Investigation of the data distribution

After all the data is converted into numerical values, one can proceed with the exploration of the characteristics of the available dataset. One important characteristic which helps to understand the appearance of data and plan further feature extraction and analysis, is the distribution of the variables values [4,17].

For categorical values, the data distribution is the range of values and the frequency (or relative frequency) of the occurrence of each category, often presented in a table.

If the data are numerical, first step is to visualize them by plotting the histogram. This can provide first impression of the range and relative quantity of the variable values. To describe the distribution, we can calculate the center, spread, modality, and shape, as well as the presence of outliers.

It is important to remember that what we have as the dataset, is called sample distribution in statistical analysis. If one repeats the same process of data collection many times, the particular values of the variable will be different, due to selection of the random realization of the underlying processes of data generation. We can use the sample statistics as characteristics of the general population only in case we can accept the assumption of stationarity and (in some cases) ergodicity. And we should recognize the fact that if such assumptions barely hold at least for one variable, not only the description of the dataset may be not correct, but also the generalization ability of the algorithms trained with machine learning may be jeopardized.

If we can accept the assumption about the repeatability of the experiments, it is safe to measure *sample statistics* to describe the variables based on the available data.

To understand where on the numeric scale the values are located, one can estimate the *central tendency* of the distribution, by sample (arithmetic) *mean* value. Also, if there is no prominent center in the distribution, the *median* value can be defined, which as the middle value after all the values are arranged in ascending order. Median is preferred if the distribution appears to be skewed, or there are many outliers.

The *spread* of the distribution can show how far away from the center the data are scattered. It can be measured by variance, standard deviation, or inter-quartile range. *Variance* is the average of the squared deviations of each value from the mean value, and the *standard deviation* is the squared root of the variance.

Another useful measure of the distribution spread is the *inter-quartile range* (IQR) visualized using boxplot [18] (Fig. 2). Quartiles of the distribution are the three values (Q1, Q2, and Q3) which divide the distribution into four parts, so in each part there is the same number of values: one fourth of the values are less than Q1, one fourth lies between Q1 and Q2, one fourth is between Q2 and Q3, and the last 25% of values are larger than Q3. Depending on the variable distribution, the quartiles may have different values and be close to each other (in case of very narrow distribution) or be apart (if the distribution is flat). The Q2 value is the same as median value.

IQR is the difference between Q3 and Q1. From definition of quartiles, the 50% of values will fall within the IQR. If it is large, the distribution is quite spread, and vice versa: for very narrow distribution IQR is small. IQR is quite robust characteristic of the distribution. If there occur some very large or small outlier values at the tails, this will almost not affect the IQR. If the distribution is normal, then IQR is approximately 4/3 of the standard deviation.

Additionally, there are two more parameters of the distribution: skewness and kurtosis. *Skewness* measured the degree of the asymmetry in the distribution with respect to the mean value. *Kurtosis* is the measure of the "peakedness"—the tendency of the data to group more around the mean value than the normally distributed data with the same variance would do.

2.2.4 Binning

If the variable takes continuous numerical values, before plotting the histograms we need to bin the values into groups [19]. Bins are the ranges of variable values to be represented as one group: all values falling within one bin will be treated together as a group. There are plenty methods of selecting the bin number [20],

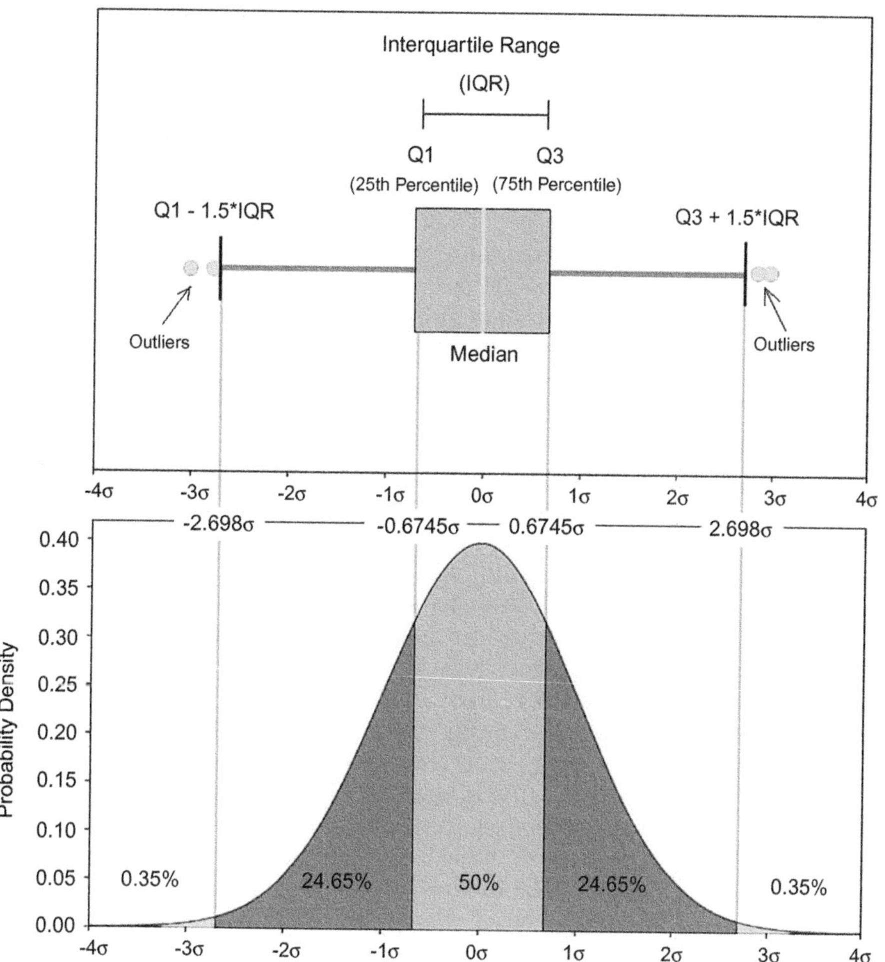

Fig. 2 Boxplot with the explained quantiles, and its corresponding normal distribution.

depending on the properties of the distribution and the need of the analysis.

Another application of binning in EDA and feature extraction is the creation of the categories. For example, we might want to predict the treatment outcome for subjects of different age. For that, we have to collect the dataset containing the outcomes for lot of subjects, and ideally we would want each age to be represented equally. This is often hard to achieve, but we can apply binning of the age and create age groups, e.g., pediatric (0–14 years old), youth (15–47 years old), middle-age (48–63 years old), and elderly (more than 64 years old). If we accept such binning, the number of data samples to collect should be equal per each group, not per each particular age.

2.2.5 Identifying and treatment of outliers

When we look at the variable, it is often possible to spot the tendency in its values for the dataset. The values can increase or decrease, or oscillate around some level, or group into clusters. Because of noise in measurements, there would be deviations from the tendency and grouping, but most of the data points will probably follow it. But there could be some particular datapoints which deviate substantially from the rest of the values. Such significant deviation may either be an extreme value of noisy sample, or it can be an anomaly in the data. Such an observation which appears far away from the rest of points is called *outlier* [21]. The outliers can be separated into noise and anomalies, but there is no definite way to distinguish between those; for every analysis identifying outliers is subjective. It is practical to consider as *outliers* the values which deviate from the rest significantly larger compared to the noisy values. So, outliers are anomalies larger than noise.

Outliers can emerge due to data entry or measurement errors, experiment design or sampling errors or be intentional. Such outliers have to be removed. Also, there could be natural outliers, meaning that in the underlying process which generates the variable, there could be rare values which substantially differ from the most of the values. That case requires thorough investigation and special treatment, such as collecting larger dataset, changes in the analysis strategy, or usage of the different data models.

Outliers can be broadly classified into three categories:

- *Point anomalies (global outliers)*—they are values which are different from the rest of the data,
- *Contextual or conditional outliers*—may be identified as outliers only in certain conditions, for example when comparing with the neighboring samples in the time series. If surrounding samples have similar values, the sample is considered normal, if the same sample appears surrounded by much smaller or larger values, it is considered as the contextual outlier,
- *Group or collective outliers*—is a group of values which is isolated from the rest of the data.

Outliers can increase the error variance and reduce the power of statistical tests, decrease data normality and bias the estimates of the data models. Therefore, in many cases it is desirable to remove the outliers from the dataset.

First, outliers should be detected, and there are two basic approaches:

- treat any value beyond the range of -1.5 IQR to 1.5 IQR as outlier and
- treat any values beyond certain number of standard deviations from the mean as outlier using the thresholding of the z-scored values.

There is a number of more formal outlier tests [22–24], which can be grouped by the assumptions of data distribution (normal/nonnormal), ability to detect single or multiple outliers, and if the test is for multiple outliers, should the number of outliers be specified beforehand exactly or as the upper boundary. Most common tests assume the normally distributed data, and are based on the concept "how far is the value from the mean." Grubb's test is recommended for single outlier detection, with Tietjen–Moore test generalized to more than one outlier. The generalized (extreme Studentized deviate) ESD test is used to detect one or more outliers.

After detecting outliers, they should be either removed or substituted with the new value. Essentially the procedure is the same as in case of treatment of missing values, and the appropriate approach can be used in this case.

Outlier analysis also can be a separate task for machine learning [25,26], which is called anomaly detection or novelty detection. It is applied not for the single value of the variable, but to the whole observation (characterized by many variables), to understand if the data sample is anomaly or not. In most cases, such problem can be posed as unsupervised task, and there are approaches based on probabilistic or linear models, and proximity-based approaches. Also, in case when the examples of outlier data are available, supervised outlier detection can be done. Specific methods exist for detecting outliers in time series and streaming data, in discrete sequences, in spatial data and in graphs and networks. Many methods are available in open-source frameworks [27] and specifically developed for deep learning [28].

2.2.6 Variable transformation

It is often desirable that numerical variables fit into similar ranges of values, e.g., from -1 to 1, from 0 to 1, or from 0 to 100. This is useful in case of machine learning methods employing the notion of distance are used: if the variables lie in the same ranges, their partial contribution in the distance between objects in the feature space is equal. In case if one variable inherently has values which are larger than other variables, its contribution will always be more heavy, and this could bias the decisions based on the distance. To avoid such bias, raw variables should be transformed [29]. On the other hand, we often want our data to be "nicely" distributed across specific range: e.g., have uniform, Poisson, or normal distribution, so we are able to statistically model the variable, or apply any machine learning techniques which assume the data is normally distributed. In case we do not have these properties in a distribution of raw data, we need to apply variable transformations. So, there are two types of variable transformation: scaling, when we change the range spanning by the variable values, and normalizing, when we change the distribution of the values.

2.2.7   Min–max scaling

The simplest method is to convert the values in range from $x_{\min}$ to $x_{\max}$ into the range from 0 to 1 using the following transform:

$$x_{i,\text{new}} = \frac{x_i - x_{\min}}{x_{\max} - x_{\min}}.$$

2.2.8   Logarithm transformation

In case the variable values are distributed nonsymmetrically or not equally across the range, we face the situation of the skewed distribution. Is such case there are more data samples whose values are close to each other in some narrow sub-range, while less data points span larger sub-range. Such distribution may lead to harder distinguishing between those samples from the dense regions, and the good practice is to transform the distribution so the data values span the range more equally. In many cases, the logarithmic transformation is appropriate way to do so. If the variable values are positive, the base 2 logarithm may be applied:

$$x_{i,\text{new}} = \log_2 x_i.$$

In case some values are negative, one can first shift them toward positive range to assure positiveness, and then apply previous expression, or use signed logarithm:

$$x_{i,\text{new}} = \text{sign}(x_i) \cdot \log_2(|x_i| + 1).$$

2.2.9 Centering and scaling

A very common and useful transformation is scaling variables to a common scale. In the result, every variable's values are expressed in the dimensionless "standard deviations away from the mean" standard units. Such transformation is called z-score. Given the variable x with values $x = x_1, x_2, ..., x_n$, centered around zero and scaled to standard deviation variable is:

$$z_i = \frac{x_i - \overline{x}}{SD(x)}$$

where $\overline{x}$ is mean value, and $SD(x)$ is the standard deviation.

In the result of such standardization applied to all variables in the dataset is that they are in the same comparable units and ranges. In case of normal distribution of data, the z-scores lie mainly between -3 and 3.

2.2.10 Box–Cox normalization

It is used to transform nonnormal variable to the normal distribution shape, which allows to apply many techniques of analysis implying normally distributed data. The transformation is performed in the following way:

$$x_{i,\text{new}} = \begin{cases} \dfrac{x_i^\lambda - 1}{\lambda}, & \lambda \neq 0 \\ \log x_i, & \lambda = 0 \end{cases}$$

where λ is the parameter usually in a range from -5 to 5, which is optimized so transformed values fit the normal distribution. In case the variable has both positive and negative values, it should be shifted to ensure positiveness.

3. Data vs features

3.1 Relations between data and features

The topic of feature extraction is covered in the separate chapter of this book, so we will limit ourselves by just brief summary relevant to the feature engineering tasks. The data is considered as the measurable quantities which the engineer directly receives from the object of interest by measurements. The task is to supply these quantities to the machine learning algorithm: either directly without any processing, or after processing and extraction of descriptive features. These features will serve as the representation of the object used by the algorithm [30,31].

Feature extraction usually follows the preprocessing part of the machine learning development pipeline. It starts after the noise, missing values and outliers are removed, the variables are transformed, and the distribution of the data is known.

3.2 Feature extraction methods

Feature extraction methods could be grouped in several ways. Here we mention two of them.

3.2.1 Linear vs nonlinear

Depending on the relations between input and output, the method could be linear or nonlinear. In *linear* feature extraction method, the superposition principle holds. If the input data magnitude becomes larger or smaller, the result of feature extraction also changes proportionally. Also, the features extracted from the sum of two data instances are equal to the sum of features extracted from each data instance separately. The example of the linear feature extraction method is Fourier transform: it is calculated by taking integral, which is linear function. If the signal is multiplied by some factor, the resulting spectrum is also becomes multiplied; the spectrum of the sum of two signals is equal to the sum of two spectra.

In *nonlinear* feature extraction methods, the superposition principle does not hold. The resulting feature is not proportional to the magnitude of the data instance, but depends on the other characteristics of the data. The example is the entropy of the time series (e.g., Shannon entropy): it depends on the predictability of the signal values, and does not depend on the magnitude. Also, entropies are not adding when the signals sum.

3.2.2 Multivariate vs univariate

In *univariate* methods feature is extracted from just one data instance. For example, mean values of the time series could be calculated in the sliding window and serve as feature. It describes the average characteristic of the time series, and requires only this time series. Another example of the univariate feature is spectra or entropy: one needs only one time series to extract them. On the contrary, if one has several data flows coming from the same object, *multivariate* features will describe the joint behavior of this data and require more than one data instance for calculations. For example, correlation coefficient, mutual information, phase synchronization requires two time series to extract a single feature.

3.3 Curse of dimensionality

Using the variety of feature extraction methods, it is possible to extract huge amount of features from the available data. The more features one has for an object of interest, the more characteristics of this object are reflected, and therefore the object is supposed to be described better. Usually each feature is referred to as one *dimension* in the multidimensional space where the object is represented. So when we extract features for the object, it is described as point in feature space with feature values as the coordinates. The more features one has, the higher is the dimensionality of the feature space.

It may seem that the more features are used for training the machine learning algorithm, the better result one should expect. But this is not always true, because if features are extracted from dataset which was collected not is a proper way, the researcher may be cursed by the curse of dimensionality. Comprehensive description of the object is good and promising for machine learning outcomes, but at the same time, the researcher should be cautious when extracting too many features from the dataset of limited size.

Curse of dimensionality refers to a set of problems that arise when training the machine learning models with data represented in high-dimensional feature space [32,33]. As the dimensionality increases, the classifier's performance increases until the optimal number of features is reached. Further increasing the dimensionality without increasing the number of training samples results in a decrease in classifier performance.

Curse of dimensionality consists of two problems:
– Data sparsity.
– Distance concentration.

3.3.1 *Data sparsity*

Machine learning model generalization refers to the models' ability to predict the outcome for an unseen input data accurately. The unseen input data has to come from the same distribution as the one used to train the model. An effective way to build a generalized model is to capture different possible combinations of the values of predictor variables (features) and the corresponding targets. From the data collection perspective, capturing different combinations means that in the training dataset there should be available objects with all possible characteristics, i.e., with all possible combinations of feature values.

So, as the number of dimensions of feature space increases, the number of training samples required to generalize a model also increases phenomenally (Fig. 3).

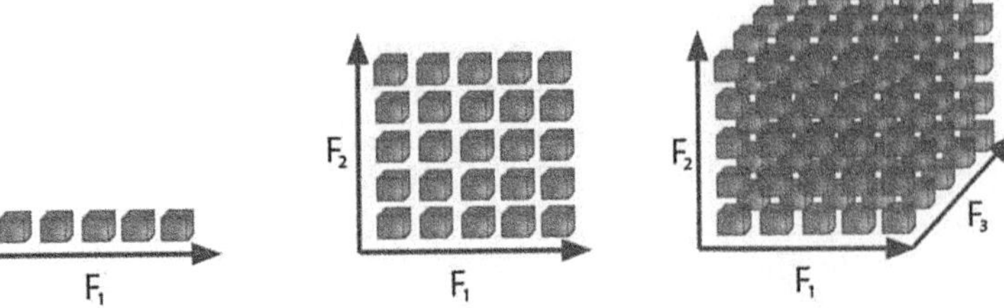

Fig. 3 Illustration of data sparsity. The more dimensions feature space has the more training data is needed to cover the feature range.

In case if the amount of available training samples is limited, they do not represent all possible features combinations for high-dimensional feature space. Such under-representative training dataset is called *sparse*—it does not cover the entire feature space. Training a model with sparse data could lead to high-variance or overfitting condition. This is because while training the model, the model has learnt from the frequently occurring combinations of the attributes and is able to predict them accurately. But the models cannot generalize to understand what should be predicted for other combinations of feature values, which are not presented in the training dataset.

3.3.2 Distance concentration

In feature spaces, mean values of features are mostly in the center of coordinate system due to data normalization. More feature values are usually concentrated around the mean, so concentration of data points is larger closer to the center than more far from the center of coordinates. If we represent the entire feature space as a hypercube, then most of the data will be spanned by the hypersphere with the center in the origin (Fig. 4). When the dimensionality of feature space is low, the volume of the hypersphere is similar to the volume of the hypercube (imagine the circle inscribed inside the square). That means that the data from the hypersphere are distributed almost equally in the hypercube and cover it almost completely. When the dimension increases, the hypersphere where most of the data live, spans less volume of the hypercube which represents all possible feature values (imagine the sphere inscribed in the cube). So more volume of a cube becomes less populated by the data points: the data are mostly around the center of origin. With further increase of dimensionality, the space becomes larger and therefore more training data will reside closer to the corners of the hypercube defining the feature space.

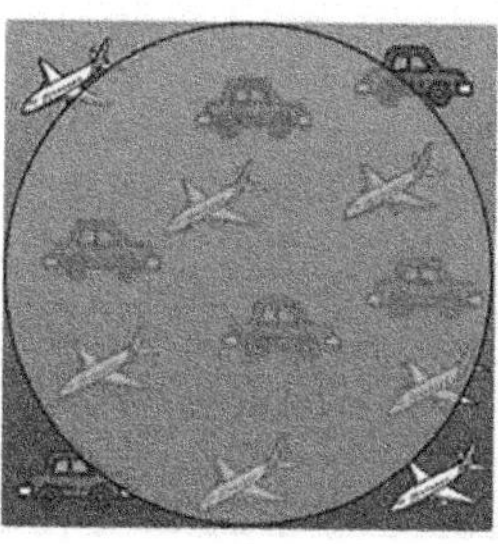 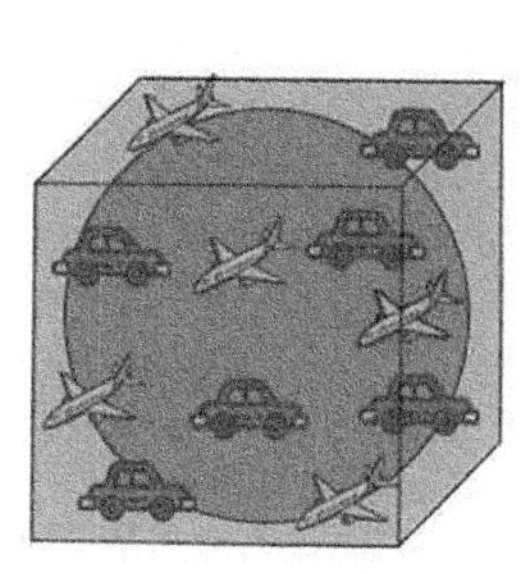 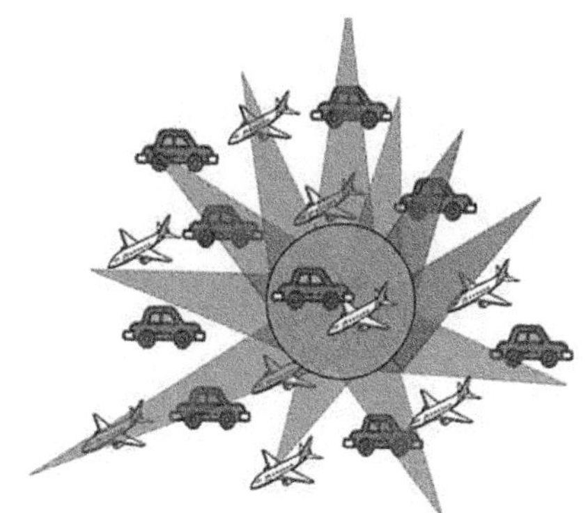

Fig. 4 Data distribution in feature space. With the increase of the dimensionality of the feature space, more data instances appear out of the central hypersphere.

When data points are scattered in the high-dimensional feature space, the distance measures between them start losing their effectiveness to measure dissimilarity. *Distance concentration* refers to the problem of all the pairwise distances between different points in the feature space converging to the same value as the dimensionality of the data increases. Due to distance concentration, the concept of proximity or similarity of the samples may not be qualitatively relevant in higher dimensions. Since classifiers often depend on these distance measures (e.g., Euclidean distance, Mahalanobis distance, Manhattan distance), classification is often easier in lower-dimensional spaces where less features are used to describe the object of interest.

3.3.3 Avoiding the curse of dimensionality

If the amount of available training data is fixed and the number of features is large, then overfitting occurs if we keep adding dimensions. Machine learning model will just remember the data, not learn the characteristics. So more features from limited data do not lead to better accuracy. To avoid this curse, we need to reduce the dimensionality (decrease number of features) while not jeopardizing the quality of machine learning models. There are three ways:
- Removing nondescriptive features,
- Removing redundant features, and
- Changing the feature space to the one with lower dimension.

The cure for avoiding the curse will be prepared in the following sections.

4. Feature reduction

Any data can be converted into features in many different ways, and researchers often use a lot of feature extraction techniques to pull the information which will be useful for machine learning. Since the cost of such feature extraction is low, the amount of features could be overwhelming. But not all features can be equally related to the target variable, so usage of all set if available features is often unnecessary and unwanted. To avoid the curse of dimensionality one needs to reduce the number of features by minimizing the number of features in a dataset [34]. This can be done by retaining the features that contain the most useful information that is needed by the model to make accurate predictions, and also by discarding features that contain little to no information.

Not useful feature can either be
- *redundant* if it contains the same information as another feature and
- *irrelevant* if it does not contain the information about the target.

Reduction of the number of features used in machine learning
- makes models more simple and interpretable,
- reduces model training time,
- reduces overfitting and increases generalization ability, and
- helps to avoid the curse of dimensionality.

There are two ways of **feature reduction**:
1. *Feature selection* is a process of selecting a subset of features that are most relevant for the modeling and business objective of the problem.
2. *Dimensionality reduction* is a process of compressing the large set of the features into the subspace of lower dimension without losing the important information.

5. Feature selection

Feature selection is the process of selecting the subset of available features which is most relevant to the task [35–37]. Feature selection can be performed in two ways:
1. *Unsupervised feature selection* does not use the target value, instead analyses the subsets of features; in this way redundant features can be removed.
2. *Supervised feature selection* takes into account the relation between feature and target variable. In this way irrelevant features can be removed.

5.1 Unsupervised feature selection

Since many available features describe the same object or process, there is a possibility that some features may bear the similar information about the target, instead of characterizing the object of interest from different perspectives. Another possibility is the two features are functionally related to each other, e.g., linearly dependent. If this is the case, usage of both features is redundant and adds unnecessary complexity to the machine learning algorithm. It is enough to use only one feature which contains the required information. To understand if there are any redundant features which can be skipped, the methods of dependency estimation are applied to initial feature set.

One of the simplest ways to understand the dependency between the pair of features, is to calculate the *correlation coefficient* [38]. If the correlation between two features is high, they are linearly dependent, and one of them can be removed.

One more method to quantify the dependency between two features is to calculate the *mutual information* between them [39]:

$$I(X; Y) = \sum_{x} \sum_{y} p(x, y) \log \frac{p(x, y)}{p(x)p(y)}$$

where $p(x)$, $p(y)$ marginal probability distributions of random variables X, Y, $p(x, y)$ joint probability distributions of random variables X, Y.

Mutual information is a quantity that measures a relationship between two random variables that are sampled simultaneously. In particular, it measures how much information is communicated, on average, in one random variable about another.

Another way of selecting the features that can be removed, is the use of *variance inflation factor*. It is the factor by which the variance in one feature is increased (inflated) when there exists the correlation among other features used in the analysis [40]. Large variance inflation factor suggests the existence of multicollinearity between features.

5.2 Supervised feature selection

In supervised feature selection, the target is not ignored, but being used to understand which features are more informative for machine learning.

5.2.1 Exhaustive search

This is the simplest method of supervised feature selection. Exhaustive search starts from creating all possible subsets of available features. Then the machine learning model is trained using each subset of features and its performance is estimated. Finally, the subsets are ranked according to the performance, and the subset yielding highest performance metric is selected for training. The obvious advantage of exhaustive search is that it is sure to find the best combination of features. Unfortunately, the obvious disadvantage is that such grid search over the all possible combinations of features is extremely time consuming, and may even be computationally intractable for all but the smallest of feature sets. Combinations of k features out of n features is defined as:

$$\binom{n}{k} = C_n^k = \frac{n!}{k!(n-k)!},$$

and the total number of possible combinations of $1..n$ out of n is $2^n - 1$. For example, if we have 10 features, the total number of combinations to test during exhaustive search is 1023.

Also, the choice of evaluation metric heavily influences the algorithm, and different subsets may be identified as optimal for different metrics.

5.2.2 Filter methods

Filter method provides another way to use the availability of target information for feature selection. It applies a statistical measure to assign a scoring to each feature based on its relation with target. Then all features are ranked and the most related are selected for model training. Depending of the type of input variable (the feature) and the output variable (the target), different metrics are used to quantify the relations in filter methods:
- If both feature and target are numerical, then Pearson or Spearman correlation coefficients could be used.
- If both feature and target are categorical, chi-squared test or mutual information can be used.
- In case when one variable is numerical, and another one is categorical, ANalysis Of Variance (ANOVA) or Kendall's rank coefficient are applied.

Filter methods are effective in computational time and robust to overfitting. The disadvantage is that it is univariate, and considers each feature independently on the other features. Therefore, filter methods tend to select redundant features because they do not consider the relationship between features.

5.2.3 Wrapper methods

The essence of this category of methods is that the classifier is run on different subsets of features of the original training set. Then a subset of features with the best performance on the training set is selected. General procedure is the following:

1. Prepare various combinations of features.
2. Train the model and evaluate it; then compare to other combinations on the basis of predictive models.
3. Assign score based on the model accuracy.
4. Based on the inference of the previous model, decide add or remove features from the subset.

Wrapper methods are computationally expensive since the model has to be trained and tested on many feature sets, also such feature selection is prone to overfitting.

There are two approaches in this class of methods:

- *inclusion* (forward selection) starts from an empty subset of features, then various features are gradually added and
- *exclusion* (backward selection) starts from the set of all features, and the features are gradually removed from it.

One of the most common wrapper method is *Recursive Feature Elimination* [41]. It works by searching for a subset of features by starting with all features in the training dataset and successfully removing features until the desired number remains. This is achieved by

- fitting the given machine learning algorithm used in the core of the model,
- ranking features by importance,
- discarding the least important features, and
- refitting the model.

This process is repeated until a specified number of features remains.

An important hyperparameter for the Recursive Feature Elimination algorithm is the number of features to select.

5.2.4 Embedded methods

These methods combine the advantages of both Filter and Wrapper methods. Embedded supervised feature selection cam be implemented by the learning algorithms that have their own built-in feature selection methods. The most common type of embedded methods of feature selection methods is regularization methods [42]. Regularization is a fine for the excessive complexity of the model, which reduces the likelihood of overtraining and eliminates signs that do not carry useful information. In case of the embedded methods, the fine is applied to the models with many features, so the models with less number of features are favored.

Different types of regularization are applied depending on the model and task, such as L1 (LASSO regularization), L2 (Ridge regularization), or Elastic nets.

6. Feature dimensionality reduction

6.1 Principal component analysis

One of the most common methods of dimensionality reduction is Principal Component Analysis (PCA) [43]. This is an unsupervised technique to find the new coordinate system in the feature space, by rotating the original coordinate system. In this new coordinate system, the data points may be presented with fewer coordinates without loss of too much information. Therefore, the dimensionality of the new representation of the object will be lower in the new coordinate system than in the previous one (Fig. 5).

To find the new coordinate system and lower dimensionality of feature space, first we need to find the correlation matrix between all N-dimensional feature vectors F_i, where $i=0,\ldots, K-1$ is the number of vectors in the training set. The correlation matrix is square positively defined N-by-N matrix. Then the eigenvectors of the correlation matrix are computed, which by definition constitute the orthogonal basis of the same dimension N that has original feature space. Now we have to pick those eigenvectors (called principal components) which will be used for low-dimensional representation of the data. These vectors will correspond to the largest eigenvalues of the correlation matrix, and their number $M<N$ is selected in order to reconstruct the large fraction of the variance of the original feature vectors. A rule of thumb is to try to keep 95% of variance while transferring data from original to new space.

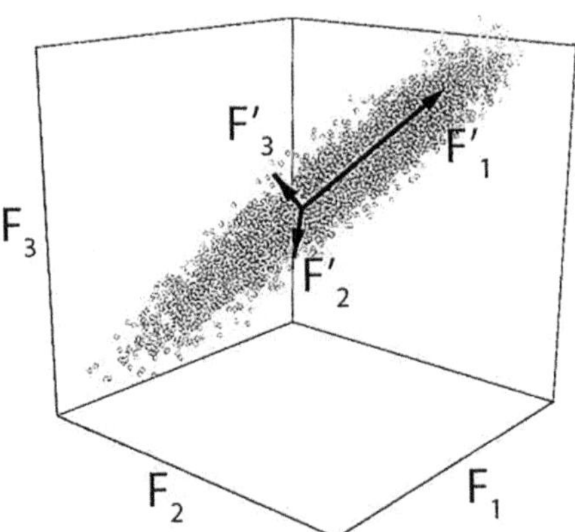

Fig. 5 Principal components F_1', F_2', F_3' in the feature space constructed by features F_1, F_2, F_3.

Finally, we map the original N-dimensional feature vectors onto the M-dimensional space of principal components. The variance of the obtained new feature vectors F_i', $i=0,\ldots,K-1$ is maximized, therefore we retain the important variability in the original data, but in the lower-dimensional space. It is important to note that the physical meaning of the new coordinates is lost after such representation. We not just select the subset of the original N coordinates (which were corresponding to the original features), but we created the new space spanned by mathematically constructed principal components. They are the optimal (in terms of retaining the variance of our dataset) subset of M vectors from N-dimensional feature space. Also, since all the eigenvectors are mutually orthogonal, principal components are orthogonal as well: the dot product of any pair of different vectors from the M-dimensional space of principal components is zero, and they are uncorrelated.

6.2 Independent component analysis

Independent Component Analysis (ICA) is an example of information-theory based algorithm [44–46]. While PCA looks for uncorrelated vectors to establish new basis in the new space (i.e., a constraint on the second-order statistics, correlation), ICA looks for *independent* vectors (i.e., a constraint on all their moments, not only second order).

In case of ICA, the problem of finding the independent vectors to constitute the new basis of smaller dimension is the problem of source separation. The available feature vectors (called *observations*) are modeled as being made of the independent components (called *sources*) after they are combined using the unknown *mixing matrix*. The source separation is finding the original sources from observations by computing the unmixing matrix given that the sources should be as independent as possible. There are a lot of approaches to ICA:
- Based on mutual information and entropy (e.g., FastICA and Infomax),
- Likelihood methods (ProdDenICA),
- Nonlinear correlation (KernelICA), etc.

6.3 Nonnegative matrix factorization

Nonnegative Matrix Factorization (NNMF) is a formal mathematical approach to dimensionality reduction [47,48]. In NNMF the original (high-dimensional) feature vectors are considered as the N-dimensional rows of the n-by-N input matrix X, where n is the number of data instances in the training set.

Dimensionality reduction is achieved by factorizing of matrix X into two matrices $X = A \cdot B$, where A is n-by-K, and B is K-by-N. In the obtained matrix A, K is the number of new features in each of n feature vectors. Since $(K < N)$, each data instance is now described in the lower-dimensional feature space. New K-dimensional feature vectors are called latent representation of original N-dimensional feature vectors. Matrix A is calculated by iterative algorithms with the requirement that its rows (feature vectors) do not contain negative values.

On contrast to PCA, the columns of matrix A are not required to be orthogonal, and the solution of the NNMF is not unique. NNMF problem is NP-hard (nondeterministic polynomial time) class, so it is solvable in polynomial time by a nondeterministic Turing machine. But there are heuristic approximations which have been proven to work well in many applications. The main problem is that it is hard to know how to choose the factorization rank (the number of dimensions K), which limits its utility in practice.

6.4   Self-organizing maps

Self-organizing map (SOM) is a type of artificial neural network that is trained using unsupervised learning to produce a low-dimensional (typically two-dimensional), discretized representation of the input space of the training samples, called a map [49]. The advantage of SOM is that for building the two-dimensional representation of high-dimensional feature vectors, it takes into account the spatial order and distance relationship in the original data. That means that in two-dimensional representation of data instances those who were close to each other in high-dimensional space, will appear close in the two-dimensional space. This facilitates a convenient inspection of the similarity relationships of the training data as well as their clustering tendency.

There are two main approaches to constructing SOMs:
- Distance-based SOM uses metric distances for finding the model whish maps data from high- to low-dimensional space.
- Dot-product SOM employs the concept of "similarity" to find the model using inner product.

6.5   Autoencoders

Autoencoders are artificial neural networks which consist of two modules (Fig. 5). *Encoder* takes the N-dimensional feature vector F as input and converts it to K-dimensional vector F. *Decoder* is attached to encoder; it takes K-dimensional vector and converts

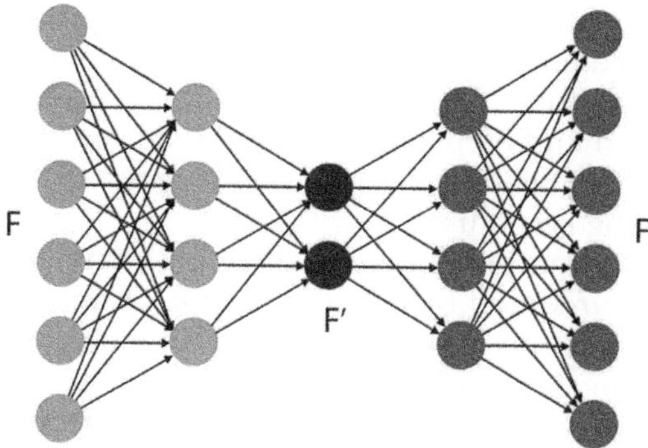

Fig. 6 Autoencoder: the deep neural network which compresses the feature vector *F* to *F′* of lower dimension, and then reconstructs from *F′* back to *F*.

it to N-dimensional vector. By converting the input N-dimensional vector into the K-dimensional vector $(K < N)$, the encoder performs the compression of the information contained in the input data, hence doing the representation in lower-dimensional space.

Autoencoder is trained to achieve the similarity between input and output N-dimensional vectors, so it is able to perfectly reconstruct the input data from compressed representation. After whole autoencoder is trained, the encoder part is used to generate the features. It is disconnected from the autoencoder, and then takes every data instance and transforms it into low-dimensional representation [50,51].

As autoencoders are deep neural networks, they require quite large training datasets to achieve good reconstruction accuracy, otherwise they are prone to overfitting (Fig. 6).

7. Concluding remarks

Feature engineering is a set of techniques to prepare the input real-world data for using in machine learning. It consists of three main steps: (1) exploration of the available measurement data and preparing it for further processing, (2) extraction of features to represent the data, and (3) selection the most informative features by retaining only nonredundant and relevant for further use.

– Feature engineering is a *valid and useful step* in machine learning, since it assures that the model will use the valid data to learn the task. The steps of feature engineering can be used in full, or partially, but the data preparation is inevitable in most of the tasks. One important exception is the usage of deep neural networks trained on huge amount of row input data. In such case the neural network can learn the features from the unprepared data and may not require feature extraction and feature reduction to be implemented by the engineer. But data exploration and preparation are still required. Also, in case if the data is not enough for training using the raw data, feature engineering is still useful.

- Important aspect of feature engineering is the *interpretability of the features* used by machine learning model to make any predictions about the target. Very often for fair and transparent usage of model it is important to understand what lead the model to the particular conclusion, and it is better to have features which could be understood by human. Most of the feature extraction methods lead to the interpretable features, computing understandable measures (such as spectral, entropy, symmetry, etc.) But after dimensionality reduction the new transformed features usually lose their physical meaning, since the features are formally transformed into abstract representations.
- To understand the features and guide the feature engineering, the *feature importance* is often useful. Defining the feature importance for the machine learning model assigns the scores to each feature which quantifies how useful it is for the machine learning model to define the target value. Knowing the feature importance helps to understand the input data, gives insights about the model, and may guide the feature selection. Also, providing feature importance may help to understand the business problem behind the machine learning task.
- When the amount of training data is not large and the model is likely to overfit, the *data augmentation* may be included in feature engineering process. This is a way to artificially increase the variability and diversity in the training dataset without actually collecting the new training data. Instead, the existing data instances are used for cropping, flipping, padding, noising, and other modifications, and then the augmented data is added to the training set.

References

[1] P. Chapman, J. Clinton, R. Kerber, T. Khabaza, T. Reinartz, C. Shearer, R. Wirth, The CRISP-DM user guide, in: 4th CRISP-DM SIG Workshop in Brussels in March, vol. 1999, 1999, March.

[2] A.I.R.L. Azevedo, M.F. Santos, KDD, SEMMA and CRISP-DM: A Parallel Overview, IADS-DM, 2008.

[3] J.S. Saczynski, D.D. McManus, R.J. Goldberg, Commonly used data-collection approaches in clinical research, Am. J. Med. 126 (11) (2013) 946–950.

[4] V. Cox, Exploratory data analysis, in: Translating Statistics to Make Decisions, Apress, Berkeley, CA, 2017, pp. 47–74.

[5] T. Milo, A. Somech, Automating exploratory data analysis via machine learning: an overview, in: Proceedings of the 2020 ACM SIGMOD International Conference on Management of Data, 2020, June, pp. 2617–2622.

[6] S.K. Yadav, S. Singh, R. Gupta, Data types, in: Biomedical Statistics, Springer, Singapore, 2019, pp. 13–16.

[7] A. Varri, B. Kemp, T. Penzel, A. Schlogl, Standards for biomedical signal databases, IEEE Eng. Med. Biol. Mag. 20 (3) (2001) 33–37.

[8] M. Soley-Bori, Dealing With Missing Data: Key Assumptions and Methods for Applied Analysis, vol. 23, Boston University, 2013, p. 20.

[9] G.E. Batista, M.C. Monard, An analysis of four missing data treatment methods for supervised learning, Appl. Artif. Intell. 17 (5–6) (2003) 519–533.

[10] P.J. García-Laencina, J.L. Sancho-Gómez, A.R. Figueiras-Vidal, Pattern classification with missing data: a review, Neural Comput. Appl. 19 (2) (2010) 263–282.

[11] B. Marlin, Missing Data Problems in Machine Learning, 2008 (Doctoral dissertation).

[12] J.M. Jerez, I. Molina, P.J. García-Laencina, E. Alba, N. Ribelles, M. Martín, L. Franco, Missing data imputation using statistical and machine learning methods in a real breast cancer problem, Artif. Intell. Med. 50 (2) (2010) 105–115.

[13] R.M. Thomas, W. Bruin, P. Zhutovsky, G. van Wingen, Dealing with missing data, small sample sizes, and heterogeneity in machine learning studies of brain disorders, in: Machine Learning, Academic Press, 2020, pp. 249–266.

[14] P. Cerda, G. Varoquaux, B. Kégl, Similarity encoding for learning with dirty categorical variables, Mach. Learn. 107 (8) (2018) 1477–1494.

[15] K. Potdar, T.S. Pardawala, C.D. Pai, A comparative study of categorical variable encoding techniques for neural network classifiers, Int. J. Comput. Appl. 175 (4) (2017) 7–9.

[16] P. Rodríguez, M.A. Bautista, J. Gonzalez, S. Escalera, Beyond one-hot encoding: lower dimensional target embedding, Image Vis. Comput. 75 (2018) 21–31.

[17] H. Kaur, H.S. Pannu, A.K. Malhi, A systematic review on imbalanced data challenges in machine learning: applications and solutions, ACM Comput. Surv. 52 (4) (2019) 1–36.

[18] C. Thirumalai, M. Vignesh, R. Balaji, Data analysis using Box and Whisker plot for lung cancer, in: 2017 Innovations in Power and Advanced Computing Technologies (i-PACT), IEEE, 2017, April, pp. 1–6.

[19] A. Zheng, A. Casari, Feature Engineering for Machine Learning: Principles and Techniques for Data Scientists, O'Reilly Media, Inc, 2018.

[20] M. Zhukov, A. Popov, Bin number selection for equidistant mutual information estimation, in: 2014 IEEE 34th International Scientific Conference on Electronics and Nanotechnology (ELNANO), IEEE, 2014, April, pp. 259–263.

[21] C.C. Aggarwal, Outlier Analysis, second ed., Springer, Cham, 2017.

[22] D.M. Hawkins, Identification of Outliers, vol. 11, Chapman and Hall, London, 1980.

[23] X. Su, C.L. Tsai, Outlier detection, Wiley Interdiscip. Rev. Data Min. Knowl. Discov. 1 (3) (2011) 261–268.

[24] S. Walfish, A review of statistical outlier methods, Pharm. Technol. 30 (11) (2006) 82.

[25] R. Domingues, M. Filippone, P. Michiardi, J. Zouaoui, A comparative evaluation of outlier detection algorithms: experiments and analyses, Pattern Recogn. 74 (2018) 406–421.

[26] S. Omar, A. Ngadi, H.H. Jebur, Machine learning techniques for anomaly detection: an overview, Int. J. Comput. Appl. 79 (2) (2013).

[27] Y. Zhao, Z. Nasrullah, Z. Li, Pyod: A Python Toolbox for Scalable Outlier Detection, 2019. arXiv preprint arXiv:1901.01588.

[28] R. Chalapathy, S. Chawla, Deep Learning for Anomaly Detection: A Survey, 2019. arXiv preprint arXiv:1901.03407.

[29] S. Patro, K.K. Sahu, Normalization: A Preprocessing Stage, 2015. arXiv preprint arXiv:1503.06462.

[30] I. Guyon, S. Gunn, M. Nikravesh, L.A. Zadeh (Eds.), Feature Extraction: Foundations and Applications, vol. 207, Springer, 2008.

[31] M. Nixon, A. Aguado, Feature Extraction and Image Processing for Computer Vision, Academic Press, 2019.

[32] F.Y. Kuo, I.H. Sloan, Lifting the curse of dimensionality, Not. Am. Math. Soc. 52 (11) (2005) 1320–1328.

[33] M. Verleysen, D. François, The curse of dimensionality in data mining and time series prediction, in: International Work-Conference on Artificial Neural Networks, Springer, Berlin, Heidelberg, 2005, June, pp. 758–770.

[34] B. Mwangi, T.S. Tian, J.C. Soares, A review of feature reduction techniques in neuroimaging, Neuroinformatics 12 (2) (2014) 229–244.

[35] G. Chandrashekar, F. Sahin, A survey on feature selection methods, Comput. Electr. Eng. 40 (1) (2014) 16–28.

[36] M. Dash, H. Liu, Feature selection for classification, Intell. Data Anal. 1 (1–4) (1997) 131–156.

[37] I. Guyon, A. Elisseeff, An introduction to variable and feature selection, J. Mach. Learn. Res. 3 (Mar) (2003) 1157–1182.

[38] I. Guyon, Practical feature selection: from correlation to causality, in: Mining Massive Data Sets for Security: Advances in Data Mining, Search, Social Networks and Text Mining, and Their Applications to Security, 2008, pp. 27–43.

[39] J.R. Vergara, P.A. Estévez, A review of feature selection methods based on mutual information, Neural Comput. Appl. 24 (1) (2014) 175–186.

[40] N. Shrestha, Detecting multicollinearity in regression analysis, Am. J. Appl. Math. Stat. 8 (2) (2020) 39–42.

[41] B.F. Darst, K.C. Malecki, C.D. Engelman, Using recursive feature elimination in random forest to account for correlated variables in high dimensional data, BMC Genet. 19 (1) (2018) 1–6.

[42] Y. Shi, J. Miao, Z. Wang, P. Zhang, L. Niu, Feature selection with $\ell_{2, 1-2}$ regularization, IEEE Trans. Neural Netw. Learn. Syst. 29 (10) (2018) 4967–4982.

[43] J. Lever, M. Krzywinski, N. Altman, Points of significance: principal component analysis, Nat. Methods 14 (7) (2017) 641–643.

[44] S.H. Hsu, L. Pion-Tonachini, J. Palmer, M. Miyakoshi, S. Makeig, T.P. Jung, Modeling brain dynamic state changes with adaptive mixture independent component analysis, Neuroimage 183 (2018) 47–61.

[45] K. Nordhausen, H. Oja, Independent component analysis: a statistical perspective, Wiley Interdiscip. Rev. Comput. Stat. 10 (5) (2018), e1440.

[46] J.V. Stone, Independent Component Analysis: A Tutorial Introduction, MIT Press, Cambridge, MA, 2004.

[47] X. Fu, K. Huang, N.D. Sidiropoulos, W.K. Ma, Nonnegative matrix factorization for signal and data analytics: identifiability, algorithms, and applications, IEEE Signal Process. Mag. 36 (2) (2019) 59–80.

[48] Z. Li, J. Tang, X. He, Robust structured nonnegative matrix factorization for image representation, IEEE Trans. Neural Netw. Learn. Syst. 29 (5) (2017) 1947–1960.

[49] S. Haykin, 9. Self-organizing maps, in: Neural Networks—A Comprehensive Foundation, second ed., Prentice-Hall, 1999.

[50] B. Eiteneuer, N. Hranisavljevic, O. Niggemann, Dimensionality reduction and anomaly detection for CPPS data using autoencoder, in: 2019 IEEE International Conference on Industrial Technology (ICIT), IEEE, 2019, February, pp. 1286–1292.

[51] E. Lin, S. Mukherjee, S. Kannan, A deep adversarial variational autoencoder model for dimensionality reduction in single-cell RNA sequencing analysis, BMC Bioinf. 21 (1) (2020) 1–11.

2

Heart rate variability

B. Dhananjay, B. Arya, N. Prasanna Venkatesh, and J. Sivaraman

Bio-signals and Medical Instrumentation Laboratory, Department of Biotechnology and Medical Engineering, National Institute of Technology Rourkela, Odisha, India

1. Introduction

Heart rate (HR) defines cardiac activity, i.e., the number of times the heart beats in a minute. The functioning of the heart largely depends upon the efficiency of heart electrophysiology. The normal limit of HR in sinus rhythm (SR) is 60–100 bpm, $\geq$100 bpm in sinus tachycardia (ST), and $\leq$60 bpm in sinus bradycardia. Generally, the variability in a healthy heart is more and decreases for the diseased heart condition. Hence, a study on heart rate variability (HRV) and its parameters are essential in determining cardiac disorders. Therefore, HRV divulges the information of heartbeats recorded over a period of time, influenced by the changes observed in the HR. HRV is a diagnostic tool that reflects the HR changes due to intrinsic and extrinsic factors [1–3]. HRV is mainly referred to as understanding the instantaneous changes occurring in HR. The HR displays a standard variability observed due to blood circulation and neural regulation [1].

The information drawn from the analysis of HRV elaborates the cardiac activity and autonomic nervous system (ANS) [2–4]. The ANS mainly influences the HR, where ANS is subdivided into the sympathetic nervous system (SNS) and parasympathetic nervous system (PNS). The SNS and PNS show contradictory behavior with respect to one another depending upon the physiological need of body. Both are modulated by different set of hormones which either stimulates the heart function or slows it down further. SNS controls the release of catecholamines, epinephrine, and norepinephrine which helps in accelerating the heart rate

Advanced Methods in Biomedical Signal Processing and Analysis. https://doi.org/10.1016/B978-0-323-85955-4.00015-6
Copyright © 2023 Elsevier Inc. All rights reserved.

during stress conditions. PNS stimulates the release of acetylcholine which leads to decreased heart rates during sleep, meditation and slow deep breaths. The degree of variation observed in the HR divulges the sensitivity of the heart in respond to changes [1–4].

Previous works [2–4] have stated that a proper understanding of the ANS is needed to diagnose any cardiac abnormality. The study on HRV in analyzing cardiac health is significant and reiterated in many works [5–12]. With the help of low-cost computers having substantial computational power, HRV signal analysis has advanced in recent times.

1.1 Effects of blood pressure on HRV

The patients under cardiovascular risk due to hypertension may develop a structural abnormality of heart due to increased blood pressure (BP) [13]. Examining the left ventricular hypertrophy (LVH) condition from the ECG signal gives information about the morbidity and mortality of the patient. In many works, reduced HRV is noted in patients undergoing abnormality such as LVH near the heart's aortic valve caused due to increased BP [14]. The arterial baroreflex consists of cardiac output and controls the activity of the cardiac vagal nerve. The sensitivity obtained in the baroreflex is directly proportional to the HRV. Previous studies stated [13–16], that patients suffering from hypertension and diabetes have significantly less HRV. This observed reduction in the sensitivity of the baroreflex is correlated with the changes observed in the LVH. Few studies [13–16] have analyzed the relation between HRV and BP, and observed fluctuations in the frequency-domain. Analyzing the relation between systolic pressure and obtained RR interval from the ECG signal using a 10 s time window showed that the systolic pressure leads the interval by more than three beats, thus forming cross-spectra. Moreover, on analyzing the respiration rate and systolic pressure, no cross-spectra variations were developed. Previous studies [14–18] have proposed a mathematical model to understand the spectrum formed by BP and HR.

1.2 Effect of myocardial infarction on HRV

The patients suffering from myocardial infarction (MI) have displayed a rise in sympathetic activity, and a corresponding decrease has been noted in the parasympathetic activity with respect to cardiac control [19]. The control of SNS on cardiac activity decreases the minimum amount of electrical stimulus required by the heart to initiate fibrillation, and also it is caused due to lack of physical activity in MI patients which further leads to ventricular fibrillation (VF). The rise of VF in MI patients due to increased sympathetic activity may lead to inappropriate tachyarrhythmias in the ventricle; thus, vagal activity tends to control it by increasing the threshold of the minimum amount of electrical stimulus [20,21]. The respiration rate of MI patients is directly proportional to parasympathetic activity [22,23], and can play a role as indicator to diagnose MI patients. Few studies [24,25] have reported that the HRV decreases linearly with the severity of the MI. A study [26] compared the clinical HRV parameters in two phases. The first phase denoted the MI patients, and the second phase displayed the MI patients under physical stress and concluded that there is no change in clinical aspects of HRV. The HRV parameters, SDNN and HF power, are used to understand the imbalance of sympathetic activity in MI patients leading to left ventricular dysfunction.

1.3 Relation between HRV and cardiac arrhythmia

The dynamics of the cardiovascular system are well understood by hypothesizing the nature of a nonlinear system. Many previous studies [27,28] have focused on analyzing the HRV of disease patients with nonlinear techniques. Various studies [25–28] have developed nonlinear systems and methods for detailed analysis of HRV. A study [28] observed mechanical activity of the heart with the help of a wavelet transform application on the ECG signal in a VF patient. In a study [29], a nonlinear model was designed and developed to detect and classify different cardiac arrhythmias. Acharya et al. [30–33] have developed other nonlinear techniques, and with the help of recent trends in artificial intelligence, they have classified HRV signals. In a study [34], the autoregressive model was used to classify NSR and six arrhythmia classes including VF, premature ventricular contraction, ventricular tachycardia (VT), supraventricular tachycardia, and atrial premature contraction. Results stated a sensible high accuracy of cardiac arrhythmia detection with 93.2%–100% using generalized linear model-based classification algorithm.

1.4 Relation between HRV, age, and gender

Studies have stated the relation between HRV and physiological parameters such as age, and sex. HRV analysis was done on old and young women and found that young, active women depicted an increase in HRV parameters [35,36]. A study [37] on analyzing the variations observed in HR among newborn males and females concluded that it is lower in males than females. In healthy adults (20–70 years), the HRV decreased with the prolongation of age and also noted that the HR variation was predominantly high in females compared to males [38]. The relationship between gender and age has been quantified in previous studies [39,40], and further analysis in the time and frequency parameters of HRV were performed. They noted variations in time and spectral domain during HRV signal analysis performed in each healthy volunteer at different times.

An increase in the sympathetic control of the ANS leads to increase in HRV, which in turn is affected by gestational age [41]. Few studies [32,33] suggested a decrease in HRV parameters with the advancing age, and this decline begins from juvenile stage itself and gradually reaches to very low variations in old age [42]. Similar result was also noted in a previous study [43] that newborn babies display an increased sympathetic activity that normally decreases with age (5–10 years). A study of HRV parameters in young volunteers states that fixed breathing in a standing posture incites HRV [42]. In adults, it is observed that as age increases, respiratory sinus arrhythmia decreases [44,45]. Comparative study on the effects of coronary artery disease (CAD) in men and women shows that men are at higher risk of CAD [46].

1.5 Effects of drugs, alcohol, and smoking on HRV parameters

The patients suffering from hypertension lead to calcium channel blockade, affecting the HRV [47–49]. The spectral analysis can help in understanding the effects of therapeutic drugs for cardiac disorders treatment on the HRV. In volunteers having normal BP, the HR fluctuations are augmented due to nifedipine and placebo [50]. A study [48] was conducted on hypertension volunteers to understand the response of acebutolol. They concluded that high and low-frequency components of the HRV analysis were inversely proportional to each other; thus, a decline in sympathetic control activity was observed. The decrease in sympathetic activity was also noted in patients suffering from heart failure and postinfarction [47,48]. Therefore, it is necessary to understand that beta-blockers restore the balance between sympathetic and parasympathetic activity during cardiovascular disorder. The effects of drug with ethyl-esters groups on the clinical aspects of HRV were also studied on MI patients [51], where the results in the time domain quantified that ethyl-ester as a drug can be used to treat MI patients. A study [52] was conducted on the effect of drugs that work on adrenalin to treat asthma patients with the help of the ratio of low frequency to high-frequency HRV parameters.

An analysis of HRV parameters in smokers has concluded a reduction of vagal activity and simultaneous increase in sympathetic activity, as the HRV is reduced due to smoking. The ANS loses its coordination with the peripheral nervous system due to the impairment caused by smoking [53–55]. Tobacco smoke in the environment can also adversely affect cardiovascular activity, including HRV [56]. The HRV decreases in volunteer with a continuous long duration of tobacco smoke exposure, thus leading to cardiac disease susceptibility. Few studies [56,57] where the effect of cigarette smoke exposure on the fetuses has concluded that the fetus neurobehavioral function may get affected due to decreased HRV. Heavy smokers tend to lose control of the vagal modulation on cardiac activity. A study also noted that cigarette smoking can act as a potent negative catalyst for the loss of autonomic control of the heart [57].

In a study [58], the response of HRV in alcohol-induced individuals was observed by the decrease of parasympathetic activity. A study [59] stated a positive correlation between the HRV parameters measured during the day and night, where the HR was monitored for 24h in volunteers with usual alcohol intake. The alcoholic volunteers displayed lower measuring values of the vagal activity when compared with healthy volunteers [58–61].

1.6 Effects of menstrual cycle on HRV parameters

The reproductive system in women undergoes various recurring changes throughout the reproduction phase compared to men, as cyclical preparation for fertilization and pregnancy [62]. One cycle with an average duration of 28 days is termed as the menstrual cycle. The broader term of the menstrual cycle is intricately classified into 2 cycles, ovarian and endometrial cycle, occurring simultaneously with the effect of changes in hormone levels [63]. The ovarian cycle is classified into follicular and luteal phases. In the follicular phase, estrogen levels increase gradually, leading to peak levels of follicular stimulating hormone and luteinizing hormone. In the luteal phase, levels of estrogen and progesterone dominate [64].

The proliferative, secretory, and menstruation phases are subdivisions of the endometrial cycle. In the proliferative phase, growth of endometrial lining occurs, facilitated by an increase in estrogens; further second phase depicts the maturation of endometrium. The ceasing of endometrial lining growth is seen with decreasing levels of estrogens. In the absence of fertilization, endometrial disintegrates due to a decrease in the level of estrogen and progesterone; hence the third and final cycle, i.e., menstruation begins.

HRV is the variations between two consecutive heartbeats. This rhythm is controlled by sinoatrial node modulated by the sympathetic and parasympathetic nervous systems [65]. Effects of hormonal fluctuations on cardiac autonomic function lead to HRV, which varies during each phase of the menstrual cycle [66].

Important time-domain parameters are SDNN, r-MSSD, NN50, and p-NN50. Two important frequency-domain parameter are low frequency component (LF; 0.04–0.15 Hz) and high frequency component (HF; >0.15 Hz) [67]. LF represents an interaction between both the sympathetic and parasympathetic nervous systems. HF represents the activity of the parasympathetic nervous system. LF/HF ratio represents the balance of the ANS. A high concentration of progesterone in the luteal phase induces sympathetic activity. However, the low concentration of steroid hormones in the menstrual cycle induces parasympathetic activity. Hence, the LF component is highest in the luteal phase, and the HF component is highest in menstrual phase [68].

Several investigations have been done with respect to change in ECG parameters at different phases of menstrual cycle. This chapter also discusses the variations in ECG parameters with respect to hormonal fluctuation at varying phases of the menstrual cycle. Also, changes in atrial and ventricular ECG components along with HRV recording at the time of lowest hormonal fluctuation (menstrual phase) and highest hormonal fluctuation (luteal or follicular phase) were investigated.

2. Literature review

2.1 Analyses of time-domain parameters

Makikallio et al. [69] analyzed the time-domain parameters of HRV among patients suffering from heart failure. The HRV parameters were recorded and analyzed on a two-channel ECG recording system for 24 h. The time-domain parameters between placebo effect and dofetilide group were analyzed for 499 volunteers and later classified as live and deceased heart failure patients. A gradual decrease in time-domain parameters was observed in patients who later died of heart failure. Agarwal et al. [70] proposed a study to determine the relationship between HRV and occurrence of atrial fibrillation (AF). The study consisted of 2 min ECG signal for 11, 715 volunteers at risk of AF.

Time-domain HRV parameters were analyzed using RR intervals, and they noted a decrease in time-domain parameters in patients with AF compared to the control group. Parsi et al. [71] concluded that time-domain parameters help to classify cardiac arrhythmias such as VF and VT. Castro et al. [72] compared the mean RR interval among depression-related patients and observed a decrease in mean RR interval. Mestanikova et al. [73], in their work, studied the parasympathetic activity response in volunteers under mental and physiological stress by analyzing the HRV parameters. On examining the time-domain parameters, control volunteers displayed a higher time-domain values when compared with depressed volunteers. Poddar et al. [74] analyzed hypertension and CAD by HRV parameters. A decrease in time-domain parameters was observed in hypertension patients compared with CAD patients.

Kallio et al. [75] studied the HRV characteristics in patients suffering from Parkinson's disease and noted that the time-domain features were minor in patients compared with the healthy volunteers. Kuppusamy et al. [76] studied the effects of HRV parameters under the control of yoga breathing (pranayama) practices in young adults. The HRV parameters were analyzed for 6 months between the yoga breathing group and volunteers not practicing yoga. It was noted that the time-domain parameters showed an increasing trend in the group practicing yoga. Sacknoff et al. [77] studied the effect on HRV while undergoing athletic exercises and concluded that the time-domain parameters of the athletes were comparatively higher than the nonathletes. Similarly, in a study done by Kiss et al. [78] concluded that the time-domain parameters of HRV are higher in athletes, and it varies with the specific sport as the ANS adjusts according to it.

2.2 Analysis of frequency-domain HRV parameters

Makikallio et al. [69] investigated the fractal analysis of HRV signals acquired from 24 h Holter ECG with left ventricular ejection fraction ($\leq$35%) and congestive heart failure (CHF) patients for 665 ± 374 days. Frequency-domain HRV parameters such as LF, HF, and the ratio of LF/HF were compared in 499 CHF patients, out of which 210 patients died after 665 days follow-up. It was noted that the patients alive from CHF showed higher frequency-domain parameters compared with the patients died of CHF. Agarwal et al. [70] concluded that the patients diagnosed with early-stage AF displayed a lower frequency-domain parameter when compared with the reference group. Castro et al. [72] analyzed the frequency-domain parameters of HRV between depressed and healthy volunteers during sleep and awake time of the day. The study did not find any significant difference in frequency-domain parameters in the volunteers. Poddar et al. [74] analyzed the different frequency parameters where the very-low-frequency parameter between hypertension and CAD patients displayed an increasing trend for the hypertension patients. In contrast, the other frequency-domain parameters presented a decreasing trend for hypertension patients compared with CAD patients.

In work done by Kallio et al. [75], the frequency-domain parameters in Parkinson's patients were analyzed, and they noted lesser values compared with healthy individuals. Kuppusamy et al. [76] studied the variation of frequency-domain parameters among yoga breathing volunteers and control volunteers for 6 months. They observed that the low-frequency parameter decreased in the yoga breathing group by the end of 6 months, whereas the control group showed a rise in the low-frequency parameter by the end of 6 months. The high-frequency parameter in the control group decreased at the end of 6 months, whereas the yoga breathing group displayed a significant change. The ratio of low to high frequency expressed a negative value for the yoga breathing group. Sacknoff et al. [77] analyzed the frequency-domain parameters in athletes and nonathletes and concluded that the frequency-domain parameters showed a negative trend compared to the nonathletes.

2.3 Classification and prediction of ECG signals

Classification and prediction of different heart rhythms through machine and deep learning algorithms is the most widespread approach in the current scenario of increased cases of cardiac diseases. Through various model-based prediction, the automated analysis of even complex indicators has become efficient and fast. Chang et al. [79] designed and developed a long short-term memory (LSTM) based model to classify 12 cardiac rhythm classes using 12 lead ECG signals as the inputs from 38,899 patients collectively for all classes. He noted the accuracy of LSTM classification as 0.982 and the values of prediction and recall as 0.692–0.625. Seera et al. [80] have classified ECG signals using nine machine learning classifiers. In this study, the test data were corrupted by the noise and training dataset were unaffected. It was noted that logistic regression model achieved highest sensitivity rate of 96% and random forest (RF) model produced highest specificity rate 94% for noise-free data set. Pandey et al. [81] in their work, classified four heartbeats i.e., normal, supraventricular ectopic beat, ventricular ectopic beat and fusion supraventricular and ventricular ectopic arrhythmias. The dataset was retrieved from the MIT-BIH arrhythmia database. To classify the ECG signals based on heartbeats, Pandey et al. [81] developed a support vector machine (SVM) model, and the results of the model were compared with other classifiers such as RF, K-nearest neighbor and LSTM and concluded that SVM produced best overall accuracy of 94.4%. Kumari et al. [82] classified ECG signals by the SVM model, where the input features were extracted from the ECG signals using discrete wavelet transform. Acharya et al. [83] classified ventricular arrhythmias by designing and developing a convolutional neural network (CNN) model of 11 layers, validated by 10-fold cross-validation. Mitra et al. [84] classified different cardiac rhythms by designing and developing an incremental back propagation neural network where the features from the ECG signal were determined by correlation. Yildirim et al. [85] designed and developed LSTM model to classify arrhythmia based on heartbeats. The arrhythmic ECG signals were further preprocessed using autoencoders to extract features. Mathews et al. [86] classified a single-lead ECG signal by designing and developing a restricted Boltzmann machine combining a deep belief network. Many studies [87–95] have used statistical models such as ARX and ARMAX to classify and predict ECG signals with HRV parameters as the feature set and noted the increased HRV in sinus rhythm condition whereas HRV parameters decreased in tachycardia condition. Dhananjay et al. [96] developed a CatBoost model to classify heart rate and studied the importance of the specific features required for classifying different cardiac rhythm.

Kelwade et al. [97] developed a neural network based on the radial function to predict eight different cardiac arrhythmias. The input to the designed and developed neural network was the time series data of the ECG signal. Krittanawong et al. [98] concluded that the machine learning algorithms could predict cardiovascular events, and machine learning algorithms like SVM and other boosting algorithms should be used, especially for prediction. Raghunath et al. [99] designed and developed a deep neural network to predict the patient's mortality within a year. The data recording period was 34 years, and the developed model's input features were the time series data acquired from the 12 leads of the ECG instrument. Chen et al. [100] developed a DNN model which can predict more than one cardiac arrhythmia in a single ECG signal and noted that lead aVR and V1 are the important single leads for arrhythmia prediction. Wang et al. [101] suggested a deep learning model that can rearrange the input feature set to predict cardiac abnormality. Kundella et al. [102] proposed a robust CNN to predict the ECG signals, which was compared with the LSTM and DNN, and they found that the proposed model outperformed.

3. Results

3.1 Statistical analysis

Joint plots are bivariate graphical representations where they display a relationship between two features. Fig. 1 depicts the joint plot of average RR interval and standard deviation of RR intervals (SDNN). The line graph of average RR interval and SDNN is also represented in Fig. 1. The x-axis represents the average RR interval, and the y-axis represents the SDNN. The graph has been plotted according to the types of volunteers considered for the study. The types of volunteers are represented in the target where "0" represents SR volunteers and "1" represents the ST volunteers. The information obtained from Fig. 1 is that SDNN is directly

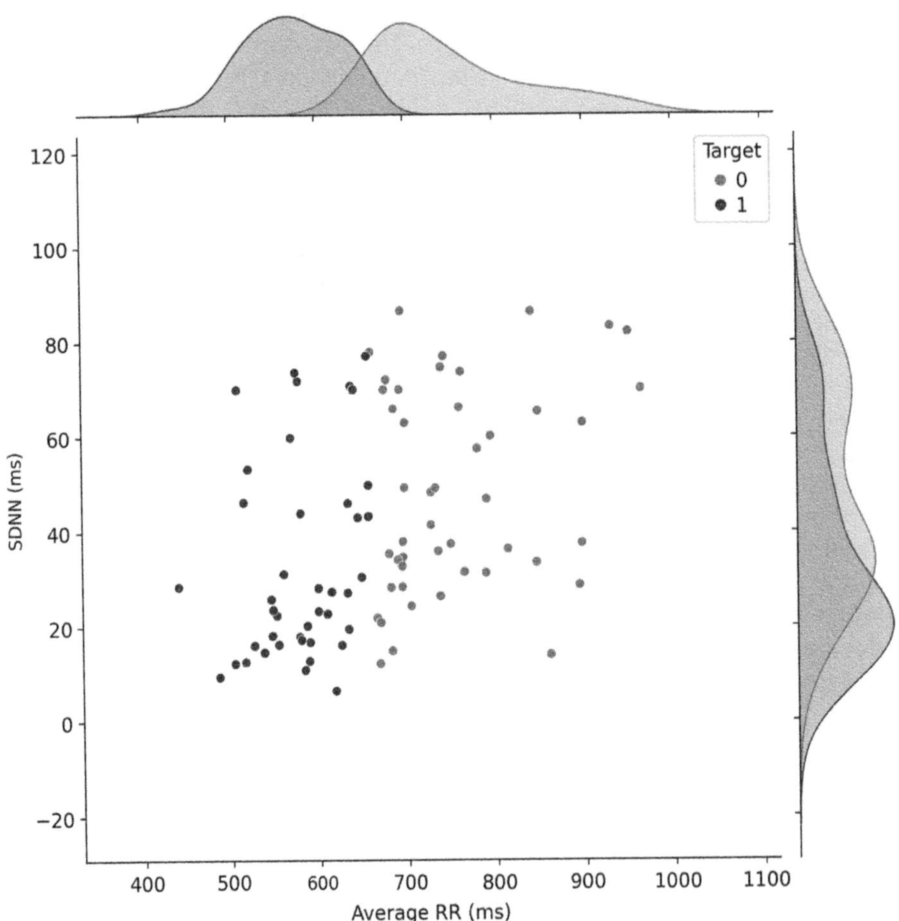

Fig. 1 The joint plot of average RR interval and SDNN.

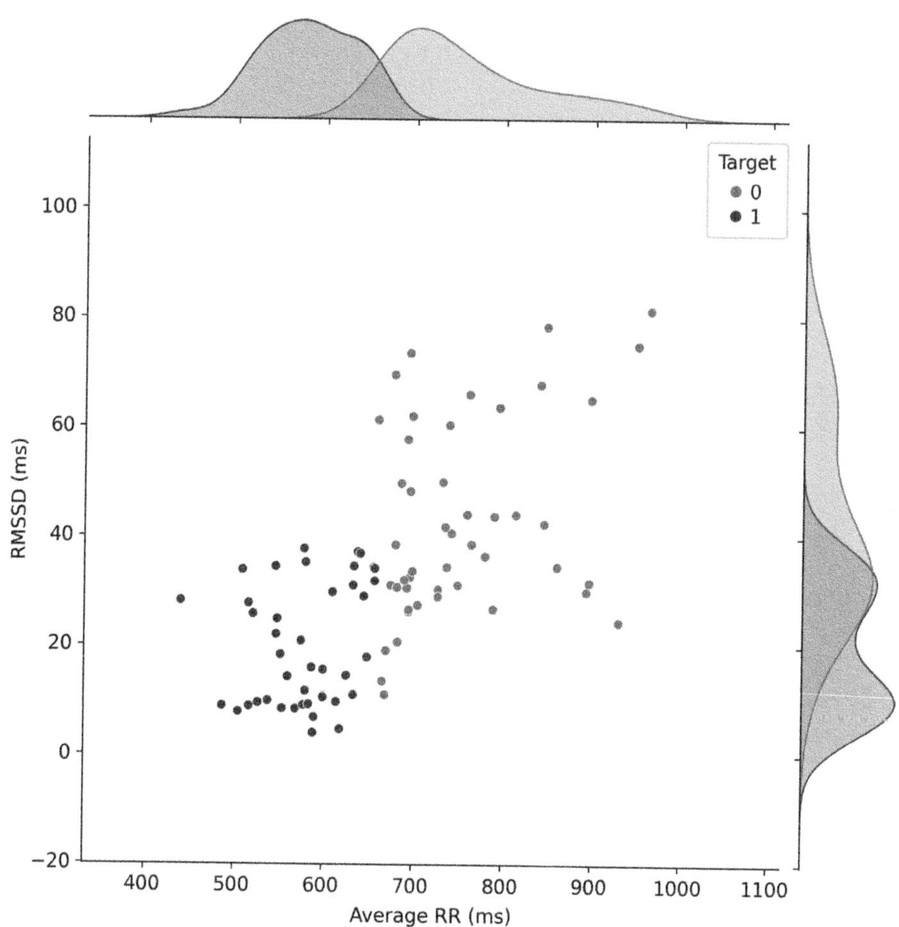

Fig. 2 The joint plot of average RR interval and RMSSD.

proportional to the increase in the length of the RR intervals. Fig. 2 represents the joint plot of the average RR interval and root mean square of successive differences of RR interval (RMSSD). The line graph is also represented for average RR interval and RMSSD.

The x-axis represents the average RR interval, and the y-axis represents the RMSSD. Fig. 2 divulges the information that RMSSD is directly proportional to the increase in the cycle length of the RR interval. Fig. 3 showcases the joint plot of the average RR interval on x-axis and NN50. The y-axis represents the difference between two RRs greater than 50 ms (NN50). The inference drawn from Fig. 3 states that the difference between consecutive RR intervals of more than 50 ms is primarily observed in SR compared to ST volunteers. Fig. 4 denotes the joint plot between the average

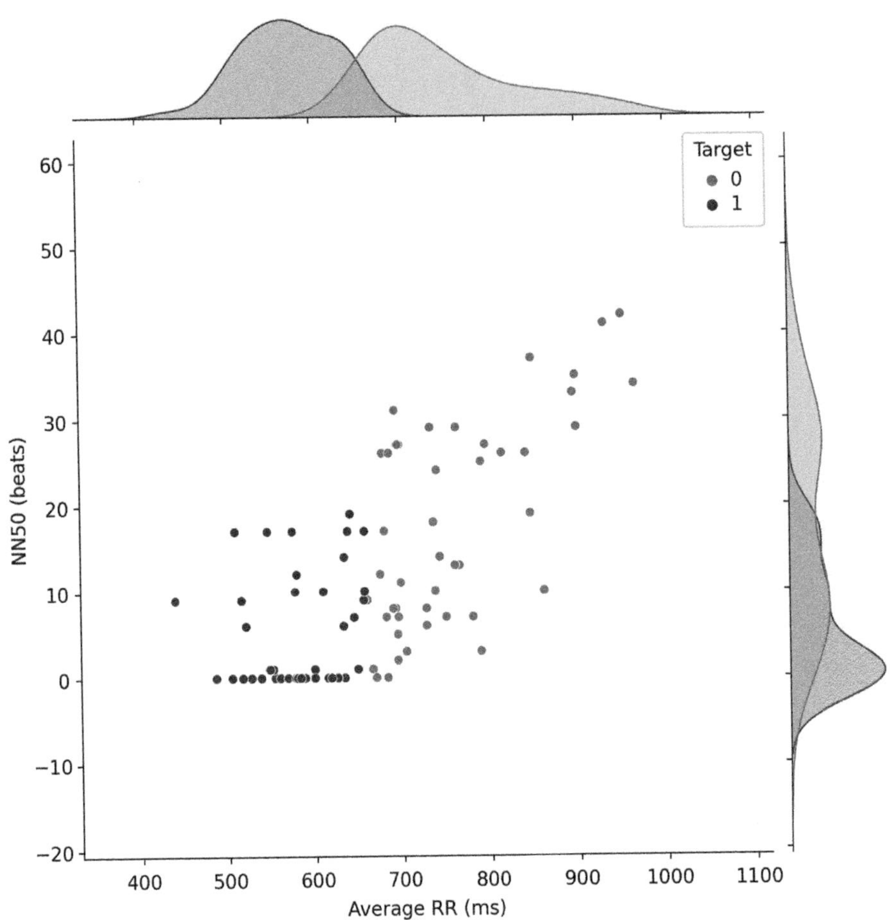

Fig. 3 The joint plot of average RR interval and NN50.

RR interval and the percentage of the consecutive RR intervals more than 50 ms (pNN50). The line graph of average RR interval and pNN50 is also represented in Fig. 4. The x-axis represents the average RR intervals, whereas the y-axis represents the pNN50. From Fig. 4, it is noted that the pNN50 is directly proportional to the increase in cycle length of the RR interval. Fig. 5 represents the joint plot between average RR interval and total power. Total power is a feature in the frequency-domain of the HRV analysis. The line graph of average RR interval and total power is also displayed in Fig. 5 which signifies that the total power is predominantly high in ST volunteers. Fig. 6 depicts the joint plot and line graph of average RR interval on x-axis and the low frequency to

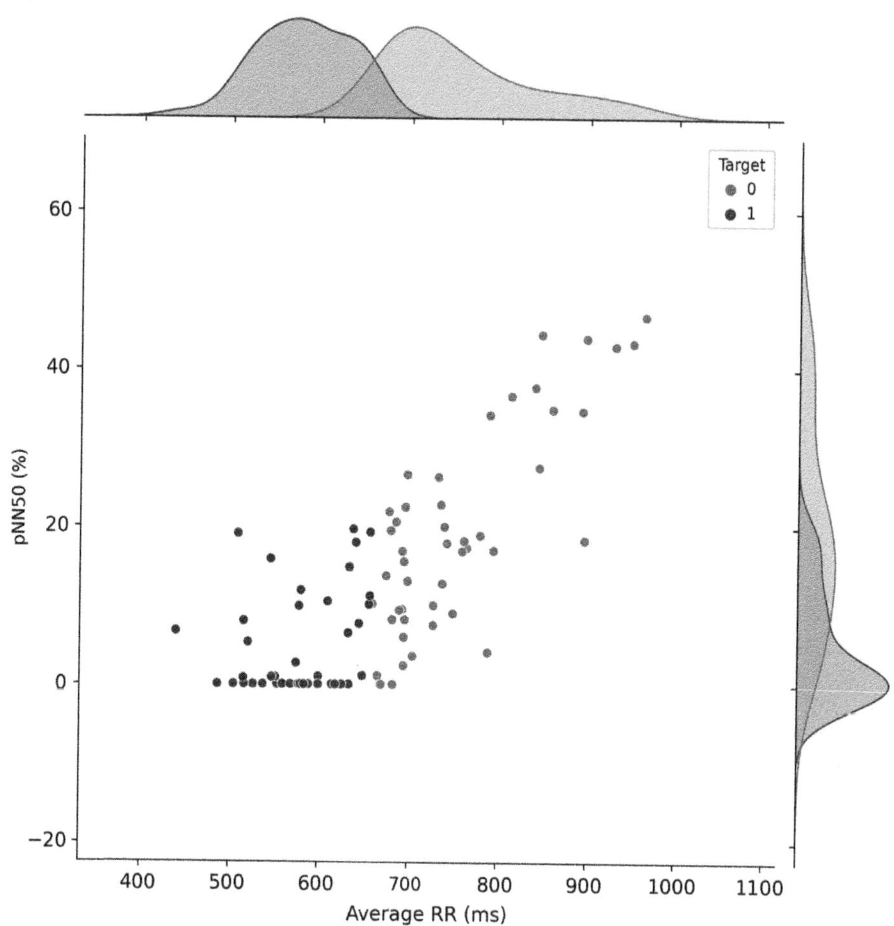

Fig. 4 The joint plot of average RR interval and pNN50.

high frequency (LF/HF) ratio on *y*-axis. Fig. 6 shows that LF/HF is high for ST volunteers compared to SR volunteers.

3.2 Machine learning results

Fig. 7 represents the confusion matrix of the extra trees (ET) classifier. As in Fig. 1, the representation of "0" and "1" are SR and ST volunteers, respectively. The *x*-axis and *y*-axis of the confusion matrix represent the predicted class and true class, respectively. Out of 17 SR volunteers, the ET classifier has accurately classified 16 data volunteers, and 1 was misclassified as ST. In the case of ST volunteers data provided to the ET classifier, all

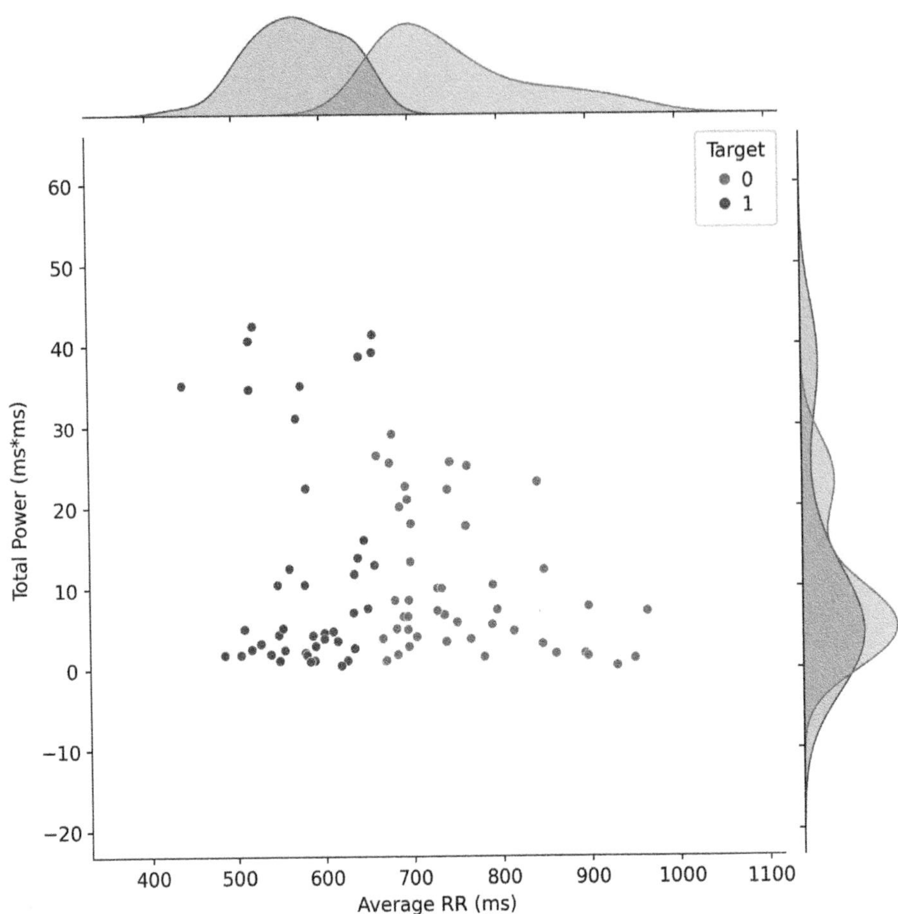

Fig. 5 The joint plot of average RR interval and total power.

11 data volunteers were classified accurately. Fig. 8 represents the feature importance plot of the ET classifier. The x-axis represents the importance of the variable, whereas the y-axis represents the ranking of the features. According to the ET classifier, the essential feature utilized to classify SR and ST data after heart rate is RMSSD, and the least important feature is SDNN. Fig. 9 represents the decision boundary of the ET classifier. The x-axis and y-axis represent the first two critical features according to the feature importance plot generated by the ET classifier. The x-axis and the y-axis denote heart rate, and RMSSD respectively. The "0" and "1" in Fig. 9 represent the SR and ST volunteers data, respectively.

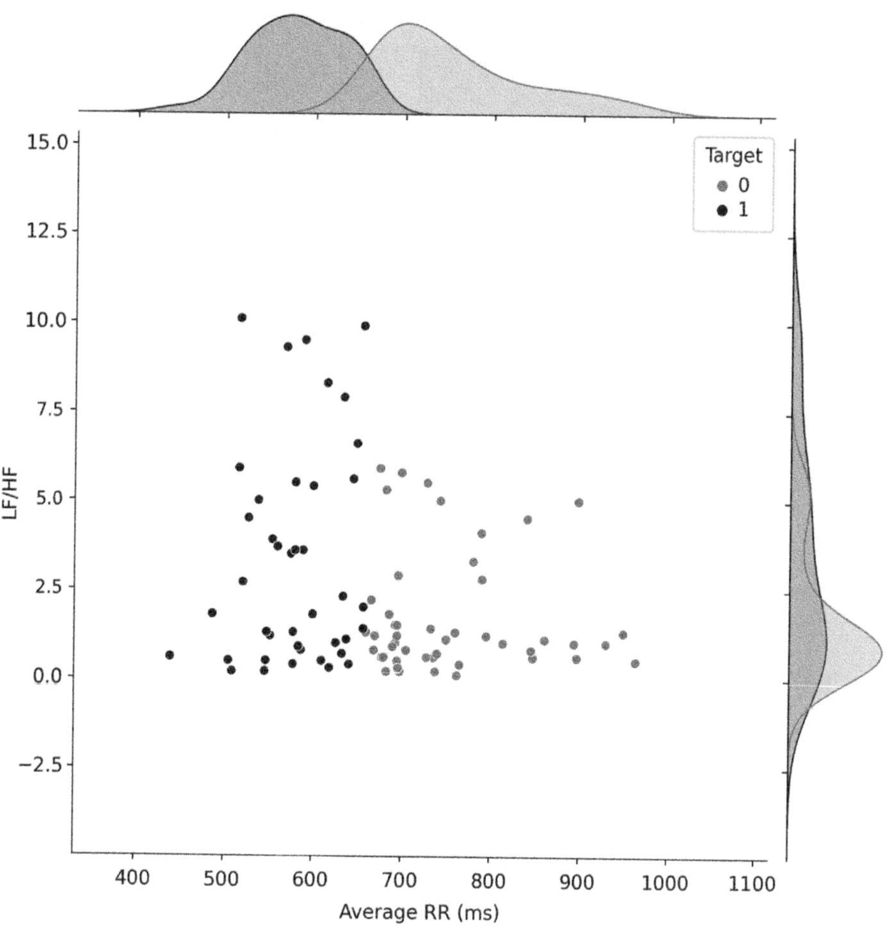

Fig. 6 The joint plot of average RR interval and the ratio of LF to HF.

3.3   Variation of HRV during the menstrual cycle

The study was conducted on 35 female volunteers in the age group of 20–25 years. Out of which, ECG was recorded in the luteal phase of the menstrual cycle in 31 females as one subset from total volunteers recruited and considered as the control group. Also, ECG was recorded during the first or second day of menstruation as the second subset of 21 females from total volunteers and considered as the study group.

No significant variation was found in the time-domain parameters of the control and study group, as shown in Table 1. Though

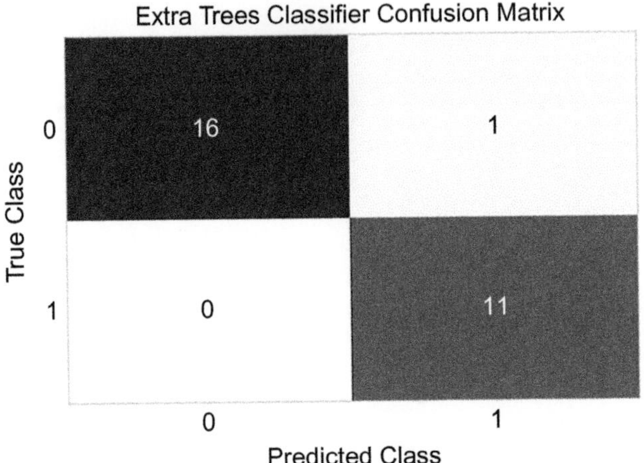

Fig. 7 Confusion matrix of ET classifier.

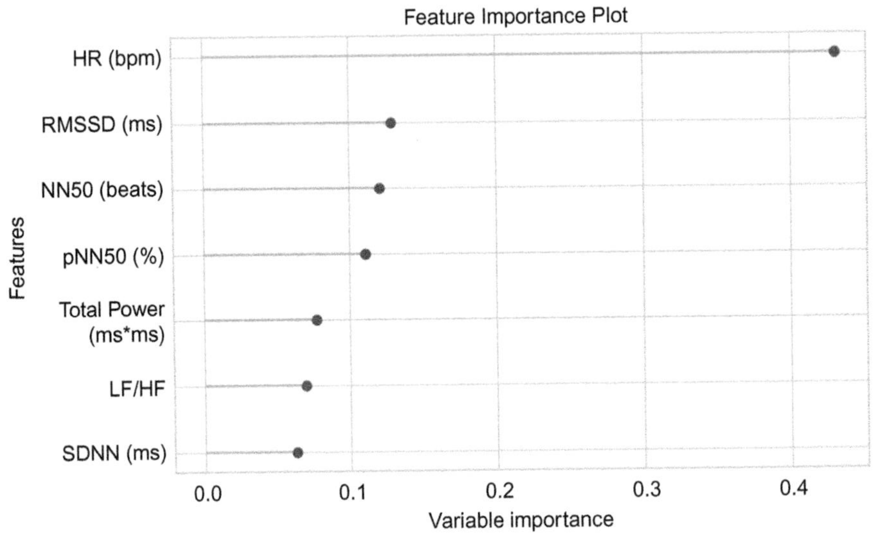

Fig. 8 Feature importance plot generated by ET classifier.

the frequency-domain parameters like LF, HF, LF/HF, total power is higher in the control group; however, not statistically significant.

No significant difference was observed in the median distribution of heart rate, average RR interval, SDNN, NN50, pNN50 value between the control and the study group, as shown in Fig. 10. However, it is noted that the median values of heart rate

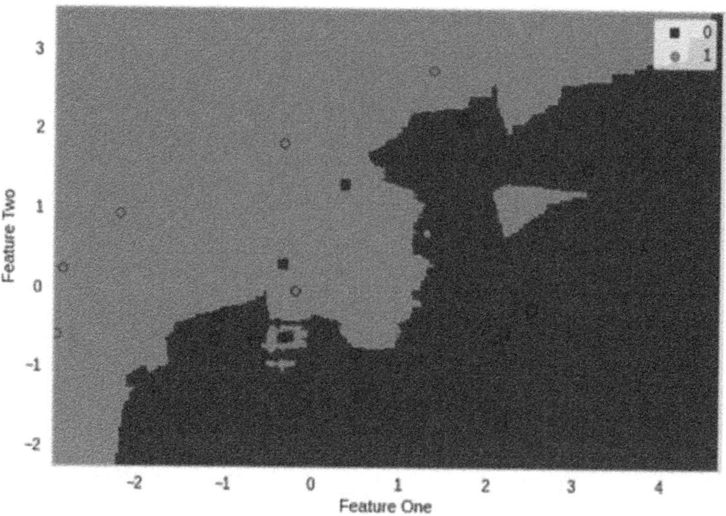

Fig. 9 Decision boundary curve of the ET classifier.

Table 1 Time and frequency-domain parameters of HRV in control and study group.

| | Group | | | | |
| | Control | | Study | | |
Parameters	Mean	SD	Mean	SD	*P*-value
Heart rate (bpm)	80	9.95	79	6.67	>0.05
Average PP interval (ms)	754	102.14	758	68.03	>0.05
Max PP interval (ms)	890	152.44	888	102.81	>0.05
Min PP interval (ms)	636	107.69	651	50.73	>0.05
SDNN	48	24.42	53	26.21	>0.05
RMSSD	48	26.38	58	49.49	>0.05
NN50	31	32.2	24	30.2	>0.05
pNN50	23	20.87	38	61.05	>0.05
LF (ms^2/Hz)	15	26.53	7	13.87	>0.05
LF norm	9	11.3	48	24.28	>0.05
HF (ms^2/Hz)	45	22.78	12	27.82	>0.05
HF norm	39	24.37	43	25.3	>0.05
LF/HF	3	3.03	2	2.28	>0.05
Total power (ms^2)	48	91.85	25	42.75	>0.05

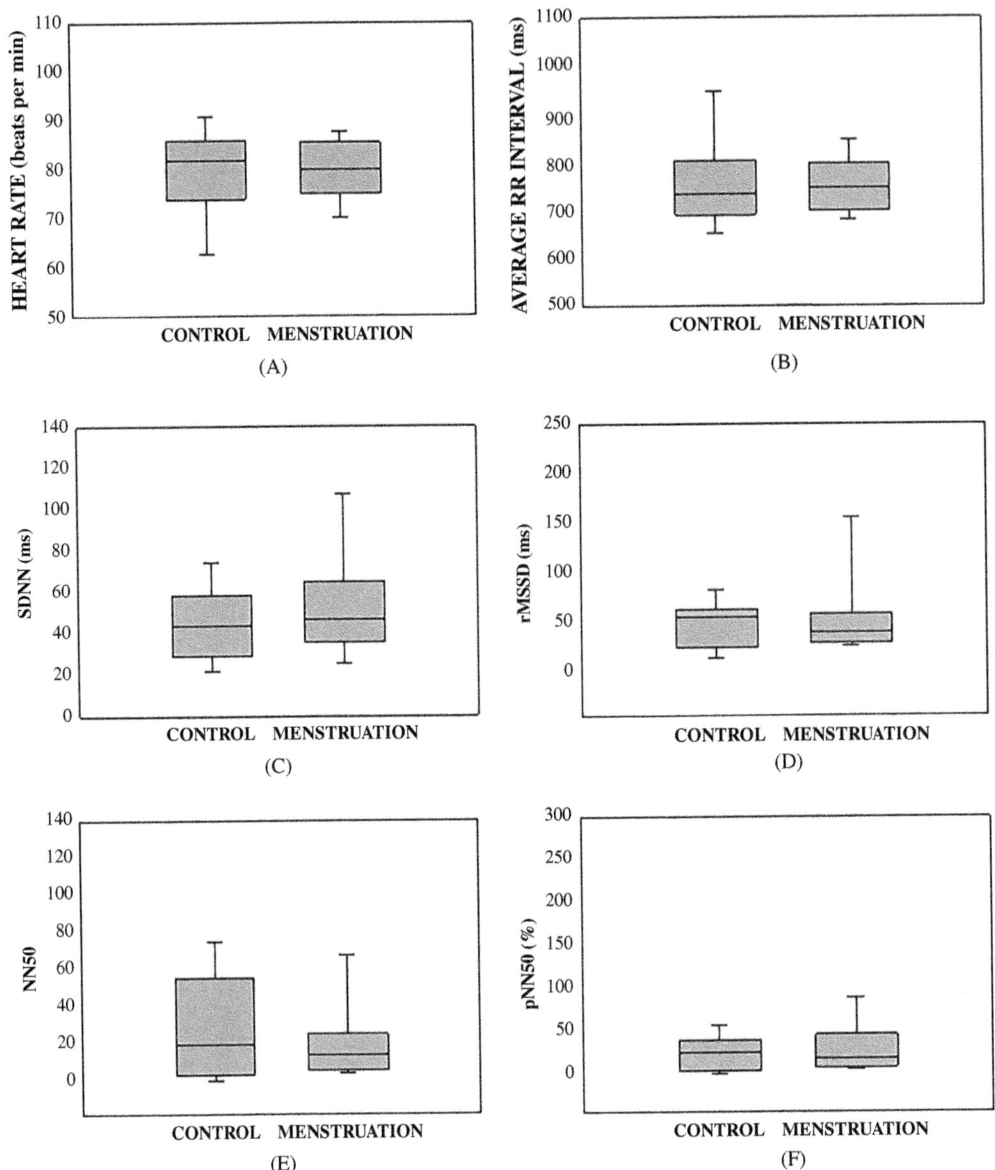

Fig. 10 Box–Whisker plot of time-domain parameters: (A) heart rate, (B) AVG RRI, (C) SDNN, (D) rMSSD, (E) NN50, and (F) pNN50 between the control and study group.

($C=82$, $S=79$), rMSSD ($C=53.996$, $S=39.094$), NN50 ($C=20$, $S=14$) and pNN50 ($C=23.9$, $S=17.5$) are higher in control group. This result contrasts with the higher median distribution value of RR interval ($C=734$, $S=745$) and SDNN ($C=43.387$, $S=46.425$) in menstruating women.

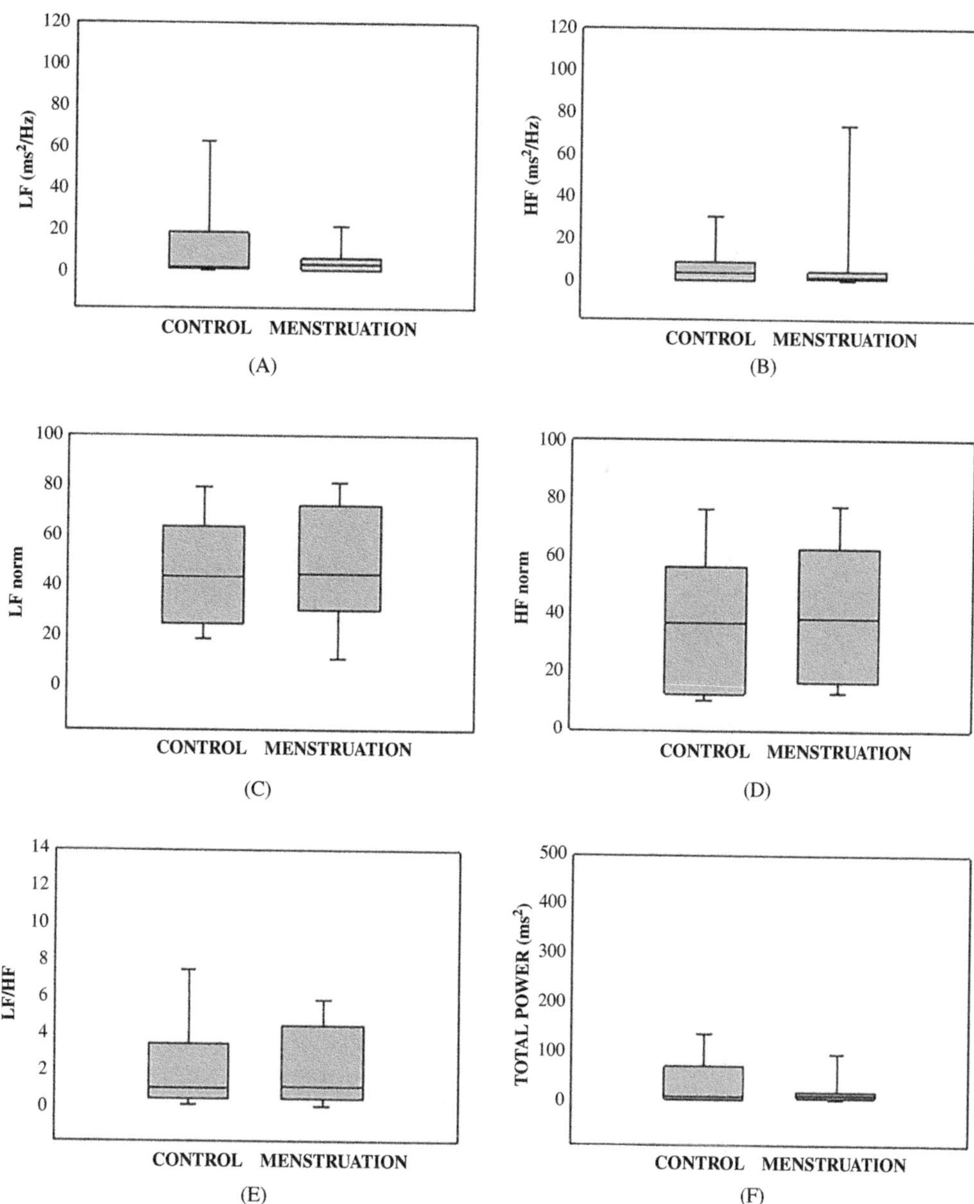

Fig. 11 Box–Whisker plot of frequency-domain parameters: (A) LF, (B) HF, (C) LF norm, (D) HF norm, (E) LF/ HF, and (F) total power.

There is no considerable change in the median distribution of all frequency-domain parameters between the control and study group, as shown in Fig. 11. Though study group have a higher median distribution for LF ($C=2.2$, $S=3.2$), LF norm ($C=43.6$, $S=44.5$), HF norm ($C=36.8$, $S=38.7$), LF/HF ($C=1.1$, $S=1.2$), total power ($C=8.6$, $S=10.9$) except HF ($C=4.2$, $S=1.8$) value of frequency-domain parameters. The interquartile range of LF and total power is higher in the control group, whereas menstruating women have a higher interquartile range for LF/HF.

4. Discussion

In the present study, the HRV parameters have been analyzed for SR and ST volunteers. The HRV parameters considered for the study were broadly divided into time and frequency-domains. The time and frequency-domain parameters are SDNN, RMSSD, NN50, pNN50, and total power and LF/HF. The HRV parameter analysis of SDNN as displayed in Fig. 1 notifies an increasing trend for SR volunteers than the ST volunteers similar to the results obtained in study [4]. Fig. 2 shows the relationship between the average RR interval and RMSSD. In SR and ST volunteers, an increasing trend of RMSSD was observed for SR compared to ST volunteers. The increasing trend was due to the fact that heart rate influences RMSSD, and similar results have been concluded in previous studies [4,103].

Fig. 3 elaborates the importance of the information of NN50 analysis in SR and ST volunteers classification. While analyzing NN50 in SR and ST volunteers, it was observed that SR volunteers showed an increasing trend because the healthy heart is more variable when compared with the stressed heart [69,70]. Fig. 4 represents the pNN50 analysis on SR and ST volunteers. The pNN50 found to be directly proportional to NN50, which increases as the cycle length of RR interval prolongs. The higher variability of pNN50 was observed in SR volunteers as the healthy heart is more dynamic, leading to increased variability in RR interval compared to ST volunteers [71,72]. In Fig. 5, the frequency-domain parameter, i.e., total power relation is expressed between SR and ST volunteer's cycle length. In many previous studies [73–76,83], total power is not analyzed as one of the frequency parameters. This work presents the analysis of total power in SR and ST volunteers, and it was observed that total power was inversely correlated to the cycle length of the RR interval. Fig. 6 displays the analysis of the LF/HF ratio in SR and ST volunteers. The LF/HF ratio displayed an increasing trend in ST volunteers when compared with SR volunteers. The higher LF/HF ratio is due to the reason that LF increases in healthy volunteers during physical training [79].

HRV is a diagnostic tool to assess the functions of ANS in various cardiac abnormalities [73]. Time-domain parameters of HRV analysis depict the activity of ANS, vagal balance, and PNS. Frequency-domain parameters mostly indicate the information of PNS activity [74,75]. It has been observed in healthy individuals that PNS is dominant while at rest. The control of parasympathetic activity decreases while performing strenuous exercises [97]. A study [94] stated that while analyzing the heart recovery cycle after exercise, it was observed that parasympathetic activity's reactivation is delayed. A study [95] stated that blocking the sympathetic activity has a significantly less impression on the heart rate. As physical activity increases, the LF also increases [96].

The sympathetic activity mainly controls the cardiac activity of patients suffering from severe myocardial infarction (MI), whereas cardiac control through PNS tends to decrease [50]. Further, MI patients may develop VF due to imbalance in SNS and PNS control of the cardiac activity [51]. Therefore, analysis of parasympathetic cardiac control can act as diagnostic tool in analyzing MI patients as it represents sinus arrhythmia [52,53]. In studies [52–55], HRV parameters tend to decrease as the occurrence of MI increases, and no optimal change can be observed in MI patients after a physical exercise.

The sinoatrial node gives rise to the sinus rate or heart rate. However, its beat-to-beat variation is influenced by the ANS, and this variation results in the formation of HRV. Study on the prediction of variations in RRI which in turn affects the HRV was performed using LSTM-RNN model [104]. Moreover, in a study [105] corrected PTaI formula was developed to determine its effect on different heart rates. Various other factors affecting HRV includes stress, age, gender, BMI, hormonal fluctuations, circadian cycle, physical activity, and other physiological and environmental parameters. Several studies presented that HRV is also influenced due to the fluctuation of hormones in females of reproductive age. Changes in the estrogen levels in menopausal women show higher sympathetic activity than premenopausal women [106]. However, few studies gave contradictory opinions on the effect of the menstrual cycle on HRV. Studies show an increase in the sympathetic dominance at the luteal phase [107–110], whereas vagal dominance increases during menstruation, while few studies show the opposite effect [111]. In contrast, other studies demonstrated no significant impact of HRV on the menstrual cycle [67,112]. Finding of this study on HRV is in agreement with previous studies showing no effect of HRV on the menstrual cycle. A study [113] shows no difference between the menstrual and control groups for atrial aspects and also no significant changes were observed in PRI, PPI. Hence, it suggests that hormonal fluctuation at the time of the menstrual cycle does not cause any effect on HRV. However, more elaborate study on large population of women during menstruation phases may provide a precise outlook on the effect of HRV on hormonal fluctuations.

5. Conclusion

HRV analysis on SR, and ST volunteers and the changes observed in HRV parameters in the menstrual cycle are discussed in this chapter. The time-domain parameters in the case of SR and ST volunteers increased with the increase in the cycle length of the RR intervals. The frequency-domain parameters showed a decreasing trend as the cycle length of the RR intervals increased in the case of SR and ST volunteers. The ET classifier was developed to classify SR and ST ECG data based on HRV features. The ET classifier achieved an accuracy of 93%. The recall, precision, and F1 score of the ET classifier were 96.66%, 92.50%, and 93.71%, respectively. Hormonal fluctuation in the menstrual cycle did not have significant effect on the HRV time and frequency-domain parameters. Further studies on a larger population are needed to figure out the normal limits of electrocardiographic parameters in women of reproductive age during menstruation.

Acknowledgments

The authors acknowledge the support from the Ministry of Education, Government of India. The present study was supported by financial grants from the Science and Engineering Research Board (SERB), Department of Science and Technology (DST), Government of India (EEQ/2019/000148).

References

[1] J.P. Saul, Beat-to-beat variations of heart rate reflect modulation of cardiac autonomic outflow, News Physiol. Sci. 5 (1990) 32–37.

[2] M.N. Levy, P.J. Schwartz, Vagal Control of the Heart: Experimental Basis and Clinical Implications, Futura Pub. Co., Armonk, New York, 1994.

[3] P.J. Schwartz, S.G. Priori, Sympathetic nervous system and cardiac arrythmias, in: D.P. Zipes, J. Jalife (Eds.), Cardiac Electrophysiology: From Cell to Bedside, W.B. Saunders, Philadelphia, 1990, pp. 330–334.

[4] A.J. Camm, M. Malik, J.T. Bigger, G. Breithardt, S. Cerutti, R.J. Cohen, et al., Heart rate variability: standards of measurement, physiological interpretation and clinical use. Task Force of the European Society of Cardiology and the North American Society of Pacing and Electrophysiology, Circulation 93 (5) (1996) 1043–1065.

[5] S. Akselrod, D. Gordon, F.A. Ubel, D.C. Shannon, A.C. Berger, R.J. Cohen, Power spectrum analysis of heart rate fluctuation: a quantitative probe of beat-to-beat cardiovascular control, Science 213 (4504) (1981) 220–222.

[6] R.D. Berger, S. Akselrod, D. Gordon, R.J. Cohen, An efficient algorithm for spectral analysis of heart rate variability, IEEE Trans. Biomed. Eng. 33 (9) (1986) 900–904.

[7] M.V. Kamath, E.L. Fallen, Power spectral analysis of heart rate variability: a non-invasive signature of cardiac autonomic function, Crit. Rev. Biomed. Eng. 21 (3) (1993) 245–311.

[8] M.V. Kamath, E.L. Fallen, Correction of the heart rate vaiability signal for ectopics and missing beats, in: M. Malik, A.J. Camm (Eds.), Heart Rate Variability, Futura Pub. Co., Armonk, 1995.

[9] M. Kobayashi, T. Musha, 1/f fluctuation of heart beat period, IEEE Trans. Biomed. Eng. 29 (6) (1982) 456–457.

[10] M. Pagani, F. Lombardi, S. Guzzetti, O. Rimoldi, R. Furlan, P. Pizzinelli, et al., Power spectral analysis of heart rate and arterial pressure variabilities as a marker of sympatho-vagal interaction in man and conscious dog, Circ. Res. 59 (2) (1986) 178–193.

[11] B. Pomeranz, R.J. Macaulay, M.A. Caudill, I. Kutz, D. Adam, D. Gordon, et al., Assessment of autonomic function in humans by heart rate spectral analysis, Am. J. Physiol. 248 (1 Pt 2) (1985) 151–153.

[12] J. Saul, R. Rea, D. Eckberg, R. Berger, R. Cohen, Heart rate and muscle sympathetic nerve variability during reflex changes of autonomic activity, Am. J. Physiol. 258 (3 Pt 2) (1990) 713–721.

[13] S. Akselrod, D. Gordon, J.B. Madwed, N.C. Snidman, D.C. Shannon, R.J. Cohen, Hemodynamic regulation: investigation by spectral analysis, Am. J. Physiol. 249 (4) (1985) H867–H875.

[14] R.W. de Boer, J.M. Karemaker, J. Strackee, Relationships between short-term blood-pressure fluctuations and heart-rate variability in resting subjects. I: a spectral analysis approach, Med. Biol. Eng. Comput. 23 (4) (1985) 352–358.

[15] R.W. de Boer, J.M. Karemaker, J. Strackee, Relationships between short-term blood-pressure fluctuations and heart-rate variability in resting subjects. II: a spectral analysis approach, Med. Biol. Eng. Comput. 23 (4) (1985) 359–364.

[16] R.W. de Boer, J.M. Karemaker, J. Strackee, Spectrum of a series of point events, generated by the integral pulse frequency modulation model, Med. Biol. Eng. Comput. 23 (2) (1985) 138–142.

[17] D. Laude, J.L. Elghozi, A. Girard, E. Bellard, M. Bouhaddi, P. Castiglioni, et al., Comparison of various techniques used to estimate spontaneous baroreflex sensitivity (the EUROVAR study), Am. J. Physiol. Regul. Integr. Comp. Physiol. 286 (1) (2004) R226–R231.

[18] B.E. Westerhof, J. Gisolf, W.J. Stok, K.H. Wesseling, J.M. Karemaker, Time-domain cross-correlation baroreflex sensitivity: performance on the EUROBAVAR data set, J. Hypertens. 22 (7) (2004) 1371–1380.

[19] M. Rothschild, A. Rothschild, M. Pfeifer, Temporary decrease in cardiac parasympathetic tone after acute myocardial infarction, Am. J. Cardiol. 62 (9) (1988) 637–639.

[20] P.J. Schwartz, M.T. La Rovere, E. Vanoli, Autonomic nervous system and sudden cardiac death. Experimental basis and clinical observations for post-myocardial infarction risk stratification, Circulation 85 (1 Suppl) (1992) I77–I91.

[21] J.M. Wharton, R.E. Coleman, H.C. Strauss, The role of the autonomic nervous system in sudden cardiac death, Trends Cardiovasc. Med. 2 (2) (1992) 65–71.

[22] P.G. Katona, F. Jih, Respiratory sinus arrhythmia: non-invasive measure of parasympathetic cardiac control, J. Appl. Physiol. 39 (5) (1975) 801–805.

[23] A. Malliani, M. Pagani, F. Lombardi, S. Cerutti, Cardiovascular neural regulation explored in the frequency domain, Circulation 84 (2) (1991) 482–492.

[24] R.M. Carney, J.A. Blumenthal, P.K. Stein, L. Watkins, D. Catellier, L.F. Berkman, Depression, heart rate variability, and acute myocardial infarction, Circulation 104 (17) (2001) 2024–2028.

[25] R.M. Carney, J.A. Blumenthal, K.E. Freedland, P.K. Stein, W.B. Howells, L.F. Berkman, Low heart rate variability and the effect of depression on post-myocardial infarction mortality, Arch. Intern. Med. 165 (13) (2005) 1486–1491.

[26] F. Duru, R. Candinas, G. Dziekan, U. Goebbels, J. Myers, P. Dubach, Effect of exercise training on heart rate variability in patients with new-onset left ventricular dysfunction after myocardial infarction, Am. Heart J. 140 (1) (2000) 157–161.

[27] J. Fell, K. Mann, J. Roschke, M.S. Gopinathan, Nonlinear analysis of continuous ECG during sleep I. Reconstruction, Biol. Cybern. 82 (2000) 477–483.

[28] K.A.R. Rao, Y.V. Kumar, D.N. Dutt, T.S. Vedavathy, Characterizing chaos in heart rate variability time series of panic disorder patients, in: Proceedings of ICBME Biovision. Bangalore, India, 2001, pp. 163–167.

[29] M.I. Owis, A.H. Abou-Zied, A.B.M. Youssef, Y.M. Kadah, Study of features on nonlinear dynamical modeling in ECG arrhythmia detection and classification, IEEE Trans. Biomed. Eng. 49 (7) (2002) 733–736.

[30] R.U. Acharya, C.M. Lim, P. Joseph, Heart rate variability analysis using correlation dimension and detrended fluctuation analysis, ITBM-RBM 23 (6) (2002) 333–339.

[31] U.R. Acharya, P.S. Bhatt, S.S. Iyengar, A. Rao, S. Dua, Classification of heart rate using artificial neural network and fuzzy equivalence relation, Pattern Recogn. 36 (1) (2003) 61–68.

[32] U.R. Acharya, N. Kannathal, S.M. Krishnan, Comprehensive analysis of cardiac health using heart rate signals, Physiol. Meas. 25 (5) (2004) 1139–1151.

[33] U.R. Acharya, N. Kannathal, O.W. Sing, L.Y. Ping, T. Chua, Heart rate analysis in normal subjects of various age groups, Biomed. Eng. Online 3 (24) (2004).

[34] D. Ge, N. Srinivasan, S.M. Krishnan, Cardiac arrhythmia classification using autoregressive modeling, Biomed. Eng. Online 1 (5) (2002).

[35] K.P. Davy, C.A. Desouza, P.P. Jones, D.R. Seals, Elevated heart rate variability in physically active young and older adult women, Clin. Sci. 94 (6) (1998) 579–584.

[36] S.M. Ryan, A.L. Goldberger, S.M. Pincus, J. Mietus, L.A. Lipsitz, gender-and age-related differences in heart rate dynamics: are women more complex than men, J. Am. Coll. Cardiol. 24 (7) (1994) 1700–1707.

[37] E. Nagy, H. Orvos, G. Bardos, P. Molnar, Gender-related heart rate differences in human neonates, Pediatr. Res. 47 (6) (2000) 778–780.

[38] H. Bonnemeier, G. Richardt, J. Potratz, U.K. Wiegand, A. Brandes, N. Kluge, et al., Circadian profile of cardiac autonomic nervous modulation in healthy subjects: differing effects of aging and gender on heart rate variability, J. Cardiovasc. Electrophysiol. 14 (8) (2003) 791–799.

[39] D. Ramaekers, H. Ector, A.E. Aubert, A. Rubens, F. van de Werf, Heart rate variability and heart rate in healthy volunteers: is the female autonomous nervous system cardioprotective? Eur. Heart J. 19 (9) (1998) 1334–1341.

[40] Y. Yamasaki, M. Kodama, M. Matsuhisa, M. Kishimoto, H. Ozaki, A. Tani, et al., Diurnal heart rate variability in healthy subjects: effects of aging and sex differences, Am. J. Physiol. 271 (1 Pt 2) (1996) H303–H310.

[41] C.M. Van Ravenswaaij, J.C. Hopman, L.A. Kollee, J.P. van Amen, G.B. Stoelinga, H.P. van Geijn, Influences on heart rate variability in spontaneously breathing preterm infants, Early Hum. Dev. 27 (3) (1991) 187–205.

[42] J.B. Schwartz, W.J. Gibb, T. Tran, Aging effects on heart rate variation, J. Gerontol. 46 (3) (1991) M99–106.

[43] J.P. Finley, S.T. Nungent, W. Hellenbrand, Heart rate variability in children. Spectral analysis of developmental changes between 5 and 24 years, Can. J. Physiol. Pharmacol. 65 (10) (1987) 2048–2052.

[44] L.A. Lipsitz, J. Mietus, G.B. Moody, A.L. Goldberger, Spectral characteristics of heart rate variability before and during postural tilt. Relations to aging and risk of syncope, Circulation 81 (6) (1990) 1803–1810.

[45] F. Weise, F. Heydenreich, S. Kropf, D. Krell, Intercorrelation analyses among age, spectral parameters of heart rate variability and respiration in human volunteers, J. Interdiscipl. Cycle Res. 21 (1) (1990) 17–24.

[46] P.W. Wilson, J.C. Evans, Coronary artery disease prediction, Am. J. Hypertens. 6 (11 Pt 2) (1993) 309S–313S.

[47] S. Bekheit, M. Tangella, A. el-Sakr, Q. Rasheed, W. Craelius, N. el-Sherif, Use of heart rate spectral analysis to study the effects of calcium channel blockers on sympathetic activity after myocardial infarction, Am. Heart J. 119 (1) (1990) 79–85.

[48] P. Coumel, J.S. Hermida, B. Wennerblom, A. Leenhardt, P. Maison-Blanche, B. Cauchemez, Heart rate variability in left ventricular hypertrophy and heart failure, and the effects of beta-blockade. A non-spectral analysis of heart rate variability in the frequency domain and in the time domain, Eur. Heart J. 12 (3) (1991) 412–422.

[49] S. Guzzetti, E. Piccaluga, R. Casati, S. Cerutti, F. Lombardi, M. Pagani, et al., Sympathetic predominance in essential hypertension: a study employing spectral analysis of heart rate variability, J. Hypertens. 6 (9) (1988) 711–717.

[50] J.E. Muller, J. Morrison, P.H. Stone, R.E. Rude, B. Rosner, R. Roberts, et al., Nifedipine therapy for patients with threatened and acute myocardial infarction: a randomized, double-blind, placebo-controlled comparison, Circulation 69 (4) (1984) 740–747.

[51] C. Pater, D. Compagnone, J. Luszick, C.N. Verboom, Effect of omacor on HRV parameters in patients with recent uncomplicated myocardial infarction—a randomized, parallel group, double-blind, placebo-controlled trial: study design, Curr. Control. Trials Cardiovasc. Med. 4 (1) (2003) 2.

[52] B. Eryonucu, K. Uzun, N. Guler, M. Bilge, Comparison of the acute effects of salbutamol and terbutaline on heart rate variability in adult asthmatic patients, Eur. Respir. J. 17 (2001) 863–867.

[53] J. Hayano, M. Yamada, Y. Sakakibara, T. Fujinami, K. Yokoyama, Y. Watanabe, et al., Short and long-term effects of cigarette smoking on heart rate variability, Am. J. Cardiol. 65 (1) (1990) 84–88.

[54] D. Luchini, F. Bertocchi, A. Malliani, M. Pagani, A controlled study of the autonomic changes produced by habitual cigarette smoking in healthy subjects, Cardiovasc. Res. 31 (4) (1996) 633–639.

[55] O.N. Niedermaier, M.L. Smith, L.A. Beightol, Z. Zukowska-Grojec, D.S. Goldstein, D.L. Eckberg, Influence of cigarette smoking on human autonomic function, Circulation 88 (2) (1993) 562–571.

[56] C.A. Pope III, D.J. Eatough, D.R. Gold, Y. Pang, K.R. Nielsen, P. Nath, et al., Acute exposure to environmental tobacco smoke and heart rate variability, Environ. Health Perspect. 109 (7) (2001) 711–716.

[57] P.S. Zeskind, J.L. Gingras, Maternal cigarette-smoking during pregnancy disrupts rhythms in fetal heart rate, J. Pediatr. Psychol. 31 (1) (2006) 5–14.

[58] S.C. Malpas, E.A. Whiteside, T.J. Maling, Heart rate variability and cardiac autonomic function in men with chronic alcohol dependence, Br. Heart J. 65 (2) (1991) 84–88.

[59] J.M. Ryan, L.G. Howes, White coat effect of alcohol, Am. J. Hypertens. 13 (10) (2000) 1135–1138.

[60] A.M. Pellizzer, P.W. Kamen, M.D. Esler, S. Lim, H. Krum, Comparative effects of mibefradil and nifedipine gastrointestinal transport system on autonomic function in patients with mild to moderate essential hypertension, J. Hypertens. 19 (2) (2001) 279–285.

[61] J. Rossinen, M. Viitasalo, J. Partanen, P. Koskinen, M. Kupari, M.S. Nieminen, Effects of acute alcohol ingestion on heart rate variability in patients with

documented coronary artery disease and stable angina pectoris, Am. J. Cardiol. 79 (4) (1997) 487–491.

[62] K.E. Barrett, H. Brooks, S. Boitano, S.M. Barman, Ganong's Review of Medical Physiology, 24th edition, Reproductive Development and Function of the Female Reproductive System, McGraw Hill, New Delhi, 2012, pp. 391–418.

[63] T.K. Brar, K.D. Singh, A. Kumar, Effect of different phases of menstrual cycle on heart rate variability (HRV), J. Clin. Diagn. Res. 9 (10) (2015) CC01–CC04.

[64] R.R. Preston, T.E. Wilson, Lippincott's Illustrated Reviews Physiology. 1st edition. Female and Male Gonads, Wolter Kluwer, New Delhi, 2013, pp. 438–448.

[65] M.H. Chung, C.C. Yang, Heart rate variability across the menstrual cycle in shift work nurses, J. Exp. Clin. Med. 3 (3) (2011) 121–125.

[66] M.P. Tarvainen, N.J. Kubois, HRV User's Guide: Version 2.1, 2012, pp. 8–12.

[67] A.S. Leicht, D.A. Hirning, G.D. Allen, Heart rate variability and endogenous sex hormones during the menstrual cycle in young women, Exp. Physiol. 88 (3) (2003) 441–446.

[68] S. Karthik, K. Balamurugesan, S. Viswanathan, V. Sivaji, Role of gender and menstrual cycle on heart rate variability, QTc and JT intervals, Int. J. Sci. Stud. 2 (12) (2015) 49–53.

[69] T.H. Makikallio, H.V. Huikuri, U. Hintze, J. Videbaek, R.D. Mitrani, A. Castellanos, et al., Fractal analysis and time-and frequency-domain measures of heart rate variability as predictors of mortality in patients with heart failure, Am. J. Cardiol. 87 (2) (2001) 178–182.

[70] S.K. Agarwal, F.L. Norby, E.A. Whitsel, E.Z. Soliman, L.Y. Chen, L.R. Loehr, et al., Cardiac autonomic dysfunction and incidence of atrial fibrillation: results from 20 years follow-up, J. Am. Coll. Cardiol. 69 (2017) 291–299.

[71] A. Parsi, D. Byrne, M. Glavin, E. Jones, Heart rate variability feature selection method for automated prediction of sudden cardiac death, Biomed. Signal Process. Control 65 (2021), 102310.

[72] M.N. Castro, D.E. Vigo, D.R. Gustafson, I. Vila-Perez, P. Massaro, C. Garcia, et al., Acute and six-month depression-related abnormalities in the sleep-wake rhythm of cardiac autonomic activity in survivors of acute coronary syndromes, J. Perinat. Med. 4 (6) (2017) 13–18.

[73] A. Mestanikova, M. Mestanik, I. Ondrejka, I. Hrtanek, D. Cesnekova, A. Jurko Jr., et al., Complex cardiac vagal regulation to mental and physiological stress in adolescent major depression, J. Affect. Disord. 249 (2019) 234–241.

[74] M.G. Poddar, A.C. Birajdar, J. Virmani, Automated classification of hypertension and coronary artery disease patients by PNN, KNN, and SVM classifiers using HRV analysis, in: Machine Learning in Bio-Signal Analysis and Diagnostic Imaging, Academic Press, 2019, pp. 99–125.

[75] M. Kallio, K. Suominen, A.M. Bianchi, T. Mäkikallio, T. Haapaniemi, S. Astafiev, et al., Comparison of heart rate variability analysis methods in patients with Parkinson's disease, Med. Biol. Eng. Comput. 40 (4) (2002) 408–414.

[76] M. Kuppusamy, D. Kamaldeen, R. Pitani, J. Amaldas, P. Ramasamy, P. Shanmugam, et al., Effects of yoga breathing practice on heart rate variability in healthy adolescents: a randomized controlled trial, Intern. Med. 9 (1) (2020) 28–32.

[77] D.M. Sacknoff, G.W. Gleim, N. Stachenfeld, N.L. Coplan, Effect of athletic training on heart rate variability, Am. Heart J. 127 (5) (1994) 1275–1278.

[78] O. Kiss, N. Sydo, P. Vargha, H. Vago, C. Czimbalmos, E. Édes, et al., Detailed heart rate variability analysis in athletes, Clin. Auton. Res. 26 (4) (2016) 245–252.

[79] K.C. Chang, P.H. Hsieh, M.Y. Wu, Y.C. Wang, J.Y. Chen, F.J. Tsai, et al., Usefulness of machine learning-based detection and classification of cardiac arrhythmias with 12-lead electrocardiograms, Can. J. Cardiol. 37 (1) (2021) 94–104.

[80] M. Seera, C.P. Lim, W.S. Liew, E. Lim, C.K. Loo, Classification of electrocardiogram and auscultatory blood pressure signals using machine learning models, Expert Syst. Appl. 42 (7) (2015) 3643–3652.

[81] S.K. Pandey, R.R. Janghel, V. Vani, Patient specific machine learning models for ECG signal classification, Procedia Comput. Sci. 167 (2020) 2181–2190.

[82] C.U. Kumari, A.S.D. Murthy, B.L. Prasanna, M.P.P. Reddy, A.K. Panigrahy, An automated detection of heart arrhythmias using machine learning technique: SVM, Mater. Today: Proc. 45 (2) (2020) 1393–1398.

[83] U.R. Acharya, H. Fujita, S.L. Oh, U. Raghavendra, J.H. Tan, M. Adam, et al., Automated identification of shockable and non-shockable life-threatening ventricular arrhythmias using convolutional neural network, Futur. Gener. Comput. Syst. 79 (3) (2018) 952–959.

[84] M. Mitra, R.K. Samanta, Cardiac arrhythmia classification using neural networks with selected features, Procedia Technol. 10 (2013) 76–84.

[85] O. Yildrium, U.B. Baloglu, R.S. Tan, E.J. Ciaccio, U.R. Acharya, A new approach for arrhythmia classification using deep coded features and LSTM networks, Comput. Methods Programs Biomed. 176 (2019) 121–133.

[86] S.M. Mathews, C. Kambhamettu, K.E. Barner, A novel application of deep learning for single-lead ECG classification, Comput. Biol. Med. 99 (2018) 53–62.

[87] J. Sivaraman, G. Uma, S. Venkatesan, M. Umapathy, V.E. Dhandapani, Normal limits of ECG measurements related to atrial activity using a modified limb lead system, Anatol. J. Cardiol. 15 (1) (2015) 2–6.

[88] J. Sivaraman, G. Uma, S. Venkatesan, M. Umapathy, K.N. Keshav, A study on atrial Ta wave morphology in healthy subjects: an approach using P wave signal-averaging method, J. Med. Imaging Health Infor. 4 (5) (2014) 675–680.

[89] J. Sivaraman, S. Venkatesan, R. Periyasamy, J. Joseph, R.M. Shanmugan, Modified limb lead ECG system effects on electrocardiographic wave amplitudes and frontal plane axis in sinus rhythm subjects, Anatol. J. Cardiol. 17 (1) (2017) 46–54.

[90] R. John, J. Sivaraman, Effects of sinus rhythm on atrial ECG components using a modified limb lead system, in: 2017 4th International Conference on Signal Processing, Computing and Control (ISPCC), Solan, India, September 21–23, 2017, pp. 527–530.

[91] S. Karimulla, J. Sivaraman, The role and significance of atrial ECG components in standard and modified lead systems, in: P.K. Mallick, P. Meher, A. Majumder, S.K. Das (Eds.), Electronic Systems and Intelligent Computing (ESIC), vol. 686, Springer, Singapore, 2020, pp. 347–355.

[92] A. Jyothsana, J. Sivaraman, A study on stability analysis of QT interval dynamics of ECG using ARMAX model, in: P.K. Mallick, P. Meher, A. Majumder, S.K. Das (Eds.), Electronic Systems and Intelligent Computing (ESIC), vol. 686, Springer, Singapore, 2020, pp. 307–316.

[93] A. Jyothsana, B. Arya, J. Sivaraman, Stability analysis on the effects of heart rate variability and premature activation of atrial ECG dynamics using ARMAX model, Phys. Eng. Sci. Med. 43 (4) (2020) 1361–1370.

[94] J. Sivaraman, G. Uma, P. Langley, M. Umapathy, S. Venkatesan, G. Palanikumar, A study on stability analysis of atrial repolarization variability using ARX model in sinus rhythm and atrial tachycardia ECGs, Comput. Methods Programs Biomed. 137 (2016) 341–351.

[95] B. Dhananjay, J. Sivaraman, The role of heart rate variability in atrial ECG components of normal sinus rhythm and sinus tachycardia subjects, in: S. Satapathy, V. Bhateja, B. Janakiramaiah, Y.W. Chen (Eds.), Intelligent System Design, Advances in Intelligent Systems and Computing, vol. 1171, Springer, Singapore, 2021, pp. 637–644.

[96] B. Dhananjay, J. Sivaraman, Analysis and classification of heart rate using CatBoost feature ranking model, Biomed. Signal Process. Control 68 (2021), 102610.

[97] J.P. Kelwade, S.S. Salankar, Radial basis function neural network for prediction of cardiac arrhythmias based on heart rate time series, in: 2016 IEEE First International Conference on Control, Measurement and Instrumentation (CMI), Kolkata, India, January 8–10, 2016, pp. 454–458.

[98] C. Krittanawong, H.U.H. Virk, S. Bangalore, Z. Wang, K.W. Johnson, R. Pinotti, et al., Machine learning prediction in cardiovascular diseases: a meta-analysis, Sci. Rep. 10 (16057) (2020) 1–11.

[99] S. Raghunath, A.E.U. Cerna, L. Jing, D.P. vanMaanen, J. Stough, N. Dustin, et al., Prediction of mortality from 12-lead electrocardiogram voltage data using a deep neural network, Nat. Med. 26 (2020) 886–891.

[100] T.M. Chen, C.H. Huang, E.S. Shih, Y.F. Hu, M.J. Hwang, Detection and classification of cardiac arrhythmias by a challenge-best deep learning neural network model, iScience 23 (3) (2020) 100886.

[101] Z. Wang, Y. Zhu, D. Li, Y. Yin, J. Zhang, Feature rearrangement based deep learning system for predicting heart failure mortality, Comput. Methods Programs Biomed. 191 (2020), 105383.

[102] S. Kundella, R. Gobinath, Robust convolutional neural network for arrhythmia prediction in ECG signals, Mater. Today Proc. (2020).

[103] A.K. Reimers, G. Knapp, C.D. Reimers, Effects of exercise on the resting heart rate: a systematic review and meta-analysis of interventional studies, J. Clin. Med. 7 (12) (2018) 503.

[104] B. Dhananjay, N.P. Venkatesh, A. Bhardwaj, J. Sivaraman, Design and development of LSTM-RNN model for the prediction of RR intervals in ECG signals, in: F. Thakkar, G. Saha, C. Shahnaz, Y.C. Hu (Eds.), Proceedings of the International e-Conference on Intelligent Systems and Signal Processing. Advances in Intelligent Systems and Computing, Springer, Singapore, 2022, p. 1370.

[105] S. Karimulla, A. Bhardwaj, J. Sivaraman, B. Dhananjay, Development of optimal corrected PTa interval formula for different heart rates, in: F. Thakkar, G. Saha, C. Shahnaz, Y.C. Hu (Eds.), Proceedings of the International e-Conference on Intelligent Systems and Signal Processing. Advances in Intelligent Systems and Computing, Springer, Singapore, 2022, p. 1370.

[106] G. Mercuro, A. Podda, L. Pitzalis, S. Zoncu, M. Mascia, G.B. Melis, et al., Evidence of a role of endogenous estrogen in the modulation of autonomic nervous system, Am. J. Cardiol. 85 (6) (2000) 787–789, A9.

[107] M. Vallejo, M.F. Márquez, V.H. Borja-Aburto, M. Cárdenas, A.G. Hermosillo, Age, body mass index, and menstrual cycle influence young women's heart rate variability: a multivariable analysis, Clin. Auton. Res. 15 (4) (2005) 292–298.

[108] N. Sato, S. Miyake, Cardiovascular reactivity to mental stress: Relationship with menstrual cycle and gender, J. Physiol. Anthropol. Appl. Human Sci. 23 (6) (2004) 215–223.

[109] P.S. McKinley, A.R. King, P.A. Shapiro, I. Slavov, Y. Fang, I.S. Chen, et al., The impact of menstrual cycle phase on cardiac autonomic regulation, Psychophysiology 49 (4) (2009) 904–911.

[110] A. Yildirir, G. Kabakci, E. Akgul, L. Tokgozoglu, A. Oto, Effects of menstrual cycle on cardiac autonomic innervation as assessed by heart rate variability, Ann. Noninvasive Electrocardiol. 7 (1) (2002) 60–63.

[111] T. Princi, S. Parco, A. Accardo, O. Radillo, F. De Seta, S. Guaschino, Parametric evaluation of heart rate variability during the menstrual cycle in young women, Biomed. Sci. Instrum. 41 (2005) 340–345.

[112] A. Weissman, L. Lowenstein, J. Tal, G. Ohel, I. Calderon, A. Lightman, Modulation of heart rate variability by estrogen in young women undergoing induction of ovulation, Eur. J. Appl. Physiol. 105 (3) (2009) 381–386.

[113] A. Padhan, A. Bhardwaj, J. Sivaraman, Effects of menstrual cycle on atrial ECG components, in: F. Thakkar, G. Saha, C. Shahnaz, Y.C. Hu (Eds.), Proceedings of the International e-Conference on Intelligent Systems and Signal Processing. Advances in Intelligent Systems and Computing, Springer, Singapore, 2022, p. 1370.

3

Understanding the suitability of parametric modeling techniques in detecting the changes in the HRV signals acquired from cannabis consuming and nonconsuming Indian paddy-field workers

Suraj K. Nayak[a], Manoja K. Majhi[a], Bikash K. Pradhan[a], Indranil Banerjee[b], Satyapriya Mohanty[c], and Kunal Pal[a]

[a]Department of Biotechnology and Medical Engineering, National Institute of Technology, Rourkela, India. [b]Department of Bioscience and Bioengineering, Indian Institute of Technology, Jodhpur, India. [c]Department of Cardiothoracic and Vascular Surgery, All India Institute of Medical Sciences (AIIMS), Bhubaneswar, India

1.　Introduction

Cannabis is an annual plant mainly found in Europe, Central Asia, and the Indian subcontinent [1]. The different parts of the plant have been explored for several potential usages, which include food, textile fiber, fuel, medicinal, and recreational applications [2,3]. However, the last few decades have witnessed a rapid increase in the recreational use of cannabis products. As per the literature, cannabis has become the third most illicit recreational product after alcohol and tobacco [4]. One of the factors contributing to the increased recreational use of cannabis is the belief of the people that it is safer than other similar products. In recent years, the legalization of recreational cannabis consumption by adults in various countries has promoted this belief [5]. However, different adverse health effects of regular cannabis consumption have been reported in the last few decades [6]. As per Martinez [7], cannabis is both a medication and a substance of abuse like

Advanced Methods in Biomedical Signal Processing and Analysis. https://doi.org/10.1016/B978-0-323-85955-4.00009-0

Copyright © 2023 Elsevier Inc. All rights reserved.

opioids, amphetamines, and ketamine [7]. This observation is promoted by the use of cannabis to treat psychiatric disorders on the one hand. On the other hand, cannabis can cause addiction and deteriorate psychiatric diseases like anxiety and psychosis. As per the report published in 2017 by the National Academies of Sciences, Engineering, and Medicine (NASEM), strong evidence is available on the enhanced symptoms of mania and hypomania in bipolar disorder patients who are regular consumers of cannabis [8]. The increased symptoms of psychosis in cannabis-consuming schizophrenia patients have also been highlighted. The NASEM report further suggested worsening of anxiety disorders due to regular cannabis consumption. Alvares et al. [9] have reported that psychiatric patients, who consume cannabis, have increased susceptibility to cardiovascular diseases that is induced due to ANS dysfunction [9]. Accordingly, there is a necessity to examine the effect of cannabis consumption on the ANS activity of regular cannabis users. Such investigation can help to divulge prognostic information about their susceptibility to psychiatric disorders followed by cardiovascular diseases.

The examination of the cardiac autonomic regulation using the analysis of the heart rate variability (HRV) signals provides a non-invasive way of estimating any alteration in the ANS physiology due to any disease or external stimulus [10]. The analysis of the HRV signals of the test and the control group of the population is performed using the time-domain, frequency-domain, and nonlinear parameters. However, researchers have also proposed the use of polynomial modeling techniques like AR, MA, ARMA, and ARIMA for the extraction of parameters from HRV signals [11,12]. Therefore, the suitability of polynomial models in detecting the HRV signal variations of cannabis users and nonusers has been examined in this study. The machine learning (ML) models are widely used nowadays for proposing automated biosignal classification systems that can aid the early diagnosis of diseases and automatic detection of external stimuli. Thus, ML models have also been developed in this study for facilitating the automatic detection of cannabis consumers.

2. Literature review on cannabis and its legal status

Cannabis refers to an annual, dioecious plant that belongs to the *Cannabaceae* family [13]. The various species of this plant that are cultivated include *Cannabis sativa*, *Cannabis indica*, and a hybrid of both. Some people believe *C. sativa* and *C. indica* to be two different species, while others believe that these are sub-species of the same type of plant. Two major psychoactive compounds, tetrahydrocannabinol (THC) and Cannabidiol (CBD), are found in the cannabis plant. The concentrations of THC and CBD are altered in the modified variants of the plant [14]. According to experts, more than 700 strains of cannabis are grown by cultivators for medical and recreational purposes.

Various parts of the cannabis plant are used to prepare psycho-active recreational products such as marijuana, hemp, hashish, ganja, weed, etc. [15]. These products have many effects on the human body due to their psychoactive properties [16]. The intensity and duration of the results depend on various factors like mode of consumption, quantity, the consumed strain, intervals between consumption, and the immunity of the consumer [17]. The smoking of cannabis products causes the psychoactive components (e.g., tetrahydrocannabinol (THC), cannabinol (CBN), and anandamide) to enter the lungs. The gaseous exchange across the alveoli transfers these psychoactive components to the bloodstream. The bloodstream carries them throughout the body. Hence, the effects are nearly instant. A sense of relaxation and euphoria are experienced when smoked in moderate amounts, along with laughter, increase in appetite, and heightened sensory perception. The effect may be attributed to the maximum plasma concentration attainment of THC within approximately 8 min after the inception of smoking [18]. Although the effects are not the same for everyone, some people experience anxiety, fear, distrust, and panic. The oral consumption of cannabis products as food or beverages takes longer to exhibit the effect [19]. This may be because the systemic absorption of THC takes place slowly, causing the maximum THC-plasma concentration attainment in 1–2 h [18].

The medical uses of cannabis remain limited due to the lack of research and legal constraints [20]. It is used for the management of specific medical conditions. Some researchers suggest using cannabis as an antinauseant in treating chemotherapy-induced nausea and vomiting (CINV) [21]. Recent literature depicts the use of cannabis for appetite stimulation in patients suffering from anorexia and wasting syndromes. The products of cannabis have also been explored as an immunosuppressant for the treatment of autoimmune diseases, including multiple sclerosis and dermatomyositis [22].

Cannabis has the altering legal status of usage for medical and recreational purposes from country to country. In the United States of America (USA), cannabis has been legalized in 36 states, four territories, and the district of Columbia for medicinal use [23].

However, it holds an illegal status at a Federal level in the USA. On the other hand, it is legally useable in the United Kingdom if it meets specific requirements or conditions [24]. A specialist medical consultant can prescribe it under circumstances where there is the availability of clear published evidence of its effectiveness, and all other medical options have been tried or exhausted. General practitioners are not permitted to prescribe it. Interestingly, the plant holds legal status in Canada for medical and recreational purposes. However, there are certain restrictions on its purchase. The notable restriction being the age of the buyer [25]. The legal age to buy cannabis in most of the country, including Canada, is 19, except Alberta and Quebec, where the legal buying age of cannabis is 18 and 21, respectively. In India, various laws are applicable in different states about the consumption of cannabis. The state of Gujarat legalized it on February 21, 2017, keeping cultural sentiments in view [26]. In Maharashtra, possession, consumption, and production of cannabis without a license are prohibited [27]. Other states like Assam and Karnataka have banned its use except for specific medical purposes [28].

3. Methods

3.1 Acquisition of the ECG signals and extraction of the HRV signals

The ECG signals (lead-I) of 5 min duration were acquired from 200 paddy-field workers of Sambalpur district, Odisha, India. The volunteers were 18–60 years old. They were not suffering from any cardiovascular diseases and were leading active life. After explaining the study protocol, the written consent of the participants was taken before participation in this study. The authorization for ECG signal acquisition was obtained from the Institute Ethical Committee (IEC) of NIT Rourkela, India (Ref.# NITRKL/IEC/FORM-2/002; dated 16/8/2017). Bhang is a recreational item derived from the cannabis plant, which is commonly consumed by people residing in villages of India. Among the 200 volunteers, 100 volunteers were regular consumers of bhang and were categorized under Category-B. The rest 100 volunteers never consumed bhang and were considered under Category-C. The sampling rate of the ECG acquisition machine (VESTA 121i ECG machine, RMS Pvt. Ltd., India) was 500.6 Hz. The ECG signals were processed using the Biomedical Workbench toolkit of LabVIEW (V2017, National Instruments, USA), and the HRV signals (also known as RR interval signals) were extracted [29]. The HRV signals were subjected to resampling at 4 Hz before further processing using parametric modeling techniques.

3.2 Parametric modeling of the HRV signals

Various parametric modeling methods like AR, MA, and ARMA have been proposed to model stationary time series signals. On the other hand, modeling techniques like ARIMA have been suggested for the nonstationary time series signals to enable their forecasting and prediction [30,31]. In our study, HRV signals of 5-s duration were extracted from the 5 min HRV signals. The stationarity of the 5-s HRV signals was examined using Augmented Dickey-Fuller (ADF) test in MATLAB software (R2020a, MathWorks Inc., USA), and all the signals were found to be stationary. After that, the HRV signals were subjected to parametric modeling techniques, namely, AR, MA, and ARMA in MATLAB software (R2020a, MathWorks Inc., USA) [12]. The development of the ARIMA model was not reported in our study because it provided the same results as the ARMA model. This can be attributed to the stationary nature of the 5-s HRV signals.

3.3 Statistical analysis

The parametric model coefficients were considered the HRV signal parameters for further analysis [12]. The nature of the distribution of the parametric model coefficients was examined using the Shapiro–Wilk test. The possibility of statistically significant variation of the model coefficients between Category-C and Category-B was analyzed using the Mann–Whitney U test method when the distribution of the coefficients was non-Gaussian in nature [32]. For the Gaussian distribution of the coefficients, the t-test was used for statistical analysis.

3.4 Development of ML classifiers

In the last few decades, the development of ML classifiers for biosignals has gained importance among researchers. Such models can help computer-aided diagnosis/identification of stimulants or diseases [33]. Therefore, ML classifiers have been developed in this study (using RapidMiner software, Educational Version 9.3, RapidMiner Inc., USA) to automate the identification of the cannabis users using the coefficients of the parametric models [34].

3.4.1 Selection of input parameters

The performance of the ML classifiers depends on the selection of suitable input parameters [35]. The appropriate inputs for the ML classifiers were chosen using the feature ranking methods and the dimensionality reduction methods in the current study. The feature ranking methods included Information Gain (IG), Information Gain Ratio (IGR), Uncertainty, Gini Index (GI), Chi-Squared Statistic (CSS), Correlation, Deviation, Relief, Rule, Tree Importance (TI), Support Vector Machine (SVM), and Component Model (CM). On the other hand, the dimension reduction methods included Principal Component Analysis (PCA), Kernel PCA, Independent Component Analysis (ICA), Singular Value Decomposition (SVD), and Self-Organizing Map (SOM)) [36].

3.4.2 Machine learning techniques

The ML classifier, namely, Naïve Bayes (NB), Generalized Linear Model (GLM), Linear Regression (LR), Deep Learning (DL), Decision Tree (DT), Random Forest (RF), Gradient Boosted Tree (GBT), Support Vector Machine (SVM), and First Large Margin (FLM) were implemented in our study [34]. A brief description of the classifiers mentioned above has been provided in Table 1. The classifiers were scrutinized for their efficiency using the performance matrices: accuracy, area under the receiver operating characteristics (ROC) curve (AUC), precision, sensitivity, F-measure, and specificity described in [46]. The best classifier was chosen by comparing the values of the performance measures and was proposed for the automatic detection of cannabis consumers.

4. Results

The AR, MA, and ARMA models are parametric polynomial models that can be employed for characterizing stationary time series signals. The 5-s HRV signals were examined using Augmented Dickey-Fuller (ADF) test and were found stationary. After that, the above-mentioned parametric models were developed from the HRV signals. The typical parametric models for Category-C and Category-B, the outcomes of the statistical analysis of the parametric model coefficients, and their suitability in developing efficient ML classifiers have been described in the following subsections.

Table 1 Brief description of ML-based classifiers.

Method	Description	References
NB	The NB classifier is based on Bayes theorem that uses a probabilistic approach for its classification purpose. It assumes that the number of input parameters used in a classification task does not depend on the number of examples considered during the classification process. This enables the classifier to show better performance with a smaller dataset	[37]
GLM	The GLM classifier is an extension of the conventional linear regression technique. It consists of three components, i.e., an error distribution, a linear predictor, and an algorithm. The error distribution may belong to one of the probability distributions: Gaussian, binomial, Poisson's, and gamma. The gamma distribution provides information regarding the pattern of the systematic effects. The algorithm estimates the maximum likelihood of the systematic effects	[38]
LR	The LR classifier is a widely used ML classifier that describes the relationship between one dependent and one or more independent variables. The classification algorithm is based on a logistic function that provides an S-shaped portrayal of the aggregate influence of dependent and independent variables. The value of the aforesaid logistic function lies within the range of 0–1. This property has led to its widespread application in many classification problems	[39]
DL	The DL classifier represents an advanced ML classifier based on the theoretical basis of artificial neural networks (ANNs). However, the amount of hidden layers makes the DL different from conventional ANNs. Further, the DL classifier uses advanced learning algorithms like the autoencoder method that are not used in classical ANNs. The DL network also potentially extracts the hidden patterns from the dataset and leads to improved performance	[40]
DT	The DT classifier recursively divides the input data into two groups and builds a tree to predict the output. The DT classifier consists of three essential components: internal nodes, branches, and child nodes or leaves. The internal node signifies a test on the input features. The child node indicates the label assigned after splitting, and the branches represent the test results. Numerous algorithms, such as IG, CSS, GI, etc., can be used to split the input data. These algorithms define variables and the threshold to segregate the input data. The splitting process continues until a full-grown tree is obtained	[41]
RF	RF belongs to the class of ensemble classifiers that is based on the principle of aggregating numerous decision trees to obtain the final prediction. Many decision trees are grown using bagging. This is achieved by feeding a subset of the training data to each tree. Further, the final prediction is made using a voting method. While designing an RF, the number of parameters involved and the aggregate of decision trees play a crucial role and must be appropriately selected	[42]

Continued

Table 1 Brief description of ML-based classifiers—cont'd

Method	Description	References
GBT	The GBT classifier is an extension of the decision tree technique, which employs an optimization algorithm called XGBoost for segregating the dataset into different groups. It is efficient in handling missing data and minimizing the loss function. This makes GBT a popular classifier and has been used in various machine learning applications	[43]
SVM	The SVM classifier finds a hyperplane in an N-dimensional space that can differentiate between two groups of data effectively. The hyperplane maximizes its distance from the support vectors or samples present on each side of the plane. The selection of the hyperplane is made by minimizing the generalized error and maximizing the gap between the hyperplane and the data points. The advantage of SVM is that a few support vectors can facilitate compact sparse illustration of the essential facts related to the training data	[44]
FLM	The FLM classifier represents a type of linear SVM. Its basis is formed by the fast-margin learner developed by Fan et al. [45]. The performance of the FLM technique is comparable to that of the classical SVM classifier. However, the advantage of the FLM technique lies in the fact that it can handle large datasets	[29]

4.1 AR modeling of the HRV signals

The AR model can be regarded as the parametric model that can predict future values of a signal based on the analysis of the past values [47]. This method is generally used when a correlation exists between the preceding and the succeeding data points. It performs the linear regression of the data points of a signal with the past values of the signal. In the AR model, the value of the output variable (Y) is dependent on the value of the predictor variable (X), similar to the simple linear regression. However, it differs from the linear regression because the output variable also needs the previous output values apart from the predictor variable to define the current output value. Mathematically, the AR model can be represented using Eq. (1) [48]

$$y_t = \sum_{i=1}^{p} \varphi_i y_{t-i} + e_t \tag{1}$$

where y_t = current sample of the time series, φ_i = AR coefficient, e_t = white noise input, and p = order of AR model.

The typical AR models of order 4, developed for HRV signals belonging to Category-C and Category-B, have been shown in

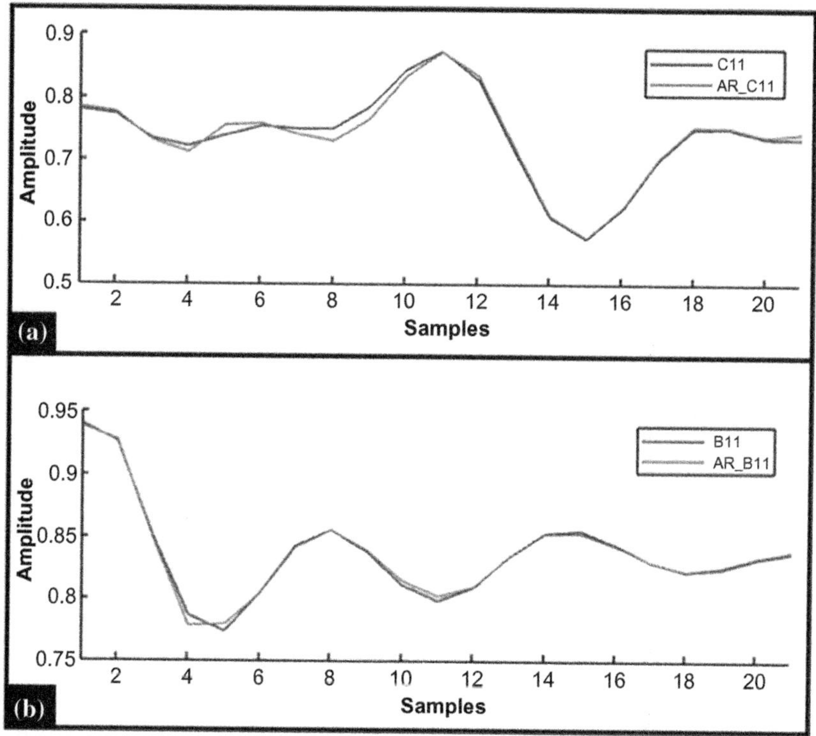

Fig. 1 Typical AR models of 5-s HRV signals: (A) Category-C and (B) Category-B.

Fig. 1. The results of the Shapiro–Wilk test suggested that all the AR model coefficients (except the second coefficient, i.e., AR_A2) exhibited a P-value of ≤ 0.05, suggesting non-Gaussian distribution. The median (MD) $\pm$ standard deviation (SD), 25th and 75th percentile values, and P-values obtained from the Shapiro–Wilk test for all the AR model coefficients have been tabulated in Table 2.

The statistical analysis of the AR model coefficients with non-Gaussian distribution was performed using the Mann–Whitney U test. On the other hand, the second coefficient of the AR model (i.e., AR_A2) was subjected to the t-test for understanding its statistical significance. However, none of the AR coefficients were identified as statistically significant by the Mann–Whitney U test or t-test. These coefficients were then used to derive new parameters using dimension reduction-based feature selection methods mentioned above. The newly derived parameters and the AR coefficients were used as input to develop nine ML-based classification models. The performance matrices of the best classifiers (out of nine generated classifiers) for each of the

Table 2 Statistical characteristics and Shapiro–Wilk test result of AR model coefficients.

Parameters	Category-C			Category-B			P-value
	MD ± SD	25th	75th	MD ± SD	25th	75th	
AR_A1	−2.749 ± 0.303	−2.931	−2.525	−2.766 ± 0.300	−2.941	−2.613	0.034
AR_A2	3.225 ± 0.588	2.774	3.587	3.256 ± 0.592	2.964	3.568	0.170
AR_A3	−1.939 ± 0.394	−2.274	−1.738	−2.012 ± 0.396	−2.250	−1.855	0.014
AR_A4	0.551 ± 0.139	0.425	0.616	0.560 ± 0.120	0.481	0.618	0.0004

parameter-selection methods have been provided in Table 3. It can be observed that the LR classifier generated using the ICA-based dimension reduction method provided the highest accuracy of 76.50% ± 7.47%.

4.2 MA modeling of the HRV signals

The MA model refers to the parametric model that can predict future values of a signal using the weighted moving average of past prediction errors, similar to the regression method [48]. Mathematically, the AR model can be represented using Eq. (2) [48]

$$y_t = \sum_{i=1}^{q} \theta_i e_{t-i} + e_t + c \tag{2}$$

where y_t = current sample of the time series, θ_i = MA coefficient, e_t = white noise input, c = constant, and q = order of the model.

In our study, the MA models of order four were generated. The typical MA models for HRV signals belonging to Category-C and Category-B have been shown in Fig. 2. The coefficients of the MA models exhibited non-Gaussian distribution as per the results of the Shapiro–Wilk test (Table 4). The median (MD) ± standard deviation (SD), 25th and 75th percentile values, and P-values obtained from the Shapiro–Wilk test for all the MA model coefficients have been provided in Table 4.

The Mann–Whitney U test suggested none of the MA model coefficients be statistically significant. The MA model coefficients were then subjected to dimension reduction-based feature selection methods mentioned above to obtain new parameters. The newly generated parameter sets and the MA model coefficients

Table 3 Performance matrices of the ML-based classification models generated from AR modeling of HRV signals.

Type of parameter selection methods	Parameter selection methods	Best classifier	Accuracy (%)	AUC	Precision (%)	F-measure (%)	Sensitivity (%)	Specificity (%)
Dimension reduction	PCA	RF	53.50% ± 7.47%	0.550 ± 0.099	53.67% ± 6.76%	60.73% ± 11.97%	77.00% ± 22.14%	30.00% ± 24.04%
	ICA	LR	76.50% ± 7.47%	0.812 ± 0.112	0.812 ± 0.112	80.21% ± 5.44%	94.00% ± 6.99%	59.00% ± 15.95%
	Kernel PCA	LR	55.50% ± 12.79%	0.480 ± 0.160	56.65% ± 13.55%	52.88% ± 13.69%	51.00% ± 16.63%	60.00% ± 18.26%
	SVD	RF	57.00% ± 7.89%	0.563 ± 0.119	54.66% ± 5.26%	65.72% ± 6.81%	83.00% ± 11.60%	31.00% ± 11.97%
	SOM	GLM	51.50% ± 10.29%	0.511 ± 0.105	50.95% ± 10.92%	48.02% ± 13.81%	47.00% ± 18.89%	56.00% ± 13.50%
All AR parameters	–	RF	56.00% ± 13.70%	0.567 ± 0.129	54.33% ± 10.00%	62.89% ± 12.51%	76.00% ± 18.97%	36.00% ± 18.38%

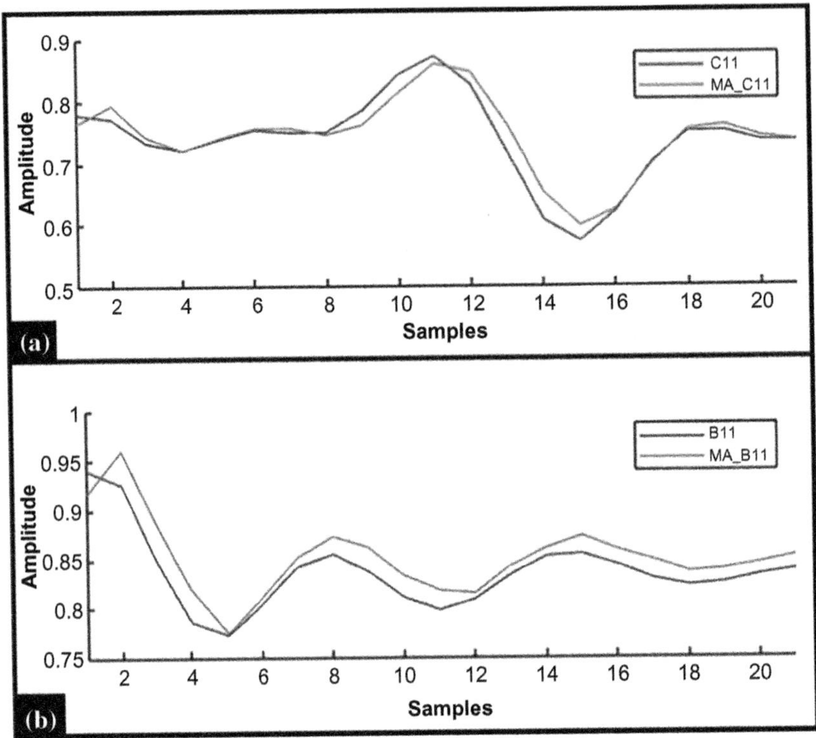

Fig. 2 Typical MA models of 5-s HRV signals: (A) Category-C and (B) Category-B.

Table 4 Statistical characteristics and Shapiro–Wilk test result of MA model coefficients.

Parameters	Category-C			Category-B			P-value
	MD ± SD	25th	75th	MD ± SD	25th	75th	
MA_C1	1.826 ± 0.572	0.872	1.963	1.839 ± 0.628	0.734	1.985	7.353E − 18
MA_C2	1.500 ± 0.748	0.224	1.500	1.500 ± 0.823	−0.088	1.500	7.619E − 21
MA_C3	1.000 ± 0.639	−0.033	1.000	0.941 ± 0.743	−0.452	1.000	2.798E − 18
MA_C4	0.411 ± 0.311	0.024	0.430	0.391 ± 0.381	−0.248	0.449	1.357E − 15

were employed to develop nine ML classifiers. The best classification models generated in each case have been given in Table 5. The results suggested that the RF classification model developed using Kernel PCA-based dimension reduction method provided the highest accuracy of 65.00% ± 11.55%.

Table 5 Performance matrices of the ML-based classification models generated from MA modeling of HRV signals.

Type of parameter selection methods	Parameter selection methods	Best classifier	Accuracy (%)	AUC	Precision (%)	F-measure (%)	Sensitivity (%)	Specificity (%)
Dimension reduction	PCA	LR	52.00% ± 12.95%	0.528 ± 0.094	55.08% ± 17.94%	46.80% ± 12.36%	42.00% ± 11.35%	62.00% ± 22.01%
	ICA	GLM	60.50% ± 12.12%	0.592 ± 0.113	58.99% ± 10.39%	62.91% ± 12.34%	68.00% ± 15.49%	53.00% ± 13.37%
	Kernel PCA	RF	65.00% ± 11.55%	0.635 ± 0.139	65.14% ± 11.94%	67.06% ± 8.96%	70.00% ± 8.16%	60.00% ± 20.00%
	SVD	RF	53.00% ± 7.53%	0.533 ± 0.083	60.88% ± 39.29%	44.05%	37.00% ± 43.98%	69.00% ± 42.02%
	SOM	NB	57.00% ± 10.33%	0.536 ± 0.114	58.45% ± 12.25%	53.77% ± 12.08%	51.00% ± 14.49%	63.00% ± 14.94%
All parameters		LR	58.50% ± 5.30%	0.587 ± 0.114	57.83% ± 5.25%	61.04% ± 5.98%	66.00% ± 12.65%	51.00% ± 14.49%

4.3 ARMA modeling of the HRV signals

The ARMA model is considered an extension of the AR model for predicting the future values of a signal that uses the past prediction errors and the past values of the signal [49]. Mathematically, the ARMA model of order (p, q) can be represented using Eq. (3) [48], where p and q indicate the order of the AR and MA polynomials, respectively

$$y_t = \sum_{i=1}^{p} \varphi_i y_{t-i} + \sum_{i=1}^{q} \theta_i e_{t-i} + e_t \tag{3}$$

where y_t=current sample of the time series, φ_i=AR coefficient, θ_i=MA coefficient, p=order of the AR polynomial, q=order of the MA polynomial, and e_t=white noise input.

The ARMA models of order (4, 4) were produced in our study. The typical ARMA models for HRV signals belonging to Category-C and Category-B have been shown in Fig. 3.

The median (MD)$\pm$standard deviation (SD), 25th and 75th percentile values, and P-values obtained from the Shapiro–Wilk test for all the ARMA model coefficients have been provided in Table 6. All of the ARMA model coefficients were found to exhibit non-Gaussian distribution according to the results of the Shapiro–Wilk test (Table 6).

Therefore, the Mann–Whitney U test was employed to determine the statistical importance of the coefficients. However, none of the ARMA model coefficients were significantly varying among Category-C and Category-B (P-value $\geq$0.05). The ARMA coefficients were subjected to dimension reduction-based feature selection methods mentioned earlier. The new parameters generated by the dimensionality reduction methods and all the ARMA coefficients were employed as input for the development of the ML-based classification models. The performance indices of the most accurate models generated in each case have been provided in Table 7 [50].

4.4 Development of ML-based classifiers using the coefficients of all the parametric models of the HRV signals

The coefficients obtained from all the models, namely AR, MA, and ARMA, were considered potential inputs for developing the ML classifiers in this attempt. This was done to understand

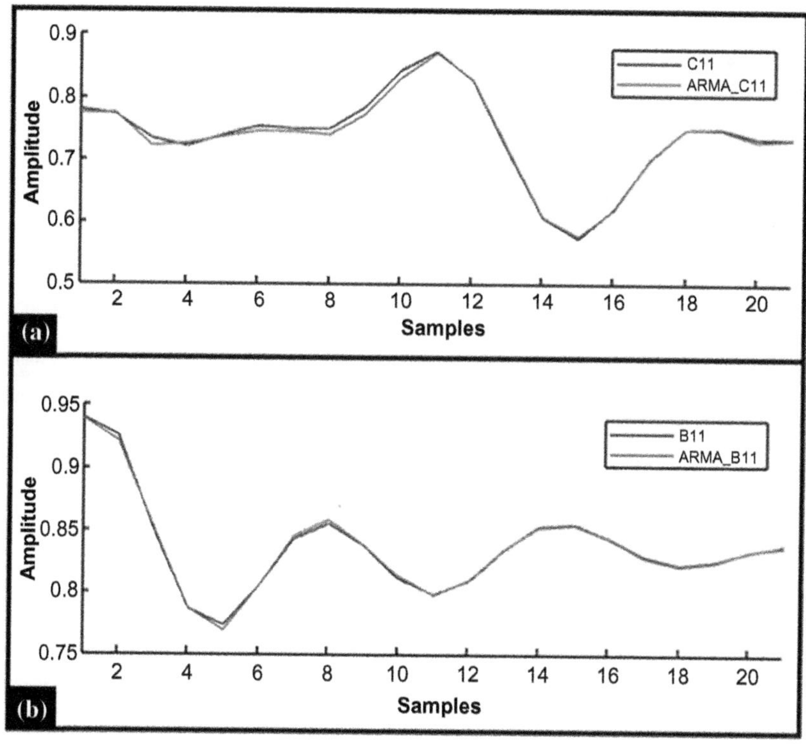

Fig. 3 Typical ARMA models of 5-s HRV signals: (A) Category-C and (B) Category-B.

the relative importance of the coefficients of all the parametric models in the development of the classifiers. The coefficients were subjected to feature ranking and dimension reduction methods. The coefficients that ranked within the top 10 by the feature ranking methods and the new parameters generated by the dimensionality reduction methods were employed as input for the development of the ML models. Finally, all the coefficients were also fed as input for the ML-based classifiers to realize the importance of the feature selection methods. The performance indices of the most accurate models generated from each feature selection method have been provided in Table 8 [50]. It is evident from Table 8 that the highest classification accuracy of 63.50% ± 10.55% was provided by the LR classifier, which was developed using the CM ICA-based feature ranking method.

Table 6 Statistical characteristics and Shapiro–Wilk test result of ARMA modeling coefficients.

Parameters	Category-C			Category-B			P-value
	MD ± SD	25th	75th	MD ± SD	25th	75th	
ARMA_A1	−2.601 ± 0.414	−2.835	−2.258	−2.627 ± 0.396	−2.874	−2.344	0.0005
ARMA _A2	2.904 ± 0.830	2.295	3.324	2.954 ± 0.781	2.407	3.518	0.0004
ARMA _A3	−1.764 ± 0.686	−2.055	−1.429	−1.874 ± 0.624	−2.123	−1.405	4.934E − 07
ARMA _A4	0.447 ± 0.279	0.317	0.539	0.465 ± 0.248	0.355	0.586	6.381E − 09
ARMA _C1	0.943 ± 0.786	0.548	1.412	1.026 ± 0.854	0.491	1.604	0.0001
ARMA _C2	0.527 ± 1.072	−0.072	1.108	0.421 ± 1.127	−0.015	1.373	7.467E − 09
ARMA _C3	0.600 ± 1.051	−0.564	1.185	0.477 ± 0.981	−0.285	1.332	0.0409
ARMA _C4	0.255 ± 0.612	−0.298	0.845	0.315 ± 0.686	−0.377	0.881	1.019E − 10

5. Discussion

Cannabis is a flowering plant that has been grown and utilized by the human race for more than 6000 years in food and medical applications [51]. However, cannabis is also used to produce illicit recreational substances like ganja and charas. As per the reported literature, the recreational use of cannabis has increased significantly worldwide in the last 5 decades [52,53]. People believe that cannabis products are safer than other illicit drugs due to their medicinal properties. This might be a significant factor in increased intake [54]. Cohen et al. [6] have revealed that the average population undergoing recreational cannabis intake is 11% in the United States, which is sufficiently higher than the global average of 4% [6]. The legalization of cannabis for recreational use by adults in various states of the United States since 2012 might have contributed in this regard. However, the incidence of different short-term and long-term adverse health issues has been reported in regular cannabis users over the last few decades, cardiovascular diseases being a major example [55,56]. Researchers have revealed that the chances of cardiovascular disease are even higher if the regular cannabis consumers have already developed psychiatric ailments [9]. However, the exact physiological mechanisms causing cardiovascular diseases in cannabis users are still under investigation [57]. Hence, there is a necessity to identify any possible alteration in cardiovascular activities in regular cannabis takers that might provide any valuable diagnostic information.

Table 7 Performance matrix of the machine learning models generated from ARMA modeling of HRV signals.

Type of parameter selection methods	Parameter selection methods	Best classifier	Accuracy (%)	AUC	Precision (%)	F-measure (%)	Sensitivity (%)	Specificity (%)
Dimension reduction	PCA	GBT	57.50% ± 8.25%	0.550 ± 0.038	57.91% ± 9.78%	56.23% ± 12.52%	58.00% ± 20.98%	57.00% ± 15.67%
	ICA	GBT	59.00% ± 15.60%	0.604 ± 0.196	57.35% ± 14.35%	58.65% ± 18.07%	61.00% ± 22.83%	57.00% ± 13.37%
	Kernel PCA	RF	65.50% ± 7.98%	0.659 = 0.084	66.20% ± 9.20%	65.72% ± 7.09%	66.00% ± 8.43%	65.00% ± 13.54%
	SVD	GBT	62.00% ± 11.60%	0.655 ± 0.116	60.89% ± 9.97%	65.20% ± 9.66%	71.00% ± 11.97%	53.00% ± 17.67%
	SOM	FLM	52.50% ± 10.07%	0.506 ± 0.100	53.29% ± 10.47%	52.39% ± 10.08%	53.00% ± 13.37%	52.00% ± 18.74%
All parameters		GBT	56.50% ± 6.26%	0.550 ± 0.099	55.69% ± 5.05%	57.50% ± 9.41%	61.00% ± 16.63%	52.00% ± 11.35%

Table 8 Performance matrix of the machine learning models generated using the combined modeling parameters (AR+MA +ARMA) of HRV signals.

Input selection methods	Feature selection methods	Classifier	Accuracy (%)	AUC	Precision (%)	*F*-measure (%)	Sensitivity (%)	Specificity (%)
Weight-based (Top 10 important parameters)	CSS	GBT	57.50% ± 8.58%	0.613 ± 0.127	56.95% ± 7.03%	58.47% ± 10.50%	62.00% ± 17.51%	53.00% ± 14.18%
	CM PCA	FLM	56.50% ± 10.29%	0.566 ± 0.115	58.28% ± 11.39%	55.31% ± 9.67%	54.00% ± 10.75%	59.00% ± 19.12%
	CM ICA	LR	63.50% ± 10.55%	0.640 ± 0.139	62.28% ± 9.51%	63.81% ± 12.46%	66.00% ± 15.78%	66.00% ± 15.78%
	CM SVD	LR	60.00% ± 6.24%	0.602 ± 0.103	61.15% ± 6.90%	57.50% ± 9.76%	56.00% ± 15.06%	64.00% ± 12.65%
	Correlation	LR	59.00% ± 9.94%	0.602 ± 0.095	59.02% ± 10.29%	59.76% ± 9.66%	61.00% ± 11.01%	57.00% ± 12.52%
	Deviation	GLM	60.50% ± 13.83%	0.583 ± 0.166	58.61% ± 17.98%	59.36% ± 19.72%	62.00% ± 23.94%	59.00% ± 15.24%
	GI	DL	57.00% ± 9.19%	0.561 ± 0.112	55.72% ± 8.88%	65.88% ± 6.35%	83.00% ± 13.37%	31.00% ± 21.83%
	IG	RF	56.00% ± 10.49%	0.584 ± 0.118	54.44% ± 13.74%	49.99% ± 19.54%	49.00% ± 24.24%	63.00% ± 14.94%
	IGR	GBT	58.50% ± 10.29%	0.568 ± 0.096	59.25% ± 12.07%	60.36% ± 8.84%	63.00% ± 11.60%	54.00% ± 19.55%
	PCA	LR	60.00% ± 12.25%	0.609 ± 0.138	61.62% ± 16.83%	60.40% ± 12.55%	61.00% ± 13.70%	59.00% ± 21.32%
	Relief	LR	56.50% ± 11.56%	0.555 ± 0.132	59.16% ± 18.36%	55.41% ± 13.87%	57.00% ± 22.14%	56.00% ± 20.66%
	Rule	GBT	58.50% ± 6.69%	0.590 ± 0.130	58.55% ± 7.42%	59.54% ± 7.46%	62.00% ± 12.29%	55.00% ± 14.34%
	SVM	RF	59.00% ± 12.87%	0.601 ± 0.164	57.04% ± 11.62%	63.20% ± 13.49%	72.00% ± 18.14%	46.00% ± 16.47%

	TI	GBT	56.50% ± 7.47%	0.612 ± 0.068	55.86% ± 6.54%	56.07% ± 11.40%	58.00% ± 17.51%	55.00% ± 11.79%
	Uncertainty	FLM	55.00% ± 8.16%	0.662 ± 0.105	59.80% ± 11.20%	59.94% ± 16.96%	62.00% ± 23.00%	61.00% ± 11.01%
Dimension reduction	PCA	RF	57.00% ± 9.78%	0.571 ± 0.101	54.67% ± 6.46%	65.64% ± 8.45%	83.00% ± 14.18%	31.00% ± 14.49%
	ICA	FLM	61.50% ± 11.56%	0.662 ± 0.105	59.80% ± 11.20%	59.94% ± 16.96%	62.00% ± 23.00%	61.00% ± 11.01%
	Kernel PCA	LR	55.50% ± 12.79%	0.480 ± 0.160	56.65% ± 13.55%	52.88% ± 13.69%	51.00% ± 16.63%	60.00% ± 18.26%
	SVD	RF	57.00% ± 10.33%	0.565 ± 0.158	54.78% ± 6.90%	66.49% ± 7.44%	85.00% ± 9.72%	29.00% ± 15.24%
	SOM	LR	53.50% ± 9.44%	0.521 ± 0.108	54.27% ± 10.96%	51.13% ± 10.27%	49.00% ± 11.01%	58.00% ± 13.98%
All parameters		LR	58.00% ± 11.11%	0.618 ± 0.128	58.67% ± 11.35%	56.25% ± 15.00%	57.00% ± 19.47%	59.00% ± 16.63%

It is a well-known fact that the ANS regulates the rhythmic contraction of the heart via its parasympathetic and sympathetic nerves [58]. Therefore, an understanding of the influence of the ANS activity on the heart using cardiac autonomic regulation (CAR) analysis divulges useful diagnostic information related to cardiovascular diseases in a noninvasive manner [59]. As per the reported literature, cannabis may cause a biphasic influence on the ANS activity, which is mainly dependent on the dose of the cannabis intake [4,29]. At a low amount of regular cannabis intake, the sympathetic nervous system gets activated and may cause tachycardia [60]. On the other hand, a high dose of regular cannabis intake enhances parasympathetic nervous system activity. It may result in bradycardia and hypotension [4,61]. The commonly used noninvasive methods of understanding a person's CAR include time and frequency methods of analysis of the HRV signals. However, recent years have witnessed studies like Pande et al. [12], where the HRV signals have been analyzed using the ARMA-based parametric models to detect any CAR activity alteration due to external stimuli [12]. Hence, the current study attempted to examine the suitability of the parametric models in detecting any possible alterations in the HRV signals due to cannabis consumption. The parametric models, namely, AR, MA, and ARMA, are used for stationary data [11]. The HRV signals of 5-s duration were extracted from the 5 min HRV signals and their stationarity was confirmed using the ADF test before subjecting them to parametric modeling. The order of the models was chosen to be four as per the recommendation of the recently reported literature [12].

The parametric model coefficients were subjected to the Shapiro–Wilk test to determine the nature of the distribution of the parameters. All the model coefficients had a P-value of ≤ 0.05 except the second coefficient of the AR model (AR_A2). This suggested the non-Gaussian behavior of all the parameters except AR_A2. Hence, the Mann–Whitney U test was performed to identify the statistically significant parameters among all the parameters except AR_A2. The statistical importance of the AR_A2 coefficient was examined using the t-test. None of the parametric model coefficients were found to be statistically different. Interestingly, our previous study observed an alteration in ANS activity from the time and frequency domain analysis of the HRV signals [29]. This suggested that the parametric model coefficients were not efficient in detecting the effect of stimulants like cannabis consumption compared to the time and frequency domain HRV parameters.

The development of ML biosignal classifiers for the early prognosis of diseases and automatic identification of external stimuli has received special attention from researchers in recent years. Thus, ML classifiers have been proposed in this study to facilitate the automatic detection of cannabis users. The complexity and computational burden during the development of the ML classifiers can be reduced by selecting appropriate parameters as inputs instead of taking all the available parameters [62]. Hence, parameter selection was performed using dimension reduction methods when coefficients of the individual parametric models were used to generate the parameter set. The weight-based ranking methods were not used in such cases as the number of parameters was less. When the coefficients from all the parametric models were combined to generate the parameter set, both dimension reduction methods and weight-based ranking methods were employed to identify the suitable parameters. The ML classifiers were developed using the chosen parameters, and 10-fold cross-validation was used to validate the classifiers [63]. It was observed that the performance of the ML classifiers generated using feature selection methods (dimension reduction and weight-based ranking) was higher as compared to the case when all the parametric model (AR, MA, and ARMA) parameters were used. This suggested the importance of parameter selection in the development of ML classifiers. The LR classifier generated from the AR model-based parameters using the ICA-based dimension reduction method provided the highest classification accuracy of 76.50% ± 7.47%. The other performance metrics of this classifier were also relatively higher as compared to the other classifiers. Hence, this model has been proposed as the best classification model for the automated detection of cannabis users.

6. Conclusion

The recreational use of cannabis products is increasing significantly worldwide nowadays. However, the incidence of cardiovascular diseases is also rising in regular cannabis users, thereby generating the necessity to understand the alterations induced by cannabis in cardiovascular physiology. Researchers have proposed various methods of analysis of the HRV signals for understanding the CAR activity. This is aimed at divulging useful diagnostic information. In this study, an attempt has been made to understand the suitability of the parametric modeling techniques in detecting significant changes in the HRV signals due to the regular consumption of cannabis. The ECG signals were acquired from 200 Indian paddy-field workers, and their HRV signals of 5-s duration were used to develop parametric models, namely, AR, MA, and ARMA. The parametric model coefficients were used as HRV signal parameters. Their statistical significance was tested using either the Mann–Whitney U test or the t-test based on the nature of their distribution as non-Gaussian or Gaussian, respectively. However, none of the coefficients could significantly differ between the cannabis users and the nonusers. Hence, the parametric models were not efficient as the time and frequency domain methods for identifying changes in the HRV signals due to the consumption of cannabis. The parametric model coefficients were further used to develop many ML classifiers. The relevance of the parameters for the development of ML-based classifiers was tested using dimension reduction and weight-based ranking methods. The developed classifiers were scrutinized based on their performance indices to propose the best model. Finally, an LR classifier obtained from AR model coefficients using the ICA-based feature selection method was chosen as the best classification model, which provided the highest classification accuracy of $76.50\% \pm 7.47\%$. However, one limitation of this study is that the enhancement in the family-wise error rate in the statistical analyses was not controlled [64]. Overall, we consider this study relatively preliminary and encourage replication.

Conflict of interest statement

The authors have no conflicts of interest to declare regarding the publication of this manuscript.

References

[1] S.A. Bonini, M. Premoli, S. Tambaro, A. Kumar, G. Maccarinelli, M. Memo, A. Mastinu, Cannabis sativa: a comprehensive ethnopharmacological review of a medicinal plant with a long history, J. Ethnopharmacol. 227 (2018) 300–315.

[2] R.C. Clarke, M.D. Merlin, Cannabis: Evolution and Ethnobotany, University of California Press, 2013.

[3] P. Pressman, R. Clemens, Introduction: cannabis in society today, Nutr. Today 54 (2) (2019) 78–83.

[4] E. Jouanjus, V. Raymond, M. Lapeyre-Mestre, V. Wolff, What is the current knowledge about the cardiovascular risk for users of cannabis-based products? A systematic review, Curr. Atheroscler. Rep. 19 (6) (2017) 26.

[5] W. Hall, M. Lynskey, Assessing the public health impacts of legalizing recreational cannabis use: the US experience, World Psychiatry 19 (2) (2020) 179–186.

[6] K. Cohen, A. Weizman, A. Weinstein, Positive and negative effects of cannabis and cannabinoids on health, Clin. Pharmacol. Ther. 105 (5) (2019) 1139–1147.

[7] D.M. Martinez, Cannabis and Cannabinoids: Weighing the Benefits and Risks in Psychiatric Patients, Medscape Psychiatry, 2020.

[8] National Academies of Sciences & Medicine, The Health Effects of Cannabis and Cannabinoids: The Current State of Evidence and Recommendations for Research, National Academies Press, 2017.

[9] G.A. Alvares, D.S. Quintana, I.B. Hickie, A.J. Guastella, Autonomic nervous system dysfunction in psychiatric disorders and the impact of psychotropic medications: a systematic review and meta-analysis, J. Psychiatry Neurosci. 41 (2) (2016) 89–104.

[10] R. Castaldo, P. Melillo, R. Izzo, N. De Luca, L. Pecchia, Fall prediction in hypertensive patients via short-term HRV analysis, IEEE J. Biomed. Health Inform. 21 (2) (2016) 399–406.

[11] U.R. Acharya, M. Sankaranarayanan, J. Nayak, C. Xiang, T. Tamura, Automatic identification of cardiac health using modeling techniques: a comparative study, Inf. Sci. 178 (23) (2008) 4571–4582.

[12] K. Pande, S. Subhadarshini, D. Gaur, S.K. Nayak, K. Pal, Analysis of ECG signals to investigate the effect of a humorous audio-visual stimulus on autonomic nervous system and heart of females, in: Design and Development of Affordable Healthcare Technologies, IGI Global, 2018, pp. 239–256.

[13] G.W. Guy, B.A. Whittle, P. Robson, The Medicinal Uses of Cannabis and Cannabinoids, Pharmaceutical Press, London, UK, 2004.

[14] D.M. Lambert, Cannabinoids in Nature and Medicine, John Wiley & Sons, 2009.

[15] J. Metrik, S.S. Bassett, E.R. Aston, K.M. Jackson, B. Borsari, Medicinal versus recreational cannabis use among returning veterans, Transl. Issues Psychol. Sci. 4 (1) (2018) 6.

[16] J.M. Ross, J.M. Ellingson, S.H. Rhee, J.K. Hewitt, R.P. Corley, J.M. Lessem, N.P. Friedman, Investigating the causal effect of cannabis use on cognitive function with a quasi-experimental co-twin design, Drug Alcohol Depend. 206 (2020), 107712.

[17] U. Bonnet, U.W. Preuss, The cannabis withdrawal syndrome: current insights, Subst. Abus. Rehabil. 8 (2017) 9.

[18] P. Sharma, P. Murthy, M.M. Srinivas Bharath, Chemistry, metabolism, and toxicology of cannabis: clinical implications, Iran. J. Psychiatry 7 (4) (2012) 149.

[19] G.B. Rasera, A. Ohara, R.J.S. de Castro, Innovative and emerging applications of cannabis in food and beverage products: from an illicit drug to a potential ingredient for health promotion, Trends Food Sci. Technol. 115 (2021) 31–41.

[20] R.S. Eisenberg, D.B. Leiderman, Cannabis for medical use, Food Drug Law J. 74 (2) (2019) 246–279.

[21] M.E. Badowski, A review of oral cannabinoids and medical marijuana for the treatment of chemotherapy-induced nausea and vomiting: a focus on pharmacokinetic variability and pharmacodynamics, Cancer Chemother. Pharmacol. 80 (3) (2017) 441–449.

[22] H. Kalant, Medicinal use of cannabis: history and current status, Pain Res. Manag. 6 (2) (2001) 80–91.

[23] D.V. Patton, A history of United States cannabis law, J. Law Health 34 (2020) 1.

[24] C. Sakal, M. Lynskey, A. Schlag, D. Nutt, Developing a real-world evidence base for prescribed cannabis in the United Kingdom: preliminary findings from project Twenty21, Psychopharmacology (2021) 1–9.

[25] S. Mahamad, E. Wadsworth, V. Rynard, S. Goodman, D. Hammond, Availability, retail price and potency of legal and illegal cannabis in Canada after recreational cannabis legalisation, Drug Alcohol Rev. 39 (4) (2020) 337–346.

[26] Bhang a Preparation Made From Cannabis Plant Is Legal in Gujarat!, 2022. Retrieved from https://ingujarat.in/information/bhang-legal-health-benefits-side-effects/.

[27] G. Kuppuram, Decriminalizing marijuana: the science and social sustainability behind the use of marijuana (Cannabis) in India, J. Assoc. Res. 26 (2) (2021) 10–27.

[28] T. Tandon, L. Collective, Drug policy in India: key developments since the UNGASS 2016, in: International Drug Policy Consortium Briefing Paper, 2019. Available from: https://idpc.net/publications/2019/02/drug-policy-in-india-key-developments-since-the-ungass-2016.

[29] S.K. Nayak, B.K. Pradhan, I. Banerjee, K. Pal, Analysis of heart rate variability to understand the effect of cannabis consumption on Indian male paddy-field workers, Biomed. Signal Process. Control 62 (2020), 102072.

[30] G.A.G. De Villa, A.J. Silvestre, G.S. de Sá e Souza, A. Carafini, A. de Oliveira Assis, A.O. Andrade, M.F. Vieira, Efficiency of AR, MA and ARMA models in prediction of raw and filtered center of pressure signals, in: Paper Presented at the XXVI Brazilian Congress on Biomedical Engineering, 2019.

[31] G. Perone, An ARIMA Model to Forecast the Spread of COVID-2019 Epidemic in Italy, arXiv preprint arXiv:2004.00382, 2020.

[32] M. Hauben, A visual aid for teaching the Mann–Whitney U formula, Teach. Stat. 40 (2) (2018) 60–63.

[33] U.R. Acharya, H. Fujita, S.L. Oh, U. Raghavendra, J.H. Tan, M. Adam, Y. Hagiwara, Automated identification of shockable and non-shockable life-threatening ventricular arrhythmias using convolutional neural network, Futur. Gener. Comput. Syst. 79 (2018) 952–959.

[34] V. Kotu, B. Deshpande, Predictive Analytics and Data Mining: Concepts and Practice with Rapidminer, Morgan Kaufmann, 2014.

[35] T. Li, M. Zhou, ECG classification using wavelet packet entropy and random forests, Entropy 18 (8) (2016) 285.

[36] R. Nisbet, J. Elder, G. Miner, Handbook of Statistical Analysis and Data Mining Applications, Academic Press, 2009.

[37] S. Xu, Bayesian Naïve Bayes classifiers to text classification, J. Inf. Sci. 44 (1) (2018) 48–59.

[38] Y. Lee, J.A. Nelder, Y. Pawitan, Generalized Linear Models With Random Effects: Unified Analysis via H-Likelihood, vol. 153, CRC Press, 2018.

[39] K. Kowsari, K. Jafari Meimandi, M. Heidarysafa, S. Mendu, L. Barnes, D. Brown, Text classification algorithms: a survey, Information 10 (4) (2019) 150.

[40] D. Ravì, C. Wong, F. Deligianni, M. Berthelot, J. Andreu-Perez, B. Lo, G.-Z. Yang, Deep learning for health informatics, IEEE J. Biomed. Health Inform. 21 (1) (2016) 4–21.

[41] Q. Zhou, H. Zhang, Z. Lari, Z. Liu, N. El-Sheimy, Design and implementation of foot-mounted inertial sensor based wearable electronic device for game play application, Sensors 16 (10) (2016) 1752.

[42] M. Belgiu, L. Drăguţ, Random forest in remote sensing: a review of applications and future directions, ISPRS J. Photogramm. Remote Sens. 114 (2016) 24–31.

[43] Y. Luo, W. Ye, X. Zhao, X. Pan, Y. Cao, Classification of data from electronic nose using gradient tree boosting algorithm, Sensors 17 (10) (2017) 2376.

[44] M.J. Zaki, W. Meira Jr., W. Meira, Data Mining and Analysis: Fundamental Concepts and Algorithms, Cambridge University Press, 2014.

[45] R.-E. Fan, K.-W. Chang, C.-J. Hsieh, X.-R. Wang, C.-J. Lin, LIBLINEAR: a library for large linear classification, J. Mach. Learn. Res. 9 (August) (2008) 1871–1874.

[46] A. Subasi, Electroencephalogram-controlled assistive devices, in: Bioelectronics and Medical Devices, Elsevier, 2019, pp. 261–284.

[47] B. Vuksanovic, M. Alhamdi, AR-based method for ECG classification and patient recognition, Int. J. Biom. Bioinforma. 7 (2) (2013) 74.

[48] S. Jain, G. Deshpande, Parametric modeling of brain signals, in: Paper Presented at the Proceedings. Eighth International Conference on Information Visualisation, 2004.

[49] A. Goshvarpour, M. Shamsi, A. Goshvarpour, Spectral and time based assessment of meditative heart rate signals, Int. J. Image Graph. Signal Process. 5 (4) (2013) 1.

[50] A. Subasi, Electromyogram-controlled assistive devices, in: Bioelectronics and Medical Devices, Elsevier, 2019, pp. 285–311.

[51] Z. Atakan, Cannabis, a complex plant: different compounds and different effects on individuals, Ther. Adv. Psychopharmacol. 2 (6) (2012) 241–254.

[52] M.A. ElSohly, S. Chandra, M. Radwan, C. Gon, J.C. Church, A comprehensive review of Cannabis potency in the USA in the last decade, Biol. Psychiatry Cogn. Neurosci. Neuroimaging 6 (2021) 603–606.

[53] W. Hall, L. Degenhardt, Adverse health effects of non-medical cannabis use, Lancet 374 (9698) (2009) 1383–1391.

[54] E. Jouanjus, V. Raymond, M. Lapeyre-Mestre, V. Wolff, What is the current knowledge about the cardiovascular risk for users of cannabis-based products? A systematic review, Curr. Atheroscler. Rep. 19 (6) (2017) 1–15.

[55] H. Goyal, H.H. Awad, J.K. Ghali, Role of cannabis in cardiovascular disorders, J. Thorac. Dis. 9 (7) (2017) 2079.

[56] S. Rezkalla, R.A. Kloner, Cardiovascular effects of marijuana, Trends Cardiovasc. Med. 29 (2018) 403–407.

[57] G. Thomas, R.A. Kloner, S. Rezkalla, Adverse cardiovascular, cerebrovascular, and peripheral vascular effects of marijuana inhalation: what cardiologists need to know, Am. J. Cardiol. 113 (1) (2014) 187–190.

[58] J.E. Hall, Guyton and Hall Textbook of Medical Physiology e-Book, Elsevier Health Sciences, 2015.

[59] I. Casier, P. Vanduynhoven, S. Haine, C. Vrints, P.G. Jorens, Is recent cannabis use associated with acute coronary syndromes? An illustrative case series, Acta Cardiol. 69 (2) (2014) 131–136.

[60] M. Echeverria-Villalobos, A.B. Todeschini, N. Stoicea, J. Fiorda-Diaz, T. Weaver, S.D. Bergese, Perioperative care of cannabis users: a comprehensive review of pharmacological and anesthetic considerations, J. Clin. Anesth. 57 (2019) 41–49.

[61] M.S.R. Patwary, K.A. Al Mamun, Drug abuse and cardiac problem, Med. Today 25 (2) (2013) 90–92.

[62] J. Cai, J. Luo, S. Wang, S. Yang, Feature selection in machine learning: a new perspective, Neurocomputing 300 (2018) 70–79.

[63] E. Guney, Revisiting cross-validation of drug similarity based classifiers using paired data, Genomics Comput. Biol. 4 (1) (2018), e100047.

[64] M.D. Moran, Arguments for rejecting the sequential bonferroni in ecological studies, Oikos 100 (2) (2003) 403–405.

4

Patient-specific ECG beat classification using EMD and deep learning-based technique

Jaya Prakash Allam[a], Saunak Samantray[b], and Samit Ari[a]
[a]*Department of Electronics and Communication Engineering, National Institute of Technology Rourkela, Rourkela, Odisha, India.* [b]*Department of ETC, IIIT Bhubaneswar, Odisha, India*

1. Introduction

Electrocardiogram (ECG) is a graphical tool utilized to record the electrical activity of the human heart. It gives detail information about function of the heart that helps doctors to provide proper medication to cardiac patients. The segments of a normal ECG signal are as follows: P, T waves, and QRS complex. Any distortions in these specific segments are observed in an ECG record for an additional investigation [1]. It is quite difficult to analyze a specific cardiac disorder by manually reviewing long-term ECG recordings. Therefore, an automated cardiac beat detection system is essential to identify disorders accurately. The performance of the automatic diagnosis tool depends on the ECG signal quality. During acquisition, however, ECG signals are contaminated with various disturbances in real time. The voltage and frequency ranges of a typical ECG signal are 1–5 mV and 0.05–150 Hz, respectively [2]. These values are not hardbound, which means that exceptions are also observed in certain ECG signals. Acquired ECG signals are classified into two types based on the duration: (i) resting ECG and (ii) ambulatory or long-term ECG. The duration of resting ECG is 5–10 min, whereas that of ambulatory ECG is 24–48 h. Ambulatory ECG acquires the signal continuously from the cardiac patients to know the working condition of the heart during daily activities. Holter monitor is used to record and monitor the ambulatory ECG. This kind of monitoring is very useful when the patient is asymptomatic with rhythm disturbances.

Advanced Methods in Biomedical Signal Processing and Analysis. https://doi.org/10.1016/B978-0-323-85955-4.00007-7
Copyright © 2023 Elsevier Inc. All rights reserved.

Since the measuring voltage and frequency are significantly small, the ECG is prone to various types of noises distorting the temporal and spectral features [1]. The most basic noise that affects an ECG signal is the baseline-wander (BW) noise, power-line interference (PLI), electrode motion artifact (EMA), and electromyographic (EMG). The harmonics of the power-line frequency sometimes prevails in the recorded signal. EMG is another type of noise in ECG signals which affect the morphology of the QRS complex in ECG. The root cause of EMG noise is muscular movements while recording the ECG. Both power-line and EMG noise are high frequency by nature [3]. BW noise is a rhythmic noise and affects the isoelectric line of the signal. This noise occurs due to the improper conduction between the skin and the electrode. The raw ECG signal with all these noises distorts the features and makes it difficult to analyze the signal. The ECG signals are generally prone to different kinds of noises. This addition of noise to the pure ECG signals may cause false predictions of the patient's condition. Some of them are as follows:

1. BW noise: BW noise is a low-frequency artifact in a subject's ECG signal recordings [1]. BW removal is crucial in ECG signal processing because BW makes it more troublesome to analyze ECG data. The patient's movement, improper electrodes, and respiration while acquiring ECG are the main causes for BW noise. This noise occurs at minimal frequencies like 0.5 Hz. Faster body movements, exercising, and stress can increase the frequency range of this noise [4].

2. PLI noise: In general, power lines are generated due to electromagnetic fields. These fields cause power-line interference to ECG signals and for any bio-electric signals. The PLI noise has a frequency range of 50–60 Hz. This noise is in the form of a sinusoidal with several harmonics. PLI noise is one of the causes of suppression of the P-wave and the T-wave [2].

3. EMA noise: The EMA characteristics are much similar to BW noise. The presence of noise in the ECG signal at the frequency range of 1–10 Hz. Hence, the spectral contents of the EMA predominantly overlap with that of the QRS complex. Electrode motion artifacts will primarily affect ambulatory ECG signals, where noise is falsely detected as QRS complex. Therefore, the removal of this noise is essential [3].

4. EMG noise: This noise is neither similar to BW like low frequency nor contains high frequency like 50 or 60 Hz. The noise is distributed throughout the P, QRS, and T waves. Hence, removing this noise is highly essential. It mainly suppresses the low-amplitude waves. Applications which deal with ECG during exercises are more prone to this noise [2].

Hence, processed ECG signals are required to identify the ECG beats effectively. As per the Association for the Advancement of Medical Instrumentation (AAMI), 16 different types of beats in the Massachusetts Institute of Technology-Beth Israel Hospital (MIT-BIH) arrhythmia database are subclassified into five types of beats [5]. They are nonectopic beats (N), supraventricular ectopic beats (S), ventricular ectopic beats (V), fusion beats (F), and unknown beats (Q) [6, 7]. Conventional techniques follow the following three steps for denoising and beat classification of the ECG signal. They are (i) preprocessing, (ii) feature extraction, and (iii) classification. Various filtering techniques are used to eliminate noise from ECG data during preprocessing. Several methods have been proposed for ECG signal denoising in the existing literature. Traditional techniques such as band-pass, Kalman, and Wiener filtering are the most commonly used techniques in preprocessing. Manual selection of frequency bands is very difficult in these traditional techniques. Hence, adaptive filters came into existence to denoise the acquired ECG signals based on a variable threshold value. Different optimization algorithms are used to control the threshold value of the adaptive filters. But sometimes, these optimization algorithms may cause oscillations in the filtered ECG signal or amplitude reduction in R-peak. To denoise the ECG signal, statistical approaches such as independent component analysis [8] and principal component analysis (PCA) [9] are utilized, which are effective in removing noise by removing the dimensions associated with noise. The mapping model, on the other hand, is extremely sensitive to noise disruptions [10]. To overcome the problems as mentioned earlier, empirical mode decomposition (EMD) [11, 12], ensemble empirical mode decomposition [13, 14], and complete ensemble empirical mode decomposition [15] are used to denoise the ECG signals effectively.

Most of the ECG beat detection systems based on deep learning follow preprocessing and classification stages. Preprocessing is the important stage to increase the quality of the ECG signal, which enhances the performance of the classification algorithm [7]. In [16], the combination of high-order synchrosqueezing transform with nonlocal means (NLM) is used to improve the quality of the ECG signals in [17]. In [18], Wiener filter and Kalman filters are independently implemented with customized windowing techniques to denoise the ECG signals. In [19], stationary wavelet transform with level thresholding (SWT-LT) is applied on ambulatory ECG to remove the effect of motion artifact. Singh et al. proposed a technique using Fourier decomposition to eliminate the basic interference in the ECG signal [20]. In [21], baseline noise is estimated and removed from the ECG signal using sparse regularization method. Discrete wavelet transform (DWT) is used to remove the unwanted frequency components from ECG signals in [22]. Several approaches are reported in the literature such as DWT [23], fast Fourier transform (FFT) [20], NLM filter [24], PCA [25], adaptive filter [26], and adaptive dual threshold filtering [27] to remove the various noises from the ECG signal.

In [16], to improve the quality of the QRS complex by denoising the ECG signal, combination of adaptive switching mean filter (ASMF) and EMD is applied in this work, where the residual high-frequency artifacts in the signal are eradicated using ASMF technique. The performance of denoising methods is estimated using MIT-BIH database. Smital et al. reported the estimation of the error-free signal by using SWT in Wiener filter [28]. The wavelet transform (WT) is widely used in various applications like handling the nonstationary signals. More information in frequency and time domain can be obtained using WT compared to Fourier transform. DWT gained popularity owing to the extensive use of computers [29]. In the tree structure of the DWT, approximated and the detailed coefficients of the input signal are extracted using low-pass filters and high-pass filter, respectively. In DWT, down samplers are also used to maintain balance in a total number of samples. The approximate coefficients carry essential feature information of the original signal. On the other hand, the original signal can be reconstructed using detail coefficients [28]. Deep learning methods have recently gained popularity for denoising ECG signals. A fully connected convolutional neural network (CNN) with a denoising auto-encoder (DAE) is successfully applied to eliminate the noise, from the corrupted signal in [30]. DAE with fully connected CNN is an artificial intelligence model that replicates the input signal approximately without noise.

CNN is a type of artificial neural network that has the unique capacity to combine both feature set extraction and classification in one stage, preventing the requirement manual feature extraction. CNN is a multilayer network that uses convolution, pooling, and fully-connected layers to learn and detect spatial data adaptively. The CNN is reported first time in 1980 for recognizing handwritten digits. The convolutional layer is a critical element of CNN that gave the name to the network as CNN. This layer performs an operation called a "convolution". It is developed for the postal department to identify the pin codes, zip codes, etc. In those days, deep learning models are known for their massive requirement of computation resources and data for getting trained and tested. Hence, the real-time applications of CNNs were limited to a specific case like postal sectors and not to the level of machine learning [16].

Over the period, Alex Krizhevsky reported ALEX-NET in 2012 that enhances the detection ability of ordinary CNN [16]. The availability of vast sets of labeled images and the emergence of the improved computing systems engrossed researchers to deep learning by bringing back the CNNs era. The CNN or ConvNet is used to analyze visual imagery. The convolution is a linear operation that performs the multiplication of two-dimensional (2D) input and a 2D filter or Kernel. It produces a 2D output with reduced size by preserving the critical features required for its identification [16]. Kernel is a vector of weights called a filter that represents specific features of the input image. The same filter can be shared with many neurons in a CNN to minimize the requirement of memory. Here, the kernel size is smaller than the input image. Convolution output is obtained by moving the kernel over the image step by step from left to right and top to bottom. On each step, multiplication is applied between the image pixel element and the respective weight element of the kernel in the overlapping patch. Further, the element-wise dot product is summed to represent the whole overlapping patch with a single value. Hence, the size of the convolution output is smaller compared to the input image. Therefore, the reduction in dimensionality increases the performance speed of the system [30].

The CNN can handle both the color and gray images, where processing the color image needs CNN with multiple planes called channels. An RGB image is represented by a pixel matrix having three planes, whereas a gray-scale image is represented with a single plane. The CNN comprises multiple layers of mathematical functions that output the two dimensional (2D) output array called feature map. Each layer of the CNN generates the feature maps that are processed in the next layer. The primary features of the input are extracted in the initial layer and processed in the next layer to extract the microlevel features and passed to the subsequent layers [7]. As the feature maps are passed on to the deeper layers, more features at the microlevel are extracted, and the image size is reduced. Finally, the reduced feature maps are fed to the dense layer called the classification layer that outputs the probability scores indicating the likelihood of the input data belonging to a particular class. For example, if a ConvNet is designated to classify cats, dogs, and horses, the dense layer outputs the probability that the input image belongs to any of those animals [9].

The spatial size of the convoluted features is reduced by the pooling layer to minimize the computational complexity. The average pooling and max pooling are the two variants of the pooling operation. In max pooling, the maximum value of a pixel from the image patch covered by the filter is picked. This process also helps in noise suppression, in discarding the noisy activation. The average of pixels from an image portion covered by the kernel is evaluated in average pooling. This pooling function also performs a reduction of spatial size and noise suppression. Although the CNNs have cons like power and resource complexity, CNNs are keen to extract microlevel features that are minute and unnoticeable by the human eye. Though the CNNs have their limitations, it made artificial intelligence revolutionized [13].

Nowadays, deep learning algorithms have become popular in classification problems also, such as CNN [31], recurrent neural network (RNN) [32], residual neural network (ResNet) [33], long short-term memory (LSTM) network [34], and deep belief network (DBN) [35]. In [34], LSTM-based auto-encoder method is proposed to classify ECG beats with a performance accuracy of 99.45%. Ding et al. proposed a technique based on DBN to classify ECG beats in AAMI standard with an accuracy of 97.30%. One-dimensional (1D)-CNN architecture is used to classify the ECG beats with the FFT feature set in [31]. The combination of CNN-LSTM approach is used to classify five different types of ECG beats in [36]. In the existing literature, raw ECG signals with noise are directly applied to the classifiers, which badly affect the detection performance. Therefore, the combination of a denoising technique with a classification algorithm is used to detect different ECG beats efficiently.

The rest of the chapter is prepared as follows: details of the dataset used in experimentation are explained in Section 2, the methodology used to classify ECG beats is in Section 3. The experimental results carried out in this work are presented in Section 4; and finally, the conclusion is presented in Section 5.

2. Database

The proposed system's performance is evaluated using the MIT-BIH arrhythmia database in this work. The literature shows that the MIT-BIH database is the benchmark in beat classification area [5]. This database consists of 48 ECG records, and each record containing 30-min duration. The total dataset consists of 1,09,000 beats. The acquired ECG signals are sampled at the rate of 360 Hz. Among these records, 23 records are recorded from the routine clinical recording. The remaining 25 records are collected from severe cardiac disorder patients. Among these files, four ECG records (102, 104, 107, and 217) are comprised paced beats; therefore, these four files are excluded from the evaluation process [37]. The individual beats are annotated with 17 different labels in Physionet. Again the 17 labels are categorized into five labels as per the AAMI standard (i.e., N, S, V, F, and Q).

3. Proposed methodology

The generalized block diagram for ECG denoising and beat classification is shown in Fig. 1. In this work, EMD-based deep learning technique is proposed for beat classification. In this system, preprocessing and classification are the two crucial stages for denoising and classification of the ECG beat [32]. Preprocessing step includes R-peak detection, beat segmentation, and EMD. R-peak detection is helpful in finding the specific QRS complex to segment the whole ECG signal into individual ECG beats. Subsequently, the EMD technique deconstructs the raw ECG beats into intrinsic mode functions (IMFs) components, and significant IMF components are added to reconstruct the noise-free ECG beat [7]. The resultant ECG beats are divided into training and testing datasets. These datasets are utilized for training and testing the deep learning model. The detailed description of the preprocessing and classification are explained in the following sections.

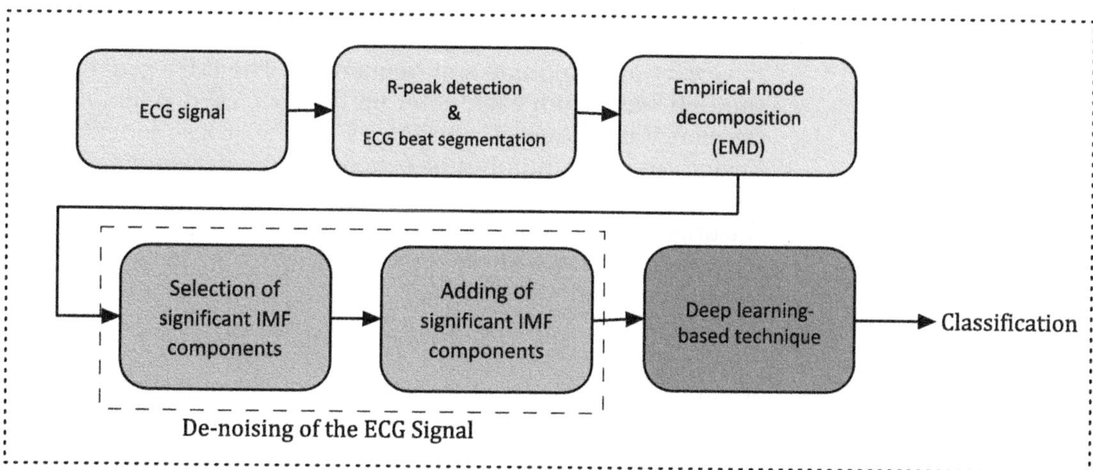

Fig. 1 Proposed methodology for ECG beat classification.

3.1 Preprocessing

The raw ECG signals are filtered in the preprocessing stage. Initially, well-known Pan-Tompkins algorithms [37] are used to identify the R-peak locations of the ECG signal. After detecting R-peak locations, every ECG beat with the length (1×256) is separated from the raw ECG signal. After successful separation, the EMD technique is applied to deconstruct the original beat into IMF components. Each IMF contains different frequency components. Among all the IMFs, significant IMFs satisfy the following two characteristics: (i) the number of maxima and the number of minimas or zero crossings are equal and (ii) the average value of the two successive envelops should be equal to zero [38].

3.1.1 Noise removal using EMD technique

EMD is a well-known method to analyze nonstationary data such as ECG, EEG, etc. Any nonstationary data can be decomposed into finite IMF components. The decomposition is based on the direct energy extraction related to the system's most critical characteristics and intrinsic time scales. In terms of the IMFs, the decomposition can alternatively be viewed as an extension of the data. This breakdown strategy is adaptable and, as a result, quite effective. The decomposition is relevant to nonlinear and nonstationary processes since it is based on the data local characteristic time scale. EMD is a powerful technique that decomposes the signal without distorting the time-domain features. It is also known as the Huang-Hilbert transform (HHT) [39]. The EMD is able to produce a different number of IMFs for applied signal. These IMFs consist of individual parts, which when added up reproduces the original signal. Each IMF can contain components that have varying amplitude and frequencies. The IMFs generated by the EMD vary from each other on the spectral domain, and the frequency decreases as one moves further. These functions are having the same number of extrema and zero crossings, along with symmetric envelopes. Two envelopes are generated from the original signal covering all the extrema and the zero-crossings using cubic spline. These upper and lower envelopes are then used to calculate the IMFs [40].

$$E_t - m_1 = P_1 \tag{1}$$

where

    m_1: mean of upper and lower envelope;

    E_t: original signal;

    P_1: proto-IMF; and

    n: number of sifting times.

The method of generating envelope from the extreme and their cubic spline is called as sifting. The IMFs are generated from the proto-IMF by extending the sifting process n times.

$$P_{1(n-1)} - mean_{1n} = P_{1n} \tag{2}$$

The sifting process is repeated several times until the original signal decomposed into n IMFs and one residue [41]. The detailed procedure of EMD is explained in Algorithm 1 [42].

The original ECG signal $ECG(t)$ represented with IMF components $S_n(t)$, and residue $res(t)$ are as follows:

$$ECG(t) = \sum_n S_n(t) + res(t) \tag{3}$$

The following conditions are used to identify significant IMF components: (i) at any point, the mean value of the envelope formed by the local maxima and the envelope defined by the local minima is zero and (ii) the number of extrema and zero-crossings must either be equal or differ by one. The crucial information of the ECG signal is located in the range of 0.05–100 Hz. High-frequency noises generally distort the ECG signal's temporal and spectral characteristics. Therefore, it is critical to remove unwanted noises without compromising the signal's fundamental properties. By rebuilding the IMFs of the signals and deleting the IMFs of noise, the EMD can minimize noise. Low-order IMFs mainly capture high-frequency components in the signal, whereas higher-order IMFs can capture low-frequency components [42]. The basic principle of denoising by EMD is to represent the denoised signal with a partial sum of the IMFs. The correlation coefficient (CC) is used to identify the significant IMFs component from the decomposed IMFs [40]. CC is calculated between original signal $ECG(t)$

Algorithm 1 Empirical mode decomposition of ECG signal.

1: **procedure** EMD (ECG signal) ◁

2:    System initialization

3:    Identifying the local minima E_{min} and maxima E_{max} of the $E(t)$.

4:    Finding the mean value of the local max and min: $Mean_1 = \frac{E_{max} + E_{min}}{2}$.

5:    The first IMF component IMF_1 is calculated as $E - m_1$.

6:    If IMF_1 is not the significant IMF, iterate on the residual mean to get new IMF.

and IMFs to obtain the particular mode, which IMF is dominated by signal rather than noise. The CC is defined as

$$
CC = \frac{\sum\limits_{i=1}^{n}(x_i - \bar{x})(y_i - \bar{y})}{\sqrt{\left[\sum\limits_{i=1}^{n}(x_i - \bar{x})^2\right]\left[\sum\limits_{i=1}^{n}(y_i - \bar{y})^2\right]}}
\tag{4}
$$

where $x = ECG(t)$, $y = IMF$, whereas $\bar{x}$ and $\bar{y}$ are the arithmetic mean of the two variables. n is the length of the variables.

CC is calculated for all the decomposed IMFs with respect to the original ECG signal. The IMFs are ranked in an ascending order based on CC values. The last two IMFs are considered for the reconstruction of the denoised ECG signal. Selected IMFs are summed and processed for ECG beat classification. Due to significant IMF selection, high-frequency noise components are removed from the ECG signal. Therefore, separating these noises from the ECG signal increases the beat detection capability of the deep learning algorithm.

3.2 Deep learning-based architecture for ECG beat classification

The proposed deep learning architecture for the detection of ECG beat classification is shown in Fig. 2. As shown in the architecture, it has six individual models to process the applied input. Each model consists of different layers as shown in Fig. 3. Every CNN block with small kernels in the architecture extracts the useful features for prediction. Then, flatten the output of the convolutional layers from three blocks and applied to the concatenate layer to generate a single feature vector. To obtain the final classification result, it is connected to the dense layers. The depth of the proposed network is increased to extract unique features from the dataset [4]. Three different datasets are prepared individually to train the three CNN blocks of the proposed network from the segmented ECG beat data. The whole segmented individual ECG beat data of size (1×256) is used to train the first CNN block (i.e., -128 to $+128$). The second CNN block is trained with the size of (1×128) by considering -128 (left side) to the R-peak location (i.e., -128 to 0). The third block of the CNN is trained with the R-peak location to $+128$ (right side) (i.e., 0 to $+128$). All three datasets are applied simultaneously to the three parallel blocks of the CNN to extract the in-detail features of the ECG beat. The detailed

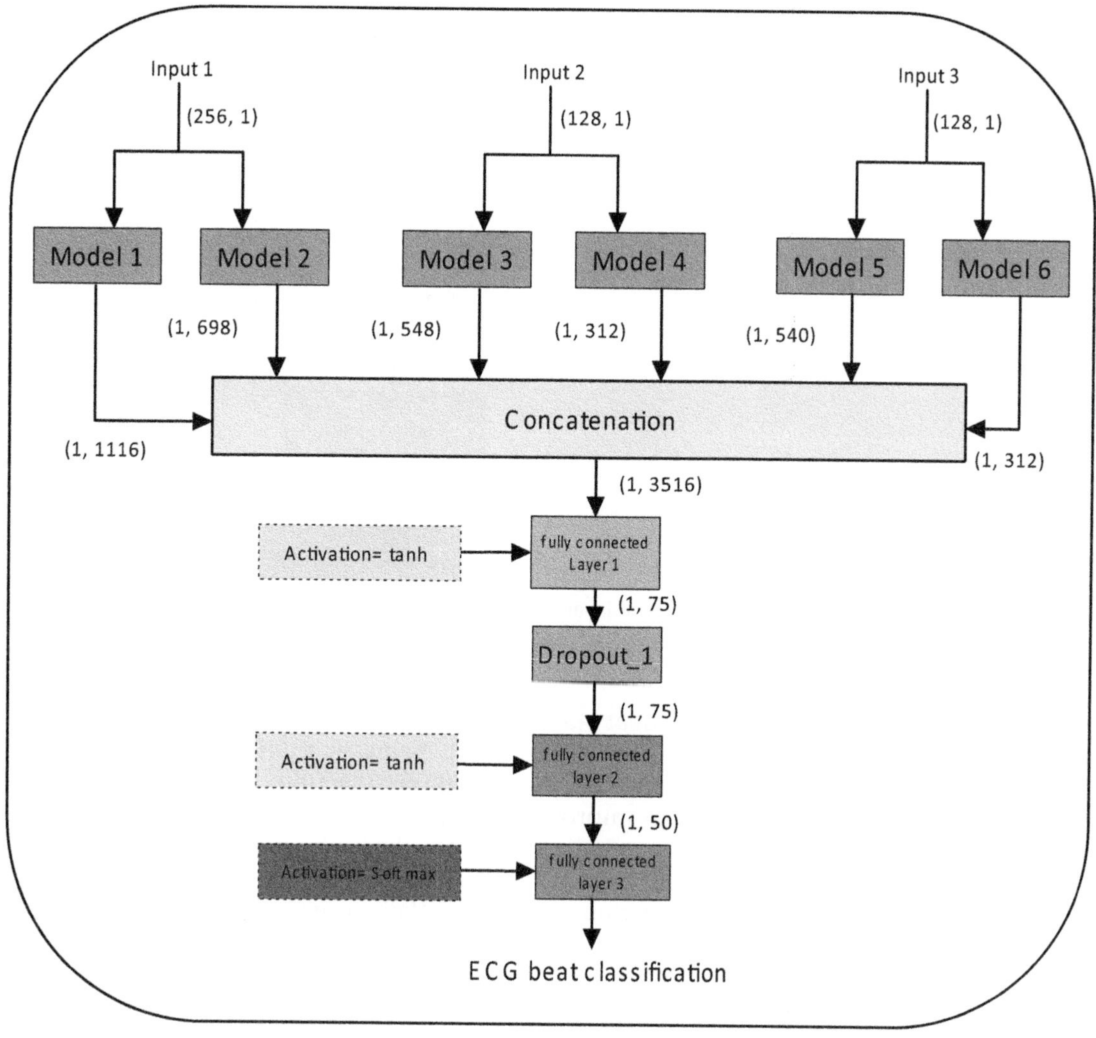

Fig. 2 Proposed CNN-based architecture for the patient-specific ECG beat classification.

architecture of the proposed deep learning model is shown in Fig. 2. In this proposed network, pooling layers are replaced by convolutional layers with strides more than one. This idea is becoming very popular in modern CNN architectures [35]. The detailed input size and output vector size of different layers in the proposed architecture is shown in Fig. 2.

Various features from ECG beat is extracted using different convolutional layers in the architecture. The first branch is mostly concentrated on the morphological nature of the QRS complex of

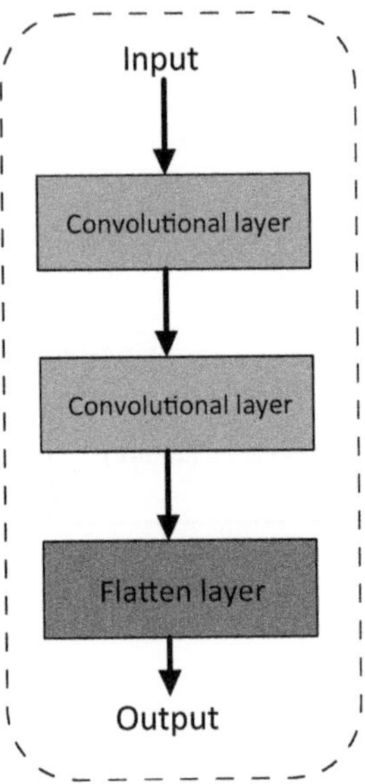

Fig. 3 Different layers in the individual model (models 1–6 as shown in Fig. 2).

the ECG beat [43, 44]. Second branch extracts the features of the P-wave, and third branch helps in finding the nature of the T-wave. Specific feature extraction from the P- and T-wave is helpful in improving the detection of S and V beats, which are clinically significant. The three branches are individually extracted features from the input data. Batch normalization and activation are sequentially executed with convolutional layers to reduce the size of the input vector. Let us say the first layer has dimensions ($32 \times 64 \times 64$) and the second layer had dimensions ($64 \times 64 \times 64$), then after concatenate, the new dimensions are ($96 \times 64 \times 64$). Therefore, to make the uniform dimension, the extracted feature data are concatenated using concatenation layer in this architecture. Finally, the dense layer implements a matrix-vector multiplication. The values in the matrix are real parameters, and these are used in training, updating through back propagation. To identify ECG beats, a densely linked layer provides learning characteristics from all the combinations of the information from the previous layer. Based on different experimentation with the deep learning network, the learning rate (η), the number of epochs (n), and batch sizes are observed as 0.001, 60, and 32 for the proposed network, respectively. The detailed tuning of the parameters related to the proposed network is discussed in Section 4.

4. Experimental results

The input data processing and modeling of the deep learning model are done in Python environment with the major libraries such as Keras, Tensorflow, and Pandas. The specification of desktop computer with NVIDIA RTX 3060 graphics card, and 32GB DDR3 RAM is used to conduct all the experiments in this work. In this EMD-based deep learning system, a standard MIT-BIH database is used to verify the performance of the proposed system. In preprocessing, ECG beats are segmented with the help of R-peak locations. After beat segmentation, noise is removed from the ECG beats using EMD technique [45]. Raw ECG signal, significant IMF components, and noise-free ECG beats are shown in Fig. 4. The significant IMF components are added to prepare noise-free dataset.

Finally, the database is prepared with 58,236 noise-free beats. A typical common training dataset is prepared randomly with 245 ECG beats, including 75 N, 75 S, 75 V beats, 13 types of F beats, and 7 type Q beats from the 100 series ECG records. In addition to this 245 beats data, 5 min of patient-specific data from 200 series ECG records is also added to the training data [46].

The remaining 25 min data in 200 series records are used to test the network, which is entirely new to the network. The detailed dataset used in this work is described in Table 1. From the table, it is concluded that the training set (TR1), testing set contains 8654 and 49,371 beats, respectively.

4.1 Performance metrics

To evaluate the performance of the proposed system, four statistical metrics are used in this work as in the previous literature [47, 48]. Those metrics are performance accuracy (*Acc*), sensitivity (*Sen*), specificity (*Spe*), and positive predictivity (*Ppr*). These parameters are calculated using a confusion matrix, which provides the classification instances information of the classifier. The four performance metrics can be calculated as

$$Acc = \frac{TP + TN}{TP + TN + FP + FN} \tag{5}$$

$$Sen = \frac{TP}{TP + FN} \tag{6}$$

$$Spe = \frac{TN}{TN + FP} \tag{7}$$

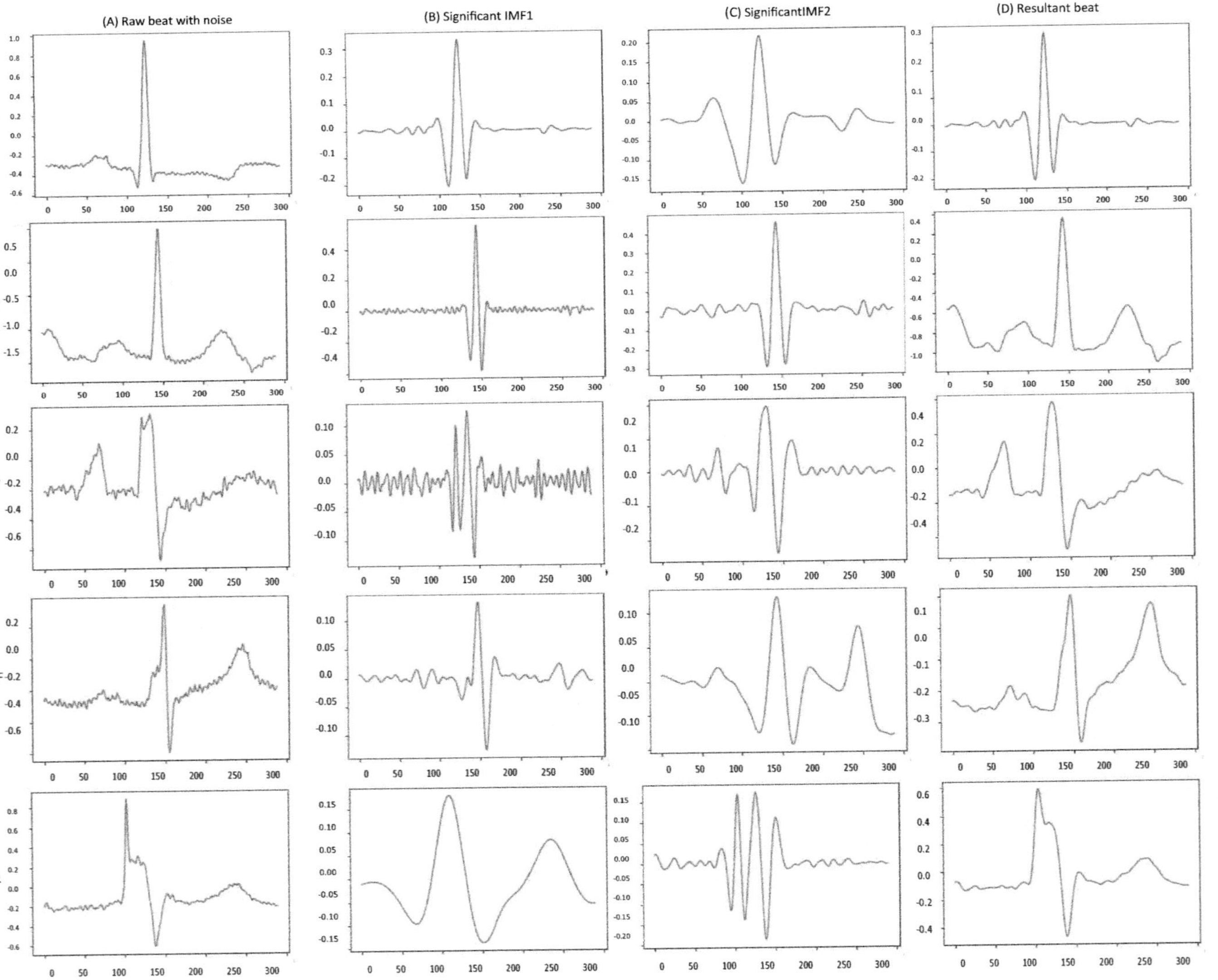

Fig. 4 N, S, V, F, and Q beats and IMF components of #100, #102, #104, #105, and #208 ECG records (number of samples are represented along the *x*-axis, whereas amplitude is shown along the *y*-axis).

Table 1 Detailed dataset description used in this work.

Class	Database	Training set (TR1)	Testing set (TS2)
N	45,981	3881	42,100
S	3837	1640	2197
V	6773	2340	4433
F	1378	754	624
Q	56	39	17

$$Ppr = \frac{TP}{TP + FP} \tag{8}$$

that is, TP, TN, FP, and FN are truly positive, truly negative, false positive, and false negative, sequentially, that is determined from the confusion matrix of the deep learning model.

4.2 Selection of hyperparameters for the proposed model

The performance of any deep learning model mainly depends upon the selection of optimized parameters. In this model, the learning rate (η) and batch size are the crucial parameters that affect the system's performance. A progression of trials is conducted to streamline these two parameters [49, 50]. At first, the network performance is tested with various learning rates while keeping the batch size constant. From this testing, it is confirmed that $\eta = 0.001$ is the ideal parameter, as presented in Table 2.

The network performance is tested with the different batch sizes by maintaining the learning rate constant, and Table 3 shows that 32 batch size is the minimum requirement for the best

Table 2 Tuning of learning rate for the proposed network.

Learning rate (η)	Batch size	Acc
0.2	16	0.9426
0.1	16	0.9635
0.01	16	0.9799
0.001	16	0.9912
0.0001	16	0.9802

Table 3 Tuning of batch size rate for the proposed network.

Learning rate (η)	Batch size	Acc
0.001	16	0.9537
0.001	32	0.9956
0.001	64	0.9654
0.001	128	0.9212
0.001	256	0.8912

performance. When the learning rate (η) and batch size are 0.001 and 32, the proposed model shows better performance.

4.3 Performance of the proposed system for ECG beat detection

The performance of the proposed system is estimated using a confusion matrix. The confusion matrix of the network is depicted in Table 4. The confusion matrix describes the performance of a classifier with correctly identified test instances. MIT-BIH dataset is applied as a test dataset to know the performance of the classifier [38]. Confusion matrix of the proposed EMD-based classifier is shown in Table 4. From the confusion matrix, it is observed that the classifier misclassified very few instances. In addition to this, the proposed algorithm can detect S and V beats accurately, which are clinically important to estimate sudden cardiac arrest. Different performance metrics in Table 5 are calculated using Table 4.

Table 4 Confusion matrix of the proposed method.

Class	N	S	V	F	Q
N	41,982	46	34	24	14
S	7	2173	0	2	15
V	12	0	4411	5	10
F	13	7	21	582	3
Q	0	2	0	0	15

Correctly classified instances detected by the proposed method is shown bold in Table 4.

Table 5 Performance metrics of the proposed method.

Class	Acc (%)	Sen (%)	Spe (%)	Ppr (%)	F-score
N	99.69	99.92	99.72	99.53	0.9982
S	99.84	97.53	98.91	99.88	0.9821
V	99.83	98.77	99.39	99.88	0.9908
F	99.85	94.94	92.97	99.94	0.9395
Q	99.90	96.82	91.59	99.91	0.9533

The proposed method provides an overall *Acc* of 99.56%, *Sen* of 99.42%, *Spe* of 99.52%, and *Ppr* of 99.49%. *F*-score is a measure of test's accuracy, and the proposed method shows an average F-score of 0.97.

The network reached stable state after 40 epochs during training, and for testing the model is taking only 0.14 s for the detection. From all the above metrics, it is concluded that the proposed detection method for identifying ECG beat type produces decent performance compared to the state-of-the-art techniques.

4.4 Comparison of the proposed framework with state-of-the-art techniques

The proposed method is compared with the latest five recent literatures based on deep learning and machine learning in Table 6. The proposed method is performed efficiently in detecting ECG beats compared to the earlier reported techniques with performance *Acc* of 99.56%. Feature extraction technique is also not needed for the proposed technique, which makes the proposed system simple. The proposed system is utilized very less amount of data for training, and converges within 60 epochs. Some of the techniques represented in Table 6 extract feature maps manually in addition to the deep learning techniques, which complicate the process.

A simple preprocessing technique is only required to remove the noise from the ECG beats. A receiver operating characteristics (ROC) curve is a graphical representation that summarizes the prediction performance of the classification model. False positive rate (FPR) versus true positive rate (TPR) is plotted as discrete ROC in Fig. 5. TPR defines as exact positive results are detected by the model among all positive samples during prediction. In contrast, FPR defines the number of incorrect positive results that occur among all negative samples available during the test.

Table 6 Performance comparison of the proposed method with literature.

Literature	Number of classes	Preprocessing	Feature extraction	Classifier	Acc (in %)
Kiranyaz et al. [31]	5	Not required	Fast Fourier transform (FFT)	1D CNN	95.58
Wang et al. [51]	2	Required	–	CNN + RNN	96.64
Oh et al. [36]	5	Not required	–	CNN-LSTM	98.10
Zhu et al. [39]	5	Required	Time and morphological domain	SVM	97.80
Asgharzadeh-Bonab et al. [52]	5	Required	–	Deep CNN	98.34
Proposed method	5	Required	–	Parallel blocks of CNN	99.56

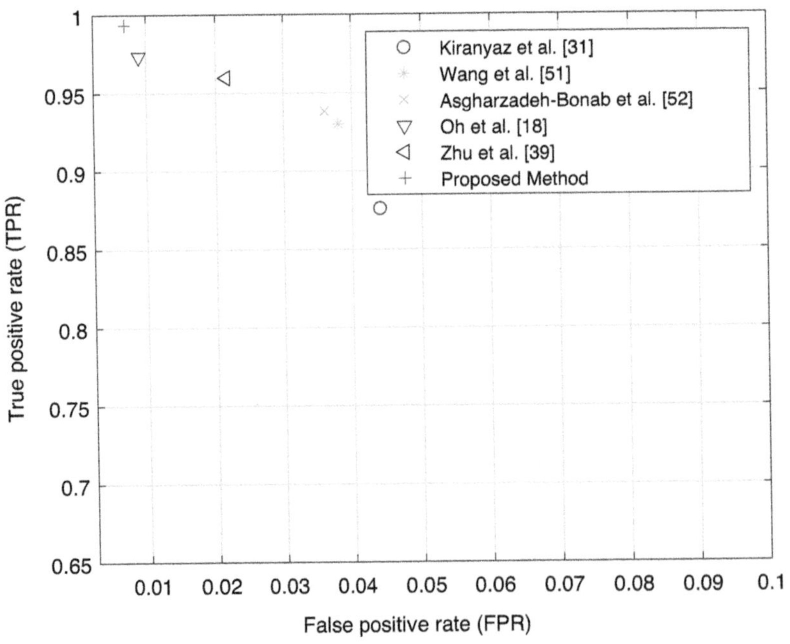

Fig. 5 Comparison of the proposed method ROC with earlier reported techniques.

The x- and y-axes of an ROC space are defined by FPR and TPR, respectively, and illustrate relative trade-offs between true positive (benefits) and false positive (costs). The ROC graph is sometimes referred as the sensitivity versus (1—specificity) plot since TPR equals sensitivity and FPR equals (1—specificity). From the discrete ROC, it is observed that the proposed method provides higher TPR and lower FPR [50].

5. Conclusions

This chapter proposes a new method for patient-specific ECG beat categorization using the deep learning technique. The proposed method is used to classify five different types of ECG beats N, S, V, F, and Q, which followed the AAMI standard. In this work, the suggested approach for beat detection consisted of two steps: preprocessing and classification. In preprocessing, applying EMD on ECG signal to extract significant IMF components is crucial to extract the relevant beat information from the signal. These significant IMF components are beneficial in removing high-frequency noise components. To extract the morphological information about the QRS complex, P-wave, and T-wave, three different datasets are prepared in this work separately. These three datasets are processed individually through three parallel CNN architectures. The experimental results show that the proposed EMD-based deep learning successfully identified ECG beats by extracting exact morphology information from the beat segments. The performance parameters of the proposed method show that it provides better performance than the earlier reported techniques. The proposed ECG beat classification system in this work has the following advantages: (i) adaptive ECG signal denoising using EMD technique, (ii) feature engineering is not required, (iii) proposed architecture of the deep learning model can achieve high accuracy with less number of epochs, and (iv) proposed algorithm can be used to deploy in automatic ECG beat classification monitoring devices.

References

[1] P. Pławiak, U.R. Acharya, Novel deep genetic ensemble of classifiers for arrhythmia detection using ECG signals, Neural Comput. Appl. 32 (15) (2020) 11137–11161.

[2] R.N.V.P.S. Kandala, R. Dhuli, P. Pławiak, G.R. Naik, H. Moeinzadeh, G.D. Gargiulo, S. Gunnam, Towards real-time heartbeat classification: evaluation of nonlinear morphological features and voting method, IEEE Sensors J. 19 (23) (2019) 5079.

[3] P. Pławiak, Novel genetic ensembles of classifiers applied to myocardium dysfunction recognition based on ECG signals, Swarm Evol. Comput. 39 (2018) 192–208.

[4] M. Faezipour, A. Saeed, S.C. Bulusu, M. Nourani, H. Minn, L. Tamil, A patient-adaptive profiling scheme for ECG beat classification, IEEE Trans. Inf. Technol. Biomed. 14 (5) (2010) 1153–1165.

[5] G.B. Moody, R.G. Mark, The impact of the MIT-BIH arrhythmia database, IEEE Eng. Med. Biol. Mag. 20 (3) (2001) 45–50.

[6] A.S. Alvarado, C. Lakshminarayan, J.C. Principe, Time-based compression and classification of heartbeats, IEEE Trans. Biomed. Eng. 59 (6) (2012) 1641–1648.

[7] P. De Chazal, R.B. Reilly, A patient-adapting heartbeat classifier using ECG morphology and heartbeat interval features, IEEE Trans. Biomed. Eng. 53 (12) (2006) 2535–2543.

[8] A.K. Barros, A. Mansour, N. Ohnishi, Removing artifacts from electrocardiographic signals using independent components analysis, Neurocomputing 22 (1–3) (1998) 173–186.

[9] I. Romero, PCA and ICA applied to noise reduction in multi-lead ECG, in: 2011 Computing in Cardiology, IEEE, 2011, pp. 613–616.

[10] A. Chacko, S. Ari, Denoising of ECG signals using empirical mode decomposition based technique, in: IEEE-International Conference on Advances in Engineering, Science and Management (ICAESM-2012), IEEE, 2012, pp. 6–9.

[11] M.A. Kabir, C. Shahnaz, Denoising of ECG signals based on noise reduction algorithms in EMD and wavelet domains, Biomed. Signal Process. Control 7 (5) (2012) 481–489.

[12] K.-M. Chang, Arrhythmia ECG noise reduction by ensemble empirical mode decomposition, Sensors 10 (6) (2010) 6063–6080.

[13] K.-M. Chang, S.-H. Liu, Gaussian noise filtering from ECG by Wiener filter and ensemble empirical mode decomposition, J. Signal Process. Syst. 64 (2) (2011) 249–264.

[14] Y. Xu, M. Luo, T. Li, G. Song, ECG signal de-noising and baseline wander correction based on CEEMDAN and wavelet threshold, Sensors 17 (12) (2017) 2754.

[15] X. Tian, Y. Li, H. Zhou, X. Li, L. Chen, X. Zhang, Electrocardiogram signal denoising using extreme-point symmetric mode decomposition and nonlocal means, Sensors 16 (10) (2016) 1584.

[16] M. Zahangir Alom, T.M. Taha, C. Yakopcic, S. Westberg, P. Sidike, M. Shamima Nasrin, B.C. Van Esesn, A.A.S. Awwal, V.K. Asari, The history began from alexnet: a comprehensive survey on deep learning approaches, arXiv Preprint arXiv:1803.01164 (2018).

[17] P. Bing, W. Liu, Z. Wang, Z. Zhang, Noise reduction in ECG signal using an effective hybrid scheme, IEEE Access 8 (2020) 160790–160801.

[18] B.R. Manju, M.R. Sneha, ECG denoising using Wiener filter and Kalman filter, Proc. Comput. Sci. 171 (2020) 273–281.

[19] D. Berwal, C.R. Vandana, S. Dewan, C.V. Jiji, M.S. Baghini, Motion artifact removal in ambulatory ECG signal for heart rate variability analysis, IEEE Sensors J. 19 (24) (2019) 12432–12442.

[20] P. Singh, I. Srivastava, A. Singhal, A. Gupta, Baseline wander and power-line interference removal from ECG signals using Fourier decomposition method, in: Machine Intelligence and Signal Analysis, Springer, 2019, pp. 25–36.

[21] H. Shi, R. Liu, C. Chen, M. Shu, Y. Wang, ECG baseline estimation and denoising with group sparse regularization, IEEE Access 9 (2021) 23595–23607.

[22] E. Ercelebi, Electrocardiogram signals de-noising using lifting-based discrete wavelet transform, Comput. Biol. Med. 34 (6) (2004) 479–493.

[23] B.N. Singh, A.K. Tiwari, Optimal selection of wavelet basis function applied to ECG signal denoising, Digital Signal process. 16 (3) (2006) 275–287.

[24] B.H. Tracey, E.L. Miller, Nonlocal means denoising of ECG signals, IEEE Trans. Biomed. Eng. 59 (9) (2012) 2383–2386.

[25] E. Gokgoz, A. Subasi, Effect of multiscale PCA de-noising on EMG signal classification for diagnosis of neuromuscular disorders, J. Med. Syst. 38 (4) (2014) 1–10.

[26] M.Z.U. Rahman, R.A. Shaik, D.V.R.K. Reddy, Efficient sign based normalized adaptive filtering techniques for cancelation of artifacts in ECG signals: application to wireless biotelemetry, Signal Process. 91 (2) (2011) 225–239.

[27] W. Jenkal, R. Latif, A. Toumanari, A. Dliou, O. El B'charri, F.M.R. Maoulainine, An efficient algorithm of ECG signal denoising using the adaptive dual threshold filter and the discrete wavelet transform, Biocybern. Biomed. Eng. 36 (3) (2016) 499–508.

[28] L. Smital, M. Vitek, J. Kozumplík, I. Provaznik, Adaptive wavelet wiener filtering of ECG signals, IEEE Trans. Biomed. Eng. 60 (2) (2012) 437–445.

[29] I.I. Christov, I.K. Daskalov, Filtering of electromyogram artifacts from the electrocardiogram, Med. Eng. Phys. 21 (10) (1999) 731–736.

[30] H.-T. Chiang, Y.-Y. Hsieh, S.-W. Fu, K.-H. Hung, Y. Tsao, S.-Y. Chien, Noise reduction in ECG signals using fully convolutional denoising autoencoders, IEEE Access 7 (2019) 60806–60813.

[31] S. Kiranyaz, T. Ince, M. Gabbouj, Real-time patient-specific ECG classification by 1-D convolutional neural networks, IEEE Trans. Biomed. Eng. 63 (3) (2015) 664–675.

[32] R.V. Andreao, B. Dorizzi, J. Boudy, ECG signal analysis through hidden Markov models, IEEE Trans. Biomed. Eng. 53 (8) (2006) 1541–1549.

[33] L. Khadra, A.S. Al-Fahoum, S. Binajjaj, A quantitative analysis approach for cardiac arrhythmia classification using higher order spectral techniques, IEEE Trans. Biomed. Eng. 52 (11) (2005) 1840–1845.

[34] B. Hou, J. Yang, P. Wang, R. Yan, LSTM-based auto-encoder model for ECG arrhythmias classification, IEEE Trans. Instrum. Meas. 69 (4) (2019) 1232–1240.

[35] J.T. Springenberg, A. Dosovitskiy, T. Brox, M. Riedmiller, Striving for simplicity: the all convolutional net, arXiv preprint arXiv:1412.6806 (2014).

[36] S.L. Oh, E.Y.K. Ng, R. San Tan, U.R. Acharya, Automated diagnosis of arrhythmia using combination of CNN and LSTM techniques with variable length heart beats, Comput. Biol. Med. 102 (2018) 278–287.

[37] M.K. Das, S. Ari, Patient-specific ECG beat classification technique, Healthcare Technol. Lett. 1 (3) (2014) 98–103.

[38] P. Pławiak, Novel methodology of cardiac health recognition based on ECG signals and evolutionary-neural system, Expert Syst. Appl. 92 (2018) 334–349.

[39] X. Chen, Y. Wang, L. Wang, Arrhythmia recognition and classification using ECG morphology and segment feature analysis, IEEE/ACM Trans. Comput. Biol. Bioinf. 16 (1) (2018) 131–138.

[40] M.M. Mukaka, A guide to appropriate use of correlation coefficient in medical research, Malawi Med. J. 24 (3) (2012) 69–71.

[41] W. Jiang, S.G. Kong, Block-based neural networks for personalized ECG signal classification, IEEE Trans. Neural Netw. 18 (6) (2007) 1750–1761.

[42] N.E. Huang, Z. Shen, S.R. Long, M.C. Wu, H.H. Shih, Q. Zheng, N.-C. Yen, C.C. Tung, H.H. Liu, The empirical mode decomposition and the Hilbert spectrum for nonlinear and non-stationary time series analysis, Proc. R. Soc. Lond. A Math. Phys. Eng. Sci. 454 (1971) (1998) 903–995.

[43] C. Ye, B.V.K. Vijaya Kumar, M.T. Coimbra, Heartbeat classification using morphological and dynamic features of ECG signals, IEEE Trans. Biomed. Eng. 59 (10) (2012) 2930–2941.

[44] M. Thomas, M.K. Das, S. Ari, Automatic ECG arrhythmia classification using dual tree complex wavelet based features, AEU-Int. J. Electron. Commun. 69 (4) (2015) 715–721.

[45] C. Wen, M.-F. Yeh, K.-C. Chang, ECG beat classification using GreyART network, IET Signal Process. 1 (1) (2007) 19–28.

[46] A. Jaya Prakash, S. Ari, SpEC: a system for patient specific ECG beat classification using deep residual network, Biocybern. Biomed. Eng. 40 (4) (2020) 1446–1457.

[47] T. Ince, S. Kiranyaz, M. Gabbouj, A generic and robust system for automated patient-specific classification of ECG signals, IEEE Trans. Biomed. Eng. 56 (5) (2009) 1415–1426.

[48] A. Kampouraki, G. Manis, C. Nikou, Heartbeat time series classification with support vector machines, IEEE Trans. Inf. Technol. Biomed. 13 (4) (2008) 512–518.

[49] A. Jaya Prakash, S. Ari, AAMI standard cardiac arrhythmia detection with random forest using mixed features, in: 2019 IEEE 16th India Council International Conference (INDICON), IEEE, 2019, pp. 1–4.

[50] A. Jaya Prakash, S. Ari, A system for automatic cardiac arrhythmia recognition using electrocardiogram signal, in: Bioelectronics and Medical Devices, Elsevier, 2019, pp. 891–911.

[51] J. Wang, C. Liu, L. Li, W. Li, L. Yao, H. Li, H. Zhang, A stacking-based model for non-invasive detection of coronary heart disease, IEEE Access 8 (2020) 37124–37133.

[52] A. Asgharzadeh-Bonab, M.C. Amirani, A. Mehri, Spectral entropy and deep convolutional neural network for ECG beat classification, Biocybern. Biomed. Eng. 40 (2) (2020) 691–700.

5

Empirical wavelet transform and deep learning-based technique for ECG beat classification

Jaya Prakash Allam[a], Saunak Samantray[b], and Samit Ari[a]

[a]Department of Electronics and Communication Engineering, National Institute of Technology Rourkela, Rourkela, Odisha, India. [b]Department of ETC, IIIT Bhubaneswar, Odisha, India

1. Introduction

Electrocardiogram (ECG) is a diagnostic test to measure the heart's rhythm, heart rate, and electrical activity. An ECG is one of the most important and common tests used to screen for certain cardiovascular diseases such as arrhythmia [1]. The ECG test shows the presence of any disorder in the heart, as it shows how fast the heart is beating and if the heart is beating normally or not. Cardiologists sometimes use this test to monitor the effect of drugs or devices, such as the pacemaker, on the heart itself. The test can measure the location and size of the heart chambers. Causes of abnormal ECG results may include damage to the heart muscle, swelling, inflammation of the heart, and other possible causes, including poor blood flow to the heart or a previous or current heart attack [2]. One of the common cardiovascular diseases is arrhythmia, which is the presence of an irregular heartbeat, where the heart may beat too fast or too slowly. This condition changes in the heart's electrical system or a short circuit in the heart, which leads to poor blood circulation in the body. Poor blood circulation in the body increases the risk of heart failure and stroke. Therefore, developing an effective system for the early detection of arrhythmia is essential.

Identifying the type of ECG beat accurately in cardiac patients is necessary for proper medication and treatment. The Association for Advancement of Medical Instrumentation (AAMI) [3] classifies the heartbeats of the arrhythmia patients into five classes: N, S, V, F,

Advanced Methods in Biomedical Signal Processing and Analysis. https://doi.org/10.1016/B978-0-323-85955-4.00006-5
Copyright © 2023 Elsevier Inc. All rights reserved.

Table 1 Categorization of ECG beats based on AAMI standard.

Beat label in AAMI standard	MIT-BIH beat type
Normal beat (N)	Atrial escape beats (e)
Left bundle branch block (LBBB)	
Nodal (junctional) escape beats (j)	
Normal (N)	
Right bundle branch block beats (RBBB)	
Supraventricular ectopic beat (S)	Aberrated atrial premature beats (a)
Atrial premature contraction (A)	
Nodal (junctional) premature beats (J)	
Supraventricular premature beats (S)	
Ventricular ectopic beat (V)	Ventricular escape beats (E)
Ventricular flutter wave (!)	
Premature ventricular contraction (PVC)	
Fusion beat (F)	Fusion of ventricular and normal beat (F)
Unclassifiable beat (Q)	Fusion of paced and normal beats (f)
Paced beats (/)	
Unclassifiable beats (Q)	

and Q. Table 1 shows the heartbeat classes contained in each class. Several types of research works were implemented in existing literature for the intelligent classification of ECG beats [2, 4–7]. From a technical aspect, there are two classification methods: conventional machine and deep learning methods [8, 9]. In general, machine learning techniques followed preprocessing, feature extraction, and classification stages. Preprocessing is used to remove the noise from the ECG signal, which is common for both machine and deep learning techniques. However, manual feature extraction techniques are required to extract the features from the ECG signal. These manually extracted features are also called as handcrafted features. If the extracted feature sets are not optimized, then optimization techniques are also necessary to optimize features. Finally, these optimized features are applied to the machine learning algorithms for further classification. Deep learning algorithms are widely popular for automatized feature extraction and classification to remove these manual feature extraction and optimization stages in machine learning. All previous results show that the classification accuracy of conventional methods is usually lower than that of deep learning methods [9]. Deep learning methods have been widely applied to classify the five-class heartbeats and deep learning approaches preprocessing and classification steps are generally followed to classify the type of ECG beats. A separate manual feature extraction technique is not required in deep learning approaches, which reduce the system's complexity. Therefore, some of the previous works based on deep learning approaches are mentioned in Section 1.1.

1.1 Related works and motivation

Most of the researchers followed convolutional neural network (CNN)-based deep learning architectures to classify ECG beats efficiently [5]. In [5], an accurate patient-specific ECG beat classification system is developed using one-dimensional (1D) CNN architecture to classify five types of ECG beats based on AAMI standard. ECG beats are segmented from the Massachusetts Institute of Technology-Beth Israel Hospital (MIT-BIH) raw ECG data and down sampled to 128 sample points from the center point of the R-peak. These samples or fast Fourier transform (FFT) of these segments are applied to the 1D CNN. The network is trained with the common 245 representative beats from all the patients and the specific patient's 5-min beat data. The remaining 25 min of data in the patient's ECG record were utilized for testing the network performance. The results of this work show that the network successfully classified all the ECG beats except S-beat. In addition, new patients wishing to use this technology must supply ECG records for 5 min and an expensive annotation process for prediction due to a patient-dependent classification system.

The combination of restricted Boltzmann machine (RBM) and deep neural network (DNN) is implemented by utilizing QRS complex, P wave, and T wave information for ECG beat classification in [10]. Important time-domain samples are extracted from ECG signal, and a sliding time window covering these sample points is also used to extract consecutive vectors. Each of these vectors holds the consecutive sample points of a complete heartbeat cycle, including the QRS complex and the P and T waves. This strategy does not require handcraft features and produces optimized ECG representation for heartbeat classification. The DNN developed in this literature classified S and V beats with descent sensitivity.

Saadatnejad et al. developed wavelet transform (WT), and multiple long short-term memory (LSTM) recurrent neural networks (RNNs)-based architecture to classify ECG beats [7]. LSTM-RNN automatically extracts features, and standard features are extracted using WT that helps to capture specific patterns in the ECG signal. In [4], two different blocks are framed for denoising and classification. Different up and down samplings are used to denoising the ECG signal, and the denoised ECG signal is applied to the HeartNetEC (customized CNN architecture) for ECG beat classification. DNN with seven hidden layers is developed to classify ECG beats using raw ECG signal in [6]. In [1], at first, ECG beats are segmented based on R-peak location, further transformed these beats into spectrograms, and finally, these spectrograms are applied to the deep residual network (ResNet) to classify five types of ECG beats in a patient-specific way. Xie et al. implemented ECG beat classification system using the combination of bidirectional RNN and CNN named as Bi-RCNN [11]. Two-dimensional (2D) gray-scale ECG beat images are applied as input to the 2D CNN for ECG beat classification and achieved 99.05% performance accuracy in [12]. In [13], a different combination of auto-encoders (AEs) and DNN is developed to classify 10 types of ECG beats. In [14], continuous WT and CNN architecture was designed to classify ECG beats based on AAMI standards. Continuous WT is utilized in this design to convert ECG beats into scalograms applied to the CNN for automatic beat identification. Different deep learning techniques such as CNN [12], LSTM [7], CNN-LSTM [15], GreyART (adaptive resonant theory) [16], and deep belief network (DBN) [17] are also popular in ECG beat classification. Machine and deep learning-based ECG beat classification systems developed in recent years are shown in Table 2. Most of the deep learning techniques successfully classified ECG beats with automatic feature extraction.

All the above-stated deep learning techniques successfully classified ECG beats when the input data are noise free. Deep learning algorithms may be misclassified when the ECG signal is contaminated with the noises during acquisition. Most of the deep learning algorithms are sensitive to the noise presented in the applied data. Hence, removing noise from the ECG signals is an important task before applying the data to the algorithm. To overcome the noise problem, a different combination of empirical wavelet transform (EWT) with customized CNN architecture is proposed in this chapter to classify ECG beats in a patient-specific way.

The remaining chapter is arranged as follows: Section 2 is devoted to the details of the dataset used in the experiments. The methodology used in the study is discussed in Section 3. The experimental results in this work are presented in Section 4, at last conclusions followed in Section 5.

2. Database

The MIT-BIH database is used to estimate the performance of the proposed system in this work. The database is extracted from the two-lead ambulatory ECG recordings. The ambulatory ECG recordings are collected from the 47 subjects: 25 male and 22 female are between 23 and 89 age. The final database is

Table 2 Existing literature on ECG beat classification.

Literature	Database	Number of ECG beats classified	Feature extraction (handcrafted/ automatic)	Classifier
Oh et al. [18]	MIT-BIH arrhythmia	5	Automatic	CNN-LSTM
Deevi et al. [4]	MIT-BIH arrhythmia	5	Automatic	CNN based HeartNet
Bidias et al. [19]	MIT-BIH arrhythmia and St. Petersburg Institute of Cardiological technics (INCART)	3	Handcrafted	Binary adaptive classifier
Abdullah et al. [20]	MIT-BIH arrhythmia	2	Handcrafted	Support vector machines (SVM)
Sahoo et al. [21]	MIT-BIH arrhythmia	5	Handcrafted	PCA and SVM
Kar et al. [22]	MIT-BIH arrhythmia	5	Handcrafted	K-NN
Yang et al. [23]	MIT-BIH arrhythmia	3	Automatic	Hybrid CNN
Van Steenkiste et al. [24]	MIT-BIH arrhythmia	5	Automatic	Parallel CNN architecture

prepared with 48 half-hour excerpts of 47 individual ambulatory recordings. Four ECG records (102, 104, 107, and 217) are exempted from the experimentation due to its poor quality. The records have been digitalized with a channel resolution of 10 mV on 360 samples per second. All recordings have raw ECG data, and two or more cardiologists have independently marked beat-by-beat annotations. A total of 108,655 heartbeats are labeled with 15 different types. These 15 different types of heartbeats are categorized into five types (N, S, V, F, and Q) as per the AAMI standard.

3. Proposed methodology

In this section, initially, the preprocessing stage is discussed. Then, the proposed architecture of the customized deep learning technique for ECG beat classification is explained. The detailed block diagram is shown in Fig. 1.

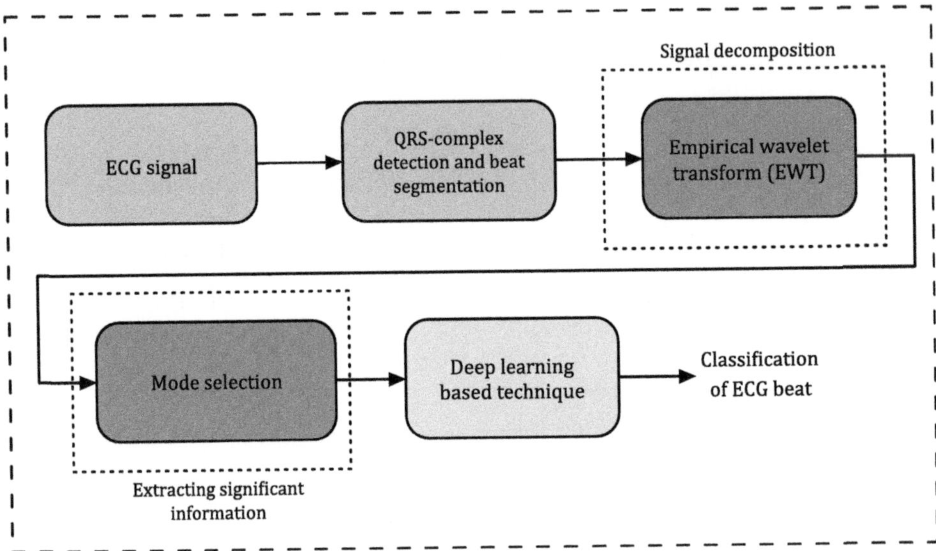

Fig. 1 Proposed methodology for ECG beat classification.

3.1 Preprocessing

In Fig. 1, preprocessing refers, removing noise from the ECG signals and extracting heartbeats from continuous ECG signals. The Pan-Tompkins algorithm [25] is used to detect exact R-peak locations in continuous ECG signals in preprocessing. The QRS complexes are identified and separated as ECG beat segments from the ECG signal with the help of detected R-peak locations. After segmentation of the ECG beats, EWT is used to eliminate the noise components. EWT is a technique that utilized to decompose the signal [26]. The goal is to extract the various modes of a signal by designing a wavelet filter bank that fits to the given signal. A family of wavelets could be built that can adapt to the particular processed signal. This method is similar to building band-pass filter banks to extract the exact information of the input signal from the spectrum. The properties of an intrinsic mode function are similar to those of a certain frequency in the analyzed signal. EWT is an advanced technique to decompose the signal better than empirical mode decomposition (EMD) [27]. EMD can also extract nonstationary information from the applied signal, but EMD is a nonlinear algorithm that has no mathematical theory, difficult to predict and understand its output. EMD is prone to noise when the signal is corrupted with some artifact noises. Ensemble EMD (EEMD) came into existence to stabilize the decomposition, but this method increases the computational

> # Algorithm 1 Empirical wavelet transform (EWT).
>
> 1: **procedure** INPUT(E, n (number of scales))
> 2:   Fourier transform of $E \to \hat{E}$
> 3:   Compute the local maxima of $\hat{E}$ in $[0, \pi]$ and find the set ω_n
> 4:   Choose $\gamma < \min_n \left(\frac{\omega_{n+1} - \omega_n}{\omega_{n+1} + \omega_n} \right)$; where γ is transition co-efficient.
> 5:   Build the filter bank
> 6:   Get decomposition by filter the input signal
> 7: **end procedure**

cost [28]. EWT is utilized in this work to overcome the problems in EMD, which combines the robustness of wavelets with the adaptability of EMD. The detailed algorithm of EWT is shown in Algorithm 1 [26].

EWT of a signal denoted as $w^e{}_f(n, t)$. The detailed coefficients are obtained by inner products with the empirical wavelets, whereas approximation coefficients (ψ_n) are obtained by the inner product of scaling function (ϕ_1). From Eqs. (1), (2), reconstruction of the original signal is obtained by Eq. (3).

$$w_f^d(nt) = \langle f . \psi_n \rangle = \int f(\tau)\psi_n(\bar{\tau} - t)d\tau = \left(\hat{f}(\omega)\overline{\psi_n}(\omega) \right)^{\vee} \tag{1}$$

$$w_f^a(0t) = \langle f . \phi_1 \rangle = \int f(\tau)\phi_1(\bar{\tau} - t)d\tau = \left(\hat{f}(\omega)\overline{\phi_1}(\omega) \right)^{\vee} \tag{2}$$

$$E(t) = w_f^a(0t)*\phi_1(t) + \sum_{n=1}^{N} w_f^d(nt)*\psi_n(t)$$
$$= \hat{w}_f^a(0\omega)*\hat{\phi}_1(\omega) + \sum_{n=1}^{N} \hat{w}_f^d(n\omega)*\hat{\psi}_n(\omega) \tag{3}$$

The different modes are extracted from the input signal using approximated and detailed coefficients of EWT. The resulting modes f_k are shown in Eqs. (4), (5). Finally, the original reconstructed ECG signal is $E(t) = \sum_{n=0}^{k} E_n(t)$ [26].

$$E_0(t) = w_f^a(0, t) * \phi_1(t) \tag{4}$$

$$E_k(t) = w_f^d(k, t) * \psi_k(t) \tag{5}$$

The number of modes is fixed to k initially; hence, EWT never overestimates the number of modes. The variable k is decided by the Fourier spectrum of the input signal [26]. It can detect the presence of modes in the spectrum and provide different components close to the original one. The EWT works in frequency space, unlike EMD, which works in temporal space. After successful decomposition of ECG signal, the specific low-frequency modes are added and form a noise-free signal. The resultant noise-free ECG beats are used as input to the customized deep learning network for further classification.

3.2   Deep learning architecture for ECG beat classification

The CNN is a deep learning technique that takes an input, time series, or image and finds relation/objects/features. It reduces the need for high preprocessing drastically, while trying to find all the possible relationships or features by itself. CNN-based deep learning architecture is proposed for ECG beat classification in this work. The detailed architecture of the deep learning method in the ECG beat classification system is shown in Fig. 2.

The deep learning architecture shown in Fig. 2 consists of three serial CNN blocks. Each CNN block consists of one convolutional layer, batch normalization, and activation. In the suggested approach, three deep convolutional blocks are employed since they exhibit a proper balance between computational efficiency and the validity of the findings. The kernel in the 1D convolutional layer is convolved with the single-dimension input vector to produce output tensor [29]. The kernel size of 40 is used in the initial layer, but gradually it is decreased to 4, which reduces the computational cost of the network. The input was managed through batch standardization. It was used to boost performance and stabilize the learning process of the deep neural network after each convolution layer and before pooling. The output of the batch normalization layer was down sampled through a 1D max-pooling layer with a pool size of 4.

Rectified linear activation unit (ReLU) activation is used in all the convolution layers, which reduce the over-fitting problem. The max-pooling in each block resizes the applied input by considering the maximum value on the window defined by the pool dimension. The pool dimension is dependent on the stride size used in convolution layers. In the final stage of the network, the average pooling performed the same operation as max pooling but with an average window value. Flatten function in the network architecture flattens the multidimensional input tensors into a single dimension. The detailed input and outsizes of the applied vector is shown in Table 3. Total trainable parameters in the proposed deep learning method are 14,197. The detailed training and testing phases of the proposed network are explained in Section 4.

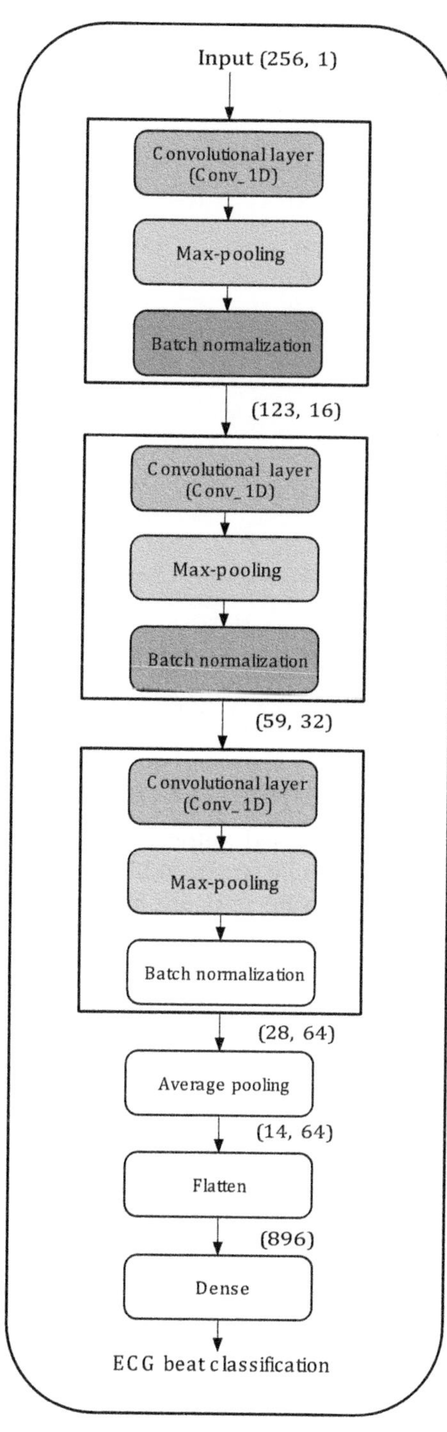

Fig. 2 Proposed CNN-based architecture for the patient-specific ECG beat classification.

Table 3 Detailed description of the proposed network.

S. no.	Layer (type)	Output shape	Parameters
1	Input	(256, 1)	0
2	Convolutional layer	(247, 16)	176
3	Max pooling	(123, 16)	0
4	Batch normalization	(123, 16)	64
5	Convolutional layer	(118, 32)	3104
6	Max pooling	(59, 32)	0
7	Batch normalization	(59, 32)	128
8	Convolutional layer	(57, 64)	6208
9	Max pooling	(28, 64)	0
10	Batch normalization	(28, 64)	256
11	Average pooling	(14, 64)	0
12	Flatten	(896)	0
13	Dense	5	4485
14	Total parameters	14,421	
15	Trainable parameters	14,197	
16	Nontrainable parameters	224	

4. Experimental results

The proposed automatic beat classification system is trained and tested on a standard MIT-BIH database. The experiments carried out in this work are implemented on a python environment using keras, tensor flow, matplotlib, and pandas libraries. The specifications of the desktop workstation used in this work are as follows: 32 GB random access memory (RAM) and NVIDIA RTX 3060 graphics card. A typical patient-specific data are prepared from the MIT-BIH to train the proposed model in this work. Preprocessing and classifications are explained in Sections 4.1 and 4.2.

4.1 Preprocessing of ECG beats using EWT technique

A common training dataset is prepared from the #100 series ECG records with 245 beats (75 of each N, S, V, 13-F, and 7-Q beats). In addition to this data, the first 5 min of data from

#200 series ECG records are also added. At first, in the ECG signal, R-peak locations are detected using the Pan-Tompkins algorithm [25]. Based on these locations, individual beats are segmented with a length of 256 samples (-128 to $+128$ around R-peak). These individual beats are further processed with EWT to remove the noise effect. EWT method is used to decompose different modes from the signal based on the frequency content. The following steps should be followed to find the number of modes in EWT:

1. Find the number of maximas and minimas in the magnitude of normalized Fourier spectrum (let R_{max} and T_{min} be the number of maximas and minimas sequentially).
2. Approximate number of modes are $R_{max} > T_{min} + n*(R_{max} - T_{min})$.

In this work, the number of maximas and minimas are 5 and 3, respectively, so $n = 2$ (number of modes) is a suitable parameter to decompose the signal into two modes (i.e., $mode_1$ and $mode_2$). Fig. 3 describes the individual beats, spectrum partition, and reconstruction of the ECG signal with selective modes. The modes are extracted based on the spectrum of the applied ECG beat. Boundaries are detected based on local maxima (S) in the spectrum and sort them in decreasing order. Let us assume S maxima are found: if $S \geq n$: these are enough maxima to define the wanted number of segments on the spectrum, then keep only the first $(n - 1)$ maxima. $S < n$: the signal has fewer modes than expected, keeps all the maxima values, and reset n to the appropriate value. In this work, $n = 2$ is considered as optimum value for the EWT, so $(n - 1)$ boundaries are located on the spectrum. Based on the preliminary information about the signal, two modes are estimated for ECG, even though the coarse histogram segmentation method is also useful with no prior information about the signal [30]. As shown in Fig. 3, two different modes, $mode_1$ and $mode_2$, are detected from each beat [31]. From the frequency spectrum and multiple experiments, it is observed that $mode_2$ alone can exactly reproduce the original signal without noise, as shown in Fig. 3. From the frequency spectrum, it is observed that $mode_1$ range is from 0 to 0.7 Hz, which is exactly similar to BW noise. Hence, $mode_1$ component is removed from the reconstruction of the original signal. The final dataset is prepared with the noise-free beats processed through EWT. The detailed information of the database used in this work is shown in Table 4.

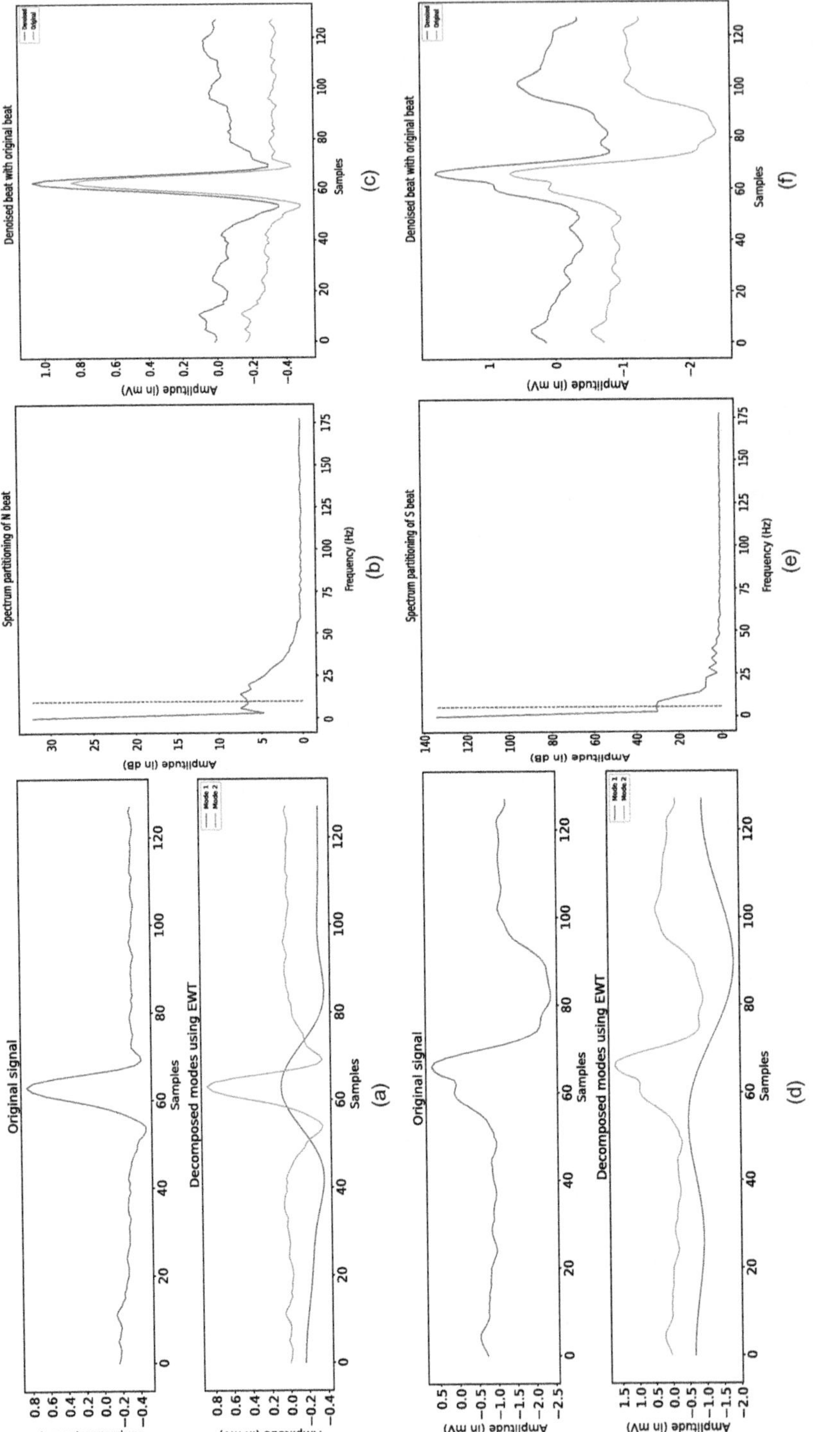

Fig. 3 N, S beat and its corresponding EWT modes, spectrum partition, and de-noised beat with the original beat for ECG record number #124 is represented as an example, from (A) to (F), respectively.

Table 4 Database description.

Dataset description	Common training set from #100 ECG records	First 5 min data from #200 ECG records	Number of testing beats from #200 ECG records
Training set (DS1)	245	8409	
Testing set (DS2)			49,371

4.2 Metrics utilized to assess the performance of the EWT-based deep learning technique

Different statistical parameters are used in this work to estimate the performance of the proposed algorithm. Mainly accuracy (*Acc*), sensitivity (*Sen*), Specificity (*Spe*), and positive predictivity (*Ppr*) are used [32]. These metrics are calculated with the help of a confusion matrix. The confusion matrix plays an important role in the field of machine and deep learning. It is also known as the error matrix. This table helps visualize the correctly classified instances among the total applied instances to the algorithm. Confusion matrix provides information about true positive (TP), true negative (TP), false positive (FP), and false negative (FN). The four metrics of the proposed deep learning technique can be evaluated as

$$Acc = \frac{TP + TN}{TP + TN + FP + FN} \tag{6}$$

$$Sen = \frac{TP}{TP + FN} \tag{7}$$

$$Spe = \frac{TN}{TN + FP} \tag{8}$$

$$Ppr = \frac{TP}{TP + FP} \tag{9}$$

In addition to these four parameters, *F*-score is also calculated, which provides the harmonic mean of *Ppr* ([or] precision (*Pre*)) and Sen. *F*-score is also called as F_1 score.

$$F-score = \frac{TP}{TP + \dfrac{(FP + FN)}{2}} \tag{10}$$

4.3 Parameters optimization of the deep learning-based model

The performance of any deep learning algorithm depends upon the optimization of its parameters. Learning rate (η), batch size (B), and the number of epochs (E) are the important parameters for better performance in classification. Several times experiments are carried out to streamline these parameters. Initially, E and η parameters are varied by keeping the batch size constant. The network Acc is observed from the above experimentation, and it is noticed that at $\eta = 0.01$, the network provides the best performance. The detailed tuning of the parameters is shown in Tables 5 and 6.

Subsequently, B and E parameters are varied as shown in Table 6, by keeping η as constant. From the experimentation, it is observed that for $B = 32$, it provides better performance. The selection of the rate of learning is a vital parameter that optimizes the efficiency of the model. The accuracy of the model is enhanced with an appropriate learning rate. High learning rates are not suitable for all the models. Low level of learning can improve the accuracy of categorization more than higher levels of learning. Still, the time needed to improve accuracy for low learning rates is more than high learning rates. We have experimented with a small range of learning rates in this investigation. From these two experiments, the final optimized parameters of the network are decided as $\eta = 0.01$, $E = 100$, and $B = 32$.

4.4 Performance of the proposed EWT-based deep learning classifier

The proposed automatic ECG beat classification system is trained with the common training data and patient-specific data (#200 ECG records). Hence, the network is tested with the #200

Table 5 Selection of learning rate for the proposed deep learning technique.

E	η	B	Acc (in %)
25	0.1	16	93.25
50	0.05	16	96.75
75	0.02	16	97.25
100	0.01	16	98.36

Table 6 Selection of batch size for the proposed deep learning technique.

E	η	B	Acc (in %)
25	0.01	4	94.95
50	0.01	8	97.27
75	0.01	16	98.38
100	0.01	32	99.75

ECG records data. The proposed automatic ECG beat classification system is trained with the common training data and patient-specific data (#200 ECG records). The total number of training beats is 8654. From this, around 20% (1730 ECG beats) of the data are used for cross-validation. After proper training cum validation, the network is tested with 49,371 ECG beats. The detailed confusion matrix of the proposed deep learning-based technique is shown in Fig. 4. Only 120 instances are misclassified by the classifier. The performance metrics of the proposed method are shown in Table 7. The overall Acc of the proposed method is 99.75%. The proposed method provides an average Acc of 99.68%, Sen of 97.42%, Spe of 99.4%, and Ppr of

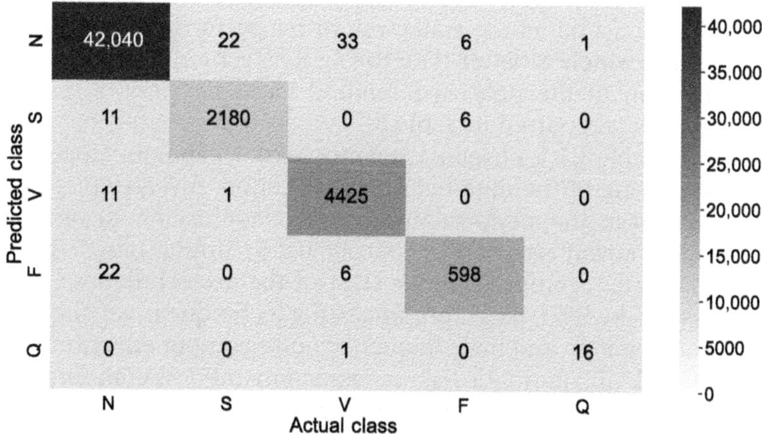

Fig. 4 Confusion matrix of the proposed methodology for ECG beat classification.

Table 7 Performance metrics of the proposed technique.

Class	Acc	Sen	Spe	Ppr	F1 score
N	0.997	0.995	0.997	0.992	0.98
S	0.998	0.986	0.992	0.998	0.99
V	0.998	0.989	0.995	0.998	0.99
F	0.998	0.978	0.992	0.994	0.95
Q	0.993	0.923	0.994	0.879	0.96

97.22%. F-score is a measure of the test's accuracy, and the proposed method shows an average of 0.974.

The deep learning model reached a constant state after 80 epochs during training, and while testing, the deep learning model took 0.12 s for classification. With the above metrics, it can be inferred that the proposed method for ECG beat classification outperforms than state-of-the-art techniques.

4.5 Performance comparison of the proposed EWT-based deep learning technique with state-of-the-art techniques

In this section, the proposed automatic ECG beat classification system performance is compared with the existing techniques in the literature. The proposed method effectively identifies applied ECG beats in a patient-specific way with a performance accuracy of 99.75%, which is better than the earlier techniques. A detailed comparison of the proposed method with the state-of-the-art techniques is reported in Table 8.

From Table 8, it is observed that most of the techniques followed preprocessing of the data before classification. Always noise-free data increase the performance of the classification algorithm. The major advantages of the proposed deep learning-based classification system compared to the state-of-the-art techniques are as follows: (i) the EWT-based preprocessing technique is very helpful in removing low- and high-frequency noise components from the ECG signal, (ii) automatic feature extraction, (iii) less computation time for the prediction, (iv) model complexity is very less, and (v) high accuracy of detection in S and V beats.

Table 8 Performance comparison of the proposed method with existing techniques.

S. no.	Literature work	Database used in the work	Technique used in preprocessing	Feature extraction	Classifier	Performance (in %)
1	Kiranyaz et al. [5]	MIT-BIH	FFT	No	1D CNN	95.58
2	Wang et al. [33]	MIT-BIH	Balance the number of beats after splitting the testing sets	No	Residual network (ResNet)	98.64
3	Dias et al. [34]	MIT-BIH	Basic filtering	RR intervals morphological high-order statistics	Linear discriminant	92.30
4	Asgharzadeh-Bonab et al. [35]	MIT-BIH	Basic filtering	No	Deep CNN	98.34
5	Proposed method	MIT-BIH	EWT	No	Three 1D CNN serial blocks	99.75

5. Conclusions

In this work, EWT-based deep learning technique is proposed to classify five types of ECG beats named N, S, V, F, and Q. The proposed automatic beat classification system has two important stages: preprocessing and classification. The proposed method can denoise and detect ECG beats effectively in the preprocessing and classification stages. The EWT successfully decomposes the ECG signal, and it can separate noisy components from the ECG signal. The proposed customized CNN can extract in-depth features automatically. The findings obtained with the MIT-BIH database in this work show better performance compared with other state-of-the-art techniques. The proposed EWT-based deep learning technique exhibits high accuracy in the classification of multiple arrhythmias. Especially, this method accurately classifies S and V beats, which clinically have high importance in finding heart conditions. Results further prove that a high-quality-aware ECG analysis system is essential to ensure the accuracy and reliability of diagnosing different arrhythmias under noisy

ECG recording conditions. The proposed EWT-based beat classification system can be also deployed for mobile-based health monitoring systems.

References

[1] A. Jaya Prakash, S. Ari, SpEC: a system for patient specific ECG beat classification using deep residual network, Biocybern. Biomed. Eng. 40 (4) (2020) 1446–1457.

[2] P. De Chazal, R.B. Reilly, A patient-adapting heartbeat classifier using ECG morphology and heartbeat interval features, IEEE Trans. Biomed. Eng. 53 (12) (2006) 2535–2543.

[3] G.B. Moody, R.G. Mark, The impact of the MIT-BIH arrhythmia database, IEEE Eng. Med. Biol. Mag. 20 (3) (2001) 45–50.

[4] S.A. Deevi, C.P. Kaniraja, V.D. Mani, D. Mishra, S. Ummar, C. Satheesh, Heart-NetEC: a deep representation learning approach for ECG beat classification, Biomed. Eng. Lett. 11 (1) (2021) 69–84.

[5] S. Kiranyaz, T. Ince, M. Gabbouj, Real-time patient-specific ECG classification by 1-D convolutional neural networks, IEEE Trans. Biomed. Eng. 63 (3) (2015) 664–675.

[6] G. Sannino, G. De Pietro, A deep learning approach for ECG-based heartbeat classification for arrhythmia detection, Futur. Gener. Comput. Syst. 86 (2018) 446–455.

[7] S. Saadatnejad, M. Oveisi, M. Hashemi, LSTM-based ECG classification for continuous monitoring on personal wearable devices, IEEE J. Biomed. Health Inf. 24 (2) (2020) 515–523, https://doi.org/10.1109/JBHI.2019.2911367.

[8] S. Sahoo, M. Dash, S. Behera, S. Sabut, Machine learning approach to detect cardiac arrhythmias in ECG signals: a survey, IRBM 41 (4) (2020) 185–194.

[9] X. Liu, H. Wang, Z. Li, L. Qin, Deep learning in ECG diagnosis: a review, Knowl. Based Syst. 227 (2021) 107187.

[10] S.S. Xu, M.-W. Mak, C.-C. Cheung, Towards end-to-end ECG classification with raw signal extraction and deep neural networks, IEEE J. Biomed. Health Inf. 23 (4) (2019) 1574–1584, https://doi.org/10.1109/JBHI.2018.2871510.

[11] P. Xie, G. Wang, C. Zhang, M. Chen, H. Yang, T. Lv, Z. Sang, P. Zhang, Bidirectional recurrent neural network and convolutional neural network (BiRCNN) for ECG beat classification, in: 2018 40th Annual International Conference of the IEEE Engineering in Medicine and Biology Society (EMBC), 2018, pp. 2555–2558, https://doi.org/10.1109/EMBC.2018.8512752.

[12] T.J. Jun, H.M. Nguyen, D. Kang, D. Kim, D. Kim, Y. Kim, ECG arrhythmia classification using a 2-D convolutional neural network, CoRR (2018). http://arxiv.org/abs/1804.06812.

[13] S. Nurmaini, R. Umi Partan, W. Caesarendra, T. Dewi, M. Naufal Rahmatullah, A. Darmawahyuni, V. Bhayyu, F. Firdaus, An automated ECG beat classification system using deep neural networks with an unsupervised feature extraction technique, Appl. Sci. 9 (14) (2019), https://doi.org/10.3390/app9142921.

[14] T. Wang, C. Lu, Y. Sun, M. Yang, C. Liu, C. Ou, Automatic ECG classification using continuous wavelet transform and convolutional neural network, Entropy 23 (1) (2021), https://doi.org/10.3390/e23010119.

[15] G. Petmezas, K. Haris, L. Stefanopoulos, V. Kilintzis, A. Tzavelis, J.A. Rogers, A.K. Katsaggelos, N. Maglaveras, Automated atrial fibrillation detection using a hybrid CNN-LSTM network on imbalanced ECG datasets, Biomed. Signal Process. Control 63 (2021) 102194.

[16] C. Wen, M.-F. Yeh, K.-C. Chang, ECG beat classification using GreyART network, IET Signal Process. 1 (1) (2007) 19–28.

[17] J.T. Springenberg, A. Dosovitskiy, T. Brox, M. Riedmiller, Striving for simplicity: the all convolutional net, arXiv Preprint arXiv:1412.6806 (2014) 1–14, https://doi.org/10.48550/arXiv.1412.6806.

[18] S.L. Oh, E.Y.K. Ng, R. San Tan, U.R. Acharya, Automated diagnosis of arrhythmia using combination of CNN and LSTM techniques with variable length heart beats, Comput. Biol. Med. 102 (2018) 278–287.

[19] J.B. Bidiasà Mougoufan, J.S.A. Eyebe Fouda, M. Tchuente, W. Koepf, Three-class ECG beat classification by ordinal entropies, Biomed. Signal Process. Control 67 (2021) 102506, https://doi.org/10.1016/j.bspc.2021.102506.

[20] D.A. Abdullah, M.H. Akpınar, A. Şengür, Local feature descriptors based ECG beat classification, Health Inf. Sci. Syst. 8 (1) (2020) 1–10.

[21] S. Sahoo, M. Mohanty, S. Sabut, Automated ECG beat classification using DWT and Hilbert transform-based PCA-SVM classifier, Int. J. Biomed. Eng. Technol. 32 (3) (2020) 287–303.

[22] N. Kar, B. Sahu, S. Sabut, S. Sahoo, Effective ECG beat classification and decision support system using dual-tree complex wavelet transform, in: Advances in Intelligent Computing and Communication, Springer, 2020, pp. 366–374.

[23] L. Yang, J. Zhu, T. Yan, Z. Wang, S. Wu, A modified convolutional neural network for ECG beat classification, J. Med. Imaging Health Inf. 10 (3) (2020) 654–660.

[24] G. Van Steenkiste, G. van Loon, G. Crevecoeur, Transfer learning in ECG classification from human to horse using a novel parallel neural network architecture, Sci. Rep. 10 (1) (2020) 1–12.

[25] J. Pan, W.J. Tompkins, A real-time QRS detection algorithm, IEEE Trans. Biomed. Eng. BME-32 (3) (1985) 230–236, https://doi.org/10.1109/TBME.1985.325532.

[26] J. Gilles, Empirical wavelet transform, IEEE Trans. Signal Process. 61 (16) (2013) 3999–4010.

[27] N.E. Huang, Z. Shen, S.R. Long, M.C. Wu, H.H. Shih, Q. Zheng, N.-C. Yen, C.C. Tung, H.H. Liu, The empirical mode decomposition and the Hilbert spectrum for nonlinear and non-stationary time series analysis, Proc. R. Soc. Lond. A Math. Phys. Eng. Sci. 454 (1971) (1998) 903–995.

[28] M.E. Torres, M.A. Colominas, G. Schlotthauer, P. Flandrin, A complete ensemble empirical mode decomposition with adaptive noise, in: 2011 IEEE International Conference on Acoustics, Speech and Signal Processing (ICASSP), IEEE, 2011, pp. 4144–4147.

[29] A. Nannavecchia, F. Girardi, P.R. Fina, M. Scalera, G. Dimauro, Personal heart health monitoring based on 1D convolutional neural network, J. Imaging 7 (2) (2021) 26.

[30] V.S. Geetikaverma, Empirical wavelet transform & its comparison with empirical mode decomposition: a review, Int. J. Appl. Eng. 4 (15) (2016) 1–5.

[31] O. Singh, R.K. Sunkaria, ECG signal denoising via empirical wavelet transform, Australas. Phys. Eng. Sci. Med. 40 (1) (2017) 219–229.

[32] U. Satija, B. Ramkumar, M.S. Manikandan, A new automated signal quality-aware ECG beat classification method for unsupervised ECG diagnosis environments, IEEE Sensors J. 19 (1) (2019) 277–286, https://doi.org/10.1109/JSEN.2018.2877055.

[33] J. Wang, X. Qiao, C. Liu, X. Wang, Y. Liu, L. Yao, H. Zhang, Automated ECG classification using a non-local convolutional block attention module, Comput. Methods Programs Biomed. 203 (2021) 106006, https://doi.org/10.1016/j.cmpb.2021.106006.

[34] F.M. Dias, H.L. Monteiro, T.W. Cabral, R. Naji, M. Kuehni, E.J.d.a.S. Luz, Arrhythmia classification from single-lead ECG signals using the inter-patient paradigm, Comput. Methods Programs Biomed. 202 (2021) 105948, https://doi.org/10.1016/j.cmpb.2021.105948.
[35] A. Asgharzadeh-Bonab, M.C. Amirani, A. Mehri, Spectral entropy and deep convolutional neural network for ECG beat classification, Biocybern. Biomed. Eng. 40 (2) (2020) 691–700.

6

Development of an internet of things (IoT)-based pill monitoring device for geriatric patients

Deepak K. Sahu[a], Bikash K. Pradhan[a], Slawomir Wilczynski[b], Arfat Anis[c], and Kunal Pal[a]

[a]*Department of Biotechnology and Medical Engineering, National Institute of Technology, Rourkela, India.* [b]*Department of Basic Biomedical Sciences, Medical University of Silesia, Katowice, Poland.* [c]*Department of Chemical Engineering, King Saud University, Riyadh, Saudi Arabia*

1. Introduction

In the last decades, there is an unexpected increase in the life expectancy of people. It has led to a rise in the population of elderly people. Further, the number of such persons is expected to double in the period between 2019 (703 million) and 2050 (1.5 billion) [1]. With an increase in age, elderly people have to deal with multiple health issues, including various age-related chronic comorbidities such as heart diseases, cancer, respiratory diseases, Alzheimer's disease, and diabetes. Nearly 84% of the elderly population suffers from two or more chronic diseases [2]. An increase in the number of patients has burdened the healthcare sector. A critical issue in managing the health of elderly patients is to provide proper and timely medication. With an increase in the number of diseases, the pill intake of the average elderly person increases. The phenomenon of advising multiple drugs to the patients is regarded as polypharmacy. Polypharmacy increases the nonadherence to medication intake [3–5]. It may trigger a reduction in the effectiveness of treatment, increased healthcare expenditure, and increased risks of morbidity and mortality [6,7]. Moreover, a gradual weakening of the physical capacity (e.g., vision and muscular) and psychological strength (e.g., logical and cognitive capabilities) makes it challenging for elderly persons to keep track of the pill dosage information [8].

Advanced Methods in Biomedical Signal Processing and Analysis. https://doi.org/10.1016/B978-0-323-85955-4.00012-0
Copyright © 2023 Elsevier Inc. All rights reserved.

Reduced vision makes it difficult to distinguish the pills of similar shape and color. These problems and forgetfulness due to dementia contribute to inappropriate medication dose intake in elderly persons [9]. Hence, there is a need for designing an automated device for monitoring medication adherence.

The rapidly increasing computing devices and the gain in computational power enable automated systems for healthcare monitoring that require less human intervention. These technologies are growing day by day, bringing continuous changes in how healthcare facilities are delivered to patients. Internet of things (IoT) is one such technology that can integrate a device, patients, and healthcare providers into one single platform [10]. An IoT-based health monitoring device mainly consists of three different layers: a perception layer, which is used to collect the healthcare data from other devices and sensors; a network layer that is used to transmit the input gathered from the perception layer; and the application layer that integrates the input information from the measuring device to provide medical services [11]. The most efficient example of IoT in medication adherence is a smart pillbox or smart pill monitoring system [8]. The smart pillbox provides medication reminders to the patients and helps them to live independently. Thus, eliminating the need for caretakers to remind the medicine dosage schedule. In recent years, many technological advancements have been incorporated into the design and application of smart pillboxes [12,13]. Commercially available smart boxes are Tricella, Pilldrill, Medofoliopillbox, E-pill-Multiplus, and E-pill-Medsmartplus [14]. These devices are being used to aid in pill intake by reminding the patients to take pills using audible and visual signals [14]. Some of these smart pillboxes rely on vision-based technology for pill counting [15,16]. They wirelessly transmit data either to the mobile phone or personal computers. Many of the vision-based systems follow continuous monitoring through video surveillance. These devices track the hand movement in front of the pillbox. It assumes that the patient has taken medicine based on hand movement tracking. Unfortunately, such devices do not ensure that the pill has been taken from the pillbox. Further, since these systems employ video surveillance, the processing of information requires a high computational cost. Many researchers have proposed computationally economical image processing-based medication monitoring systems. These devices read the weight of the medication bottle from the digital weighing machine. But, such systems can only monitor a single medication.

In this study, we propose to develop an image processing-based medication monitoring device. The pill monitoring was achieved by taking pictures of the pills at regular intervals, which reduces the proposed device's computational burden compared to vision-based surveillance methods. The software of the proposed device uses a novel template selection method to extract the color parameter of the pills in the pill tray. It enables the device to choose the correct medication. The device's display panel regularly shows the pill dosage information and promotes self-management of pills by providing reminders through the user's e-mail. This method allows the detection of pills without using expensive sensors. The IoT-based pill monitoring device is user-friendly so that elderly persons staying alone can operate the device independently.

2. Literature review

Medication adherence is resulted due to a decreased capacity in managing the dosage and time of medicine. Nonadherence in medicine and consumption of incorrect medicine may lead to deteriorated health conditions and longer treatment duration. Hence, there is a need for a medication dispenser and reminder system. Numerous studies in the past have reported the design of low-cost and easy-to-use pill monitoring devices. Recent developments in these devices primarily focus on the design, security, interface, technology, and application to specific health conditions. In [17], an intelligent pill dispenser called "MEDIC" was developed for persons who want to maintain their medication routine independently without any close supervision of a caretaker. The designed device provides the caretaker to set the prescribed medicine and the time of medication. Further, the device was incorporated with an alarm system that reminds the patient to take medicine and the caretaker to refill the medication in the pill tray. Sousa et al. (2019) has developed a portable pillbox that was easier to carry with the patient. The device also showed flexibility in adapting to the pharmacological needs of the patients [18]. The main advantage of this portable device was that it could hold capsules/tablets and liquid and powdered medicines. In another study [19], the authors reported a pill dispenser that was constructed using an Arduino IDE. The device used three micro-servo motors that can accommodate three different shapes of medication [19]. When the three motors worked simultaneously, the pill tray could dispense medicines of various sizes with 100% accuracy. Ramkumar et al. [20] have proposed a pill monitoring device with special attention to the proper intake of pills. It has been achieved through human interaction between the patient and the doctor that helps decide the appropriate dosage of the medicine. In [21], the authors designed an electronic pillbox that can dispense medication in a controlled manner with a track on the medication dosage. Herein, three alarming methods have been used: buzzing sound, phone calls, or flashing of light. Kassem et al. (2019) have also used human interaction to help elderly people to take their medicine on time. The device helped the elderly people who were more prone to memory issues and forgetfulness to avoid an accidental overdose and skip the medication [22]. Further, the alarming system notifies the caregiver when there is a missed event. The system also stored the medication record of the patients for the future reference of doctors. In [23], the authors have reported a pill dispenser equipped with mobile applications that alert healthcare professionals during a critical situation.

The last decade has witnessed substantial growth in the application of internet of things (IoT) technology in the development of pill monitoring devices. In [23], real-time AI-IoT technology has been applied for automatic pill dispensing with an effective user interface. Moise et al. (2020) have presented the application of internet of things (IoT) technology in their designed device [24]. Apart from the usual job of a pill dispenser, the device uses a system that can retrieve and store information from several pill distributors in an online database. The system reported, in this case, can be used for individual or administrative purposes. The individual mode of operation was for the persons who want to track if a patient is taking medication either at home or hospital. However, the administrative mode was used to supervise a network of pill dispensing systems. The information from the network could be availed using several microcontrollers. Rajendran et al. (2021) have developed a dispenser system that records the patient's health information (heartbeat and temperature) and medication management. Herein, the sensed data was used to open the pill container [25]. In a similar study [26], the pillbox measures the patient's information (temperature and heartbeat) using a biosensor to avoid any adverse health condition due to overdose. The device also contained six different subpill boxes that helped to organize and manage six types of pills. "SIMoP Box," a smart healthcare system, was developed, especially helpful for patients with mild memory loss. The system used a timer that alerts the patients about the timing and dosage of medication. In addition to the medication, an appropriate amount of water was also provided to the patients using a liquid dispenser. The quality of air inside the patient's room was also maintained using an air-cooling assembly. The use of an internet protocol camera enabled the remote monitoring of the patient from a distant location using a smartphone. Further, the dosage of medication could also be updated using a web application after interacting with the healthcare professionals [27].

Several recent studies have also explored integrated technology where the IoT technology was employed with other state-of-the-art technologies to achieve better performance. In [28], the authors proposed IoT and blockchain-based medication adherence systems that include device configuration, medication adherence data management, and an alarming system. Herein, the authors claimed that the inclusion of these functionality increases the degree of medication adherence of the device. Chavez et al. (2020) has also proposed an integrated architecture employing IoT and wireless sensor network for a smart pill dispenser system [29]. In [30], mobile technology has been used to add automatic operation in the pill dispenser to benefit elderly sick people from expensive in-home medical care. Mohammad et al. (2018) have used a cloud-based smart application to provide two-way communication in feedback between older patients and doctors to monitor medication adherence [31]. Some studies have also given particular importance to the security of the information of the patients. In [32], the communication between the user and the healthcare provider starts with a unique barcode, which could be later used in the nearest pill dispenser to procure the prescribed medicines. In another study [33], the dispenser system delivered the medication only at the scheduled time and after the authorized person was identified using facial recognition. However, the use of such advanced technology requires high computational costs and further increases the cost.

Despite the advancement in the field of pill dispensers, it is still far away from the reach of common people. Again, most of the studies as mentioned earlier, are limited to only research work without any commercialization. The two most typical issues for the unpopularity are cost and the ability to choose the correct medication. While many other technologies have been integrated with IoT, a few applications of image processing technology are found. The reason may be due to its associated issues, including higher data storage and computational cost. Hence, in the current study, a novel template selection method has been employed that uses the color parameter from the medicine to dispense and select the correct medication.

3. Materials and methods

3.1 Materials and softwares

Raspberry Pi 3 (Model B, 1.2 GHz, 1 GB RAM, Raspberry Pi Foundation, United Kingdom), LCD display (dimension: 7 in., resolution: 800 × 480, Waveshare Electronics, China), CMOS camera (Pi camera: 5 MP, 2592 × 1944 resolution, Raspberry Pi Foundation, United Kingdom), LM2596 buck converter (input voltage: 4.2–40 V, output voltage: 1.25–37 V), DS3231 real-time clock (frequency: 32.768 kHz), IN4007 diode (forward current: 1 A, power dissipation: 3 W), BC547 transistor (type: NPN), resistors (10 Ω, 1.5 KΩ), 1 KΩ potentiometers, LEDs (power: 1 W, color: pure-white), relay module (12 V DC), power adapter (12 V, 2A), memory card (type: MicroSDHC, size: 32 GB, SanDisk), and sandpaper sheet (grit size: 400, material: Silicon Carbide) were obtained from the local market. Raspbian Operating System (type: Linux, Debian version: 10) was installed in the memory card that was instilled in the Raspberry Pi for the functioning of the Raspberry Pi. Python programming language (version: 3.7, Python Software Foundation) was used for developing the software of the device, EAGLE PCB designing software (version: 9.5.1, Autodesk, USA) was used to design the circuit, and SolidWorks CAD software (version: 2016, Dassault Systèmes, USA) was used to design the model of the device.

3.2 Methods

3.2.1 Designing the medication monitoring system

The proposed monitoring system consisted of two components, namely, the hardware component and the software component. The hardware component consisted of an imaging system (ImS) coupled with the portable processing system (PCP; Raspberry Pi) integrated with the proposed device's casing. The software component was developed using Python programming language to acquire images from the ImS and do the computation to compute the number of pills at definite time intervals.

Designing the hardware component

The ImS consisted of an IS that allowed the user to properly illuminate the scene (in this case, the pill tray). For this purpose, a panel of three white LEDs was developed. A diffuser was attached to the LED panel. Also, a current-limiting resistor (10 Ω) and a potentiometer (10 KΩ) were connected with the LED panel. This arrangement allowed controlling the brightness of the LEDs by adjusting the rider of the potentiometer (Fig. 1). The circuit was powered using a 12 V DC power supply. Further, a relay-based switching system was introduced to power on the LEDs when the ImS captured the image. The PCP controlled the relay through the GPIO terminal. The terminal ensures that the LED glows 100 ms before the capturing of the image. A printed circuit board (PCB) for the IS was developed using the layout given in Fig. 1. The IS was used in conjunction with the ImS connected with the PCP to capture the images of the pills. The *Camera Serial Interface* Type 2 (CSI-2) protocol was used to facilitate the connection of the IS to the PCP. The proposed device consisted of three parts, namely, casing, lighting box, and pill tray. The casing provides a base to place the LCD screen in a stable position. The IS and the ImS were recognized on the top of the lighting box. The pills to be monitored by the device were kept in the pill tray. The pill tray has four compartments, which allow the device to monitor four different pills simultaneously. The sliding mechanism allows the pill tray to slide parallel to the lower edge of the lighting box. The virtual 3D model of the individual components and the entire device was conceived and designed using SolidWorks software (Fig. 2). The schematic representation of the proposed device has been shown in Fig. 3.

Development of the software for medication monitoring

A graphical user interface (GUI) based software was developed using Python programming language (Fig. 4). The initiation of the software pops up in the main window. The main window allows the user to select the number of medications to be monitored by the device. After selecting the number of medications (Fig. 5A–D), a second window was opened (Fig. 5A1–D1). The dose information was to be entered in the second window. In the first window, the lower section was further vertically divided into two subsections. The top subsection (Choose the number of pills to monitor) allows the user to select either one, two, three, or four pills. The bottom subsection has a pushbutton called "Select." The activation of the "Select" button stores the user-selected choice (i.e., the number of pills to be monitored) in the device memory. In the second window, the lower section was further vertically divided into three subsections. The top subsection (Enter the medication information) allows the user to enter the time interval between two successive pills, the total number of pills and the pills to be taken in each dose. The middle subsection (Enter the user information) allows the user to enter the person's e-mail address to whom an e-mail will be sent whenever the

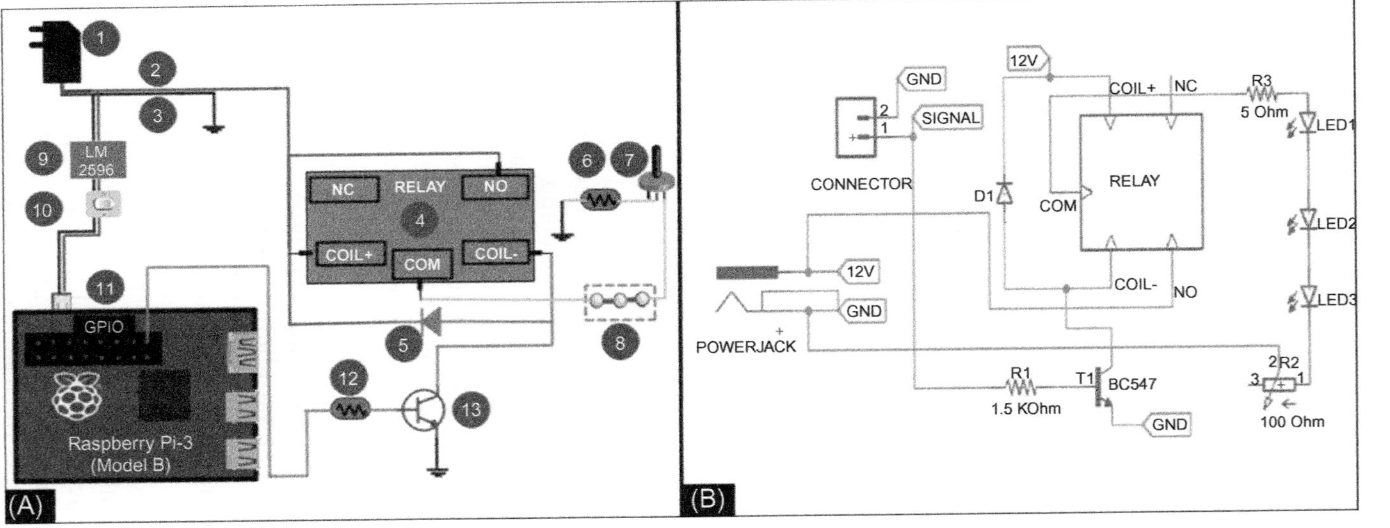

Fig. 1 Interconnectivity of the electronic components of the IS. (A) Schematic diagram and (B) schematic of the PCB developed using Eagle software. NB: (1) 12 VDC power adapter, (2) 12 V power line, (3) ground wire, (4) relay: 12 V, (5) diode: IN4007, (6) resistor: 5 W, (7) 1 KW potentiometer, (8) LED panel, (9) buck converter (LM2596, 12–5 V), (10) single-pole switch, (11) Raspberry Pi (Model 3-B), (12) 1.5 KW resistor, and (13) transistor (BC547-NPN).

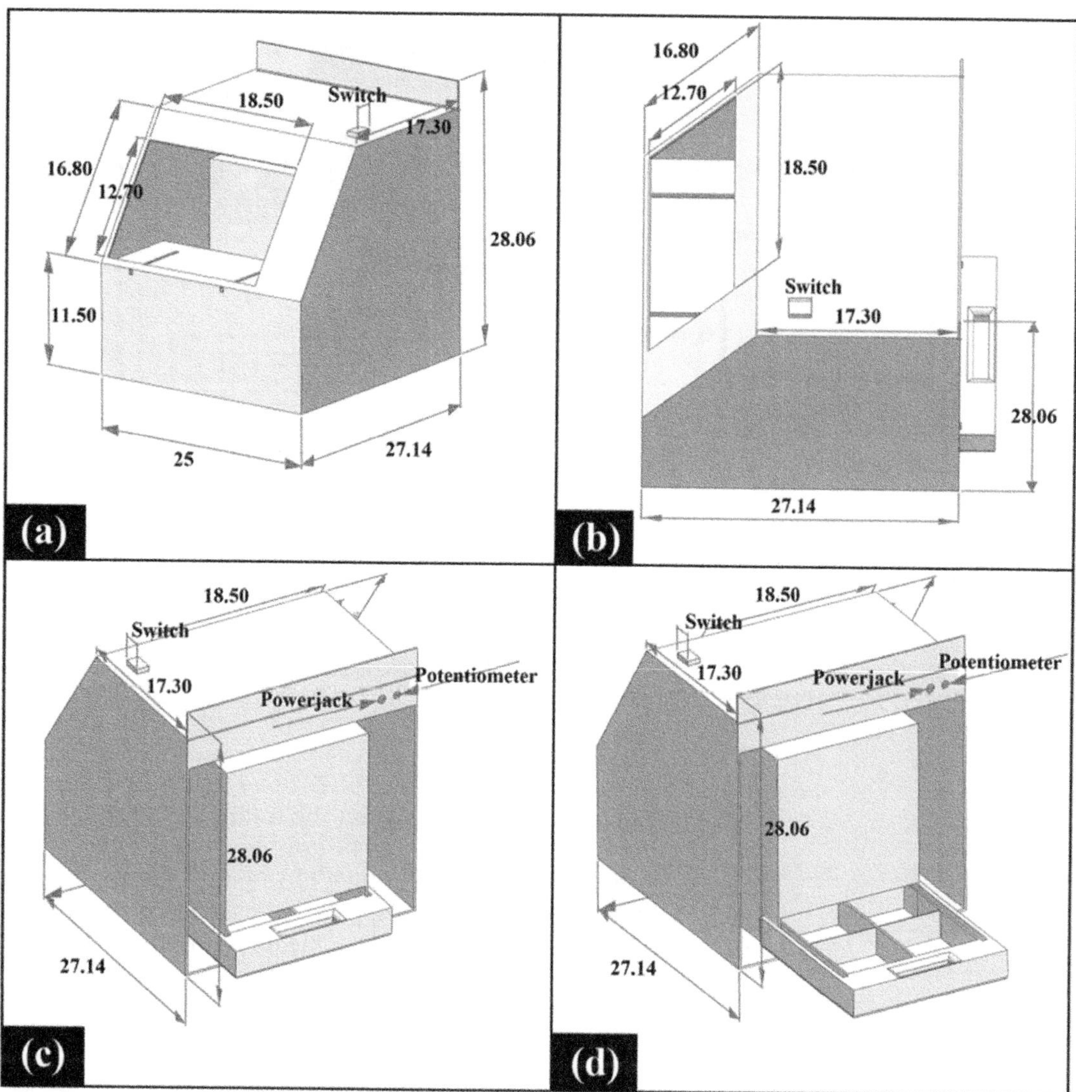

Fig. 2 Schematic diagram of the casing of the proposed device developed using Solidworks software. (A) Trimetric view of the front side, (B) bimetric view of the left side, (C) trimetric view of the backside, and (D) trimetric view of the backside with extended pill tray (all dimensions are in cm).

medication is skipped or there is an improper dose intake. The bottom subsection consisted of three pushbuttons: "Save," "Choose a template," and "Start monitoring." The "Save" button helps to store the user information in the temporary memory. The "Choose a Template" button allows the user to select the

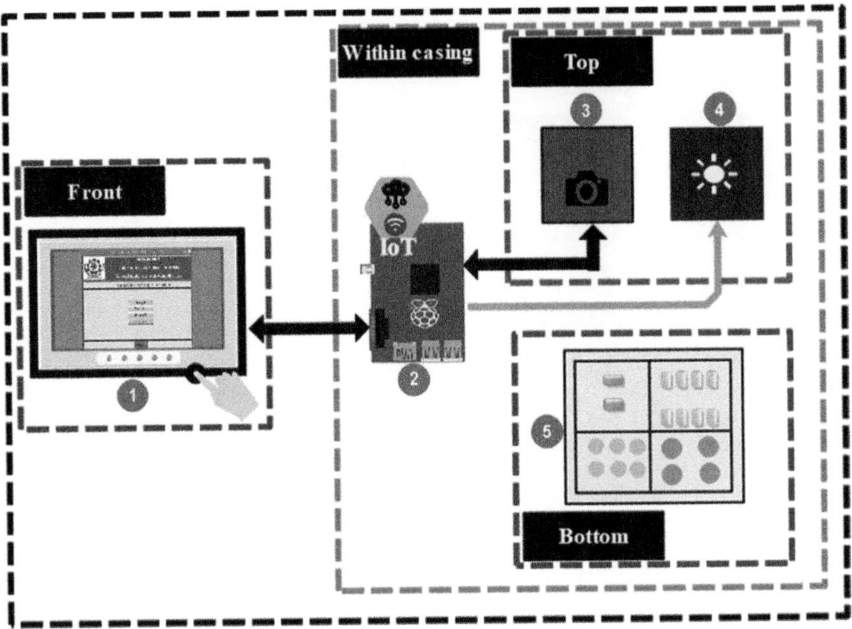

Fig. 3 Schematic diagram of the proposed device. NB: (1) 7-in. Pi touchscreen display to interact with the GUI, (2) Raspberry Pi (Model 3-B), (3) CMOS camera to capture the image of the pills, (4) LED panel to illuminate the pill tray, and (5) pill tray to store the pills.

template image, which helps count the total number of pills present in the device. Clicking this button pops up a window that shows the real-time preview image of the area captured by the CMOS camera. In our case, it displays the real-time preview image of the bottom section of the device. The image of the device's bottom section was captured by pressing the keyboard key "Q." From the captured image, the device's software requires only the image area where the pill tray was present. The software automatically crops the specific area of the pill tray from the image of the scene. The cropped image of the pill tray was further divided into four subimages, corresponding to the four pill compartments, by the software. For each of these subimages, a separate template image is to be created by the user. The template was created by cropping a rectangular region within the pill area of the subimage using the mouse pointer. The software then calculates the average RGB (Red, Green, Blue) color values for each of the four template images. The average RGB values of each template image are then converted into HSV (Hue, Saturation, Value) color values using the color conversion formula (Appendix). The upper and lower limits of the HSV values of every template image were generated by the

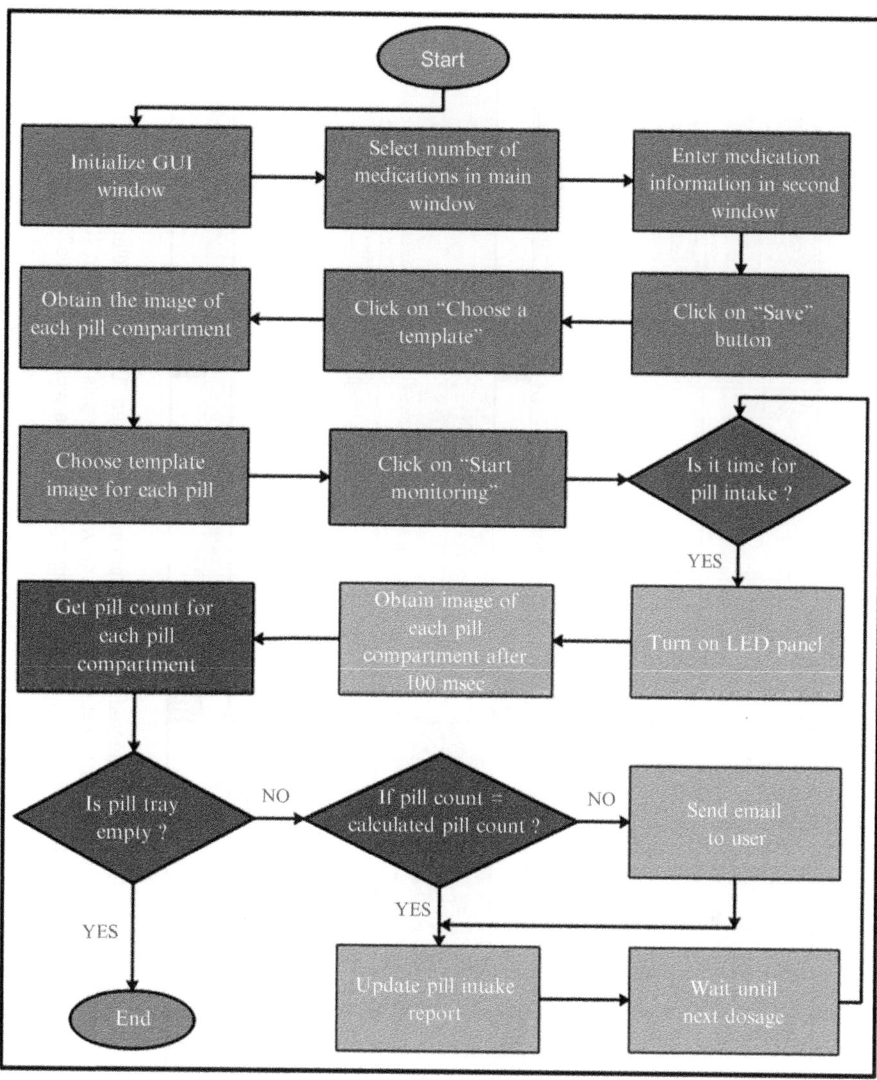

Fig. 4 The process flowchart of the software.

software. For the calculation of the upper and the lower limits of the H-value, a value of 20% of the average H-value was added and subtracted, respectively, from the calculated average H-value of the template. Similarly, for calculating the upper and lower limits of the S- and V-values, a value of 40% of average S- and V-values was added and subtracted, respectively, from the calculated average S- and V-values in the template. The number of pills was calculated before determining the upper and lower limits of the HSV

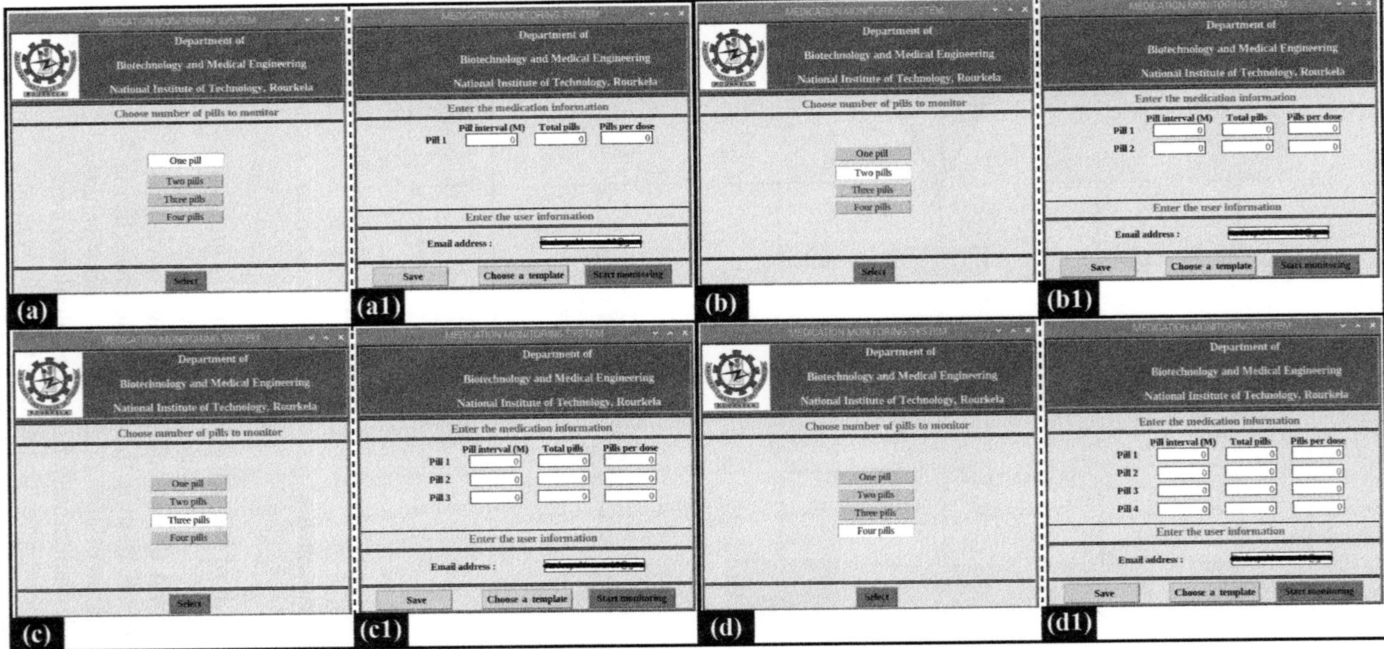

Fig. 5 GUI interface of the software. (A) Interface when "One pill" is selected, (A1) dose input interface when "One pill" is selected, (B) interface when "Two pills" is selected, (B1) dose input interface when "Two pills" is selected, (C) interface when "Three pills" is selected, (C1) dose input interface when "Three pills" is selected, (D) interface when "Four pills" is selected, and (D1) dose input interface when "Four pills" is selected.

values. Counting the pills involved two steps: extracting the color image of the pills and detecting contour and centroid for the extracted pills. Initially, the captured image was blurred (image smoothening) using a Gaussian filter with a kernel size of 5×5. This blurred image was converted to HSV color space. The pixel slicing algorithm without background was applied using the limits that have been previously calculated. This step resulted in the formation of a binary image. The binary image, so obtained, was used as the mask for further processing. On this mask, the morphological opening and closing operations were performed using an elliptical structuring element, having a size of 15×15. After that, the software performed a bit-wise "AND" operation between the mask and captured image to segment the pill area from the background. The segmented image was then converted to a grayscale image. Subsequently, the thresholding operation was performed using a constant value of 60 such that the pixels within the pill area acquired a normalized value of 1. From this normalized binary image, the outer contours were retrieved. The retrieved contours were then subjected to contour approximation. Then, the convex hull operation was performed to determine the smallest polygon that contained all the foreground pixel values. The centroids of each of the foreground areas were determined using image moments. The total number of centroids indicated the total number of pills that are present in the device. The "Start monitoring" button helps to initiate the medication monitoring process of the software. A multithreading-based approach was used in designing the process of continuous medication monitoring. A separate thread, one for each pill compartment, is responsible for parallel medication monitoring of the different pills. Each of these threads runs in the background and waits until the time of the following scheduled medication. At the time of scheduled medication, the threads initiate the process of pill counting and compare the result of the pill counting with the calculated pill count from the user's input. If a mismatch in the pill counts, the software sends an alert message by e-mail address to remind of the missed dose. The process flow chart for pill counting is represented in Fig. 6. The software generates the pill intake report of the user by regularly updating four different files (one for each medication) with information like time of pill intake, actual pill intake, and ideal pill intake. When the pill count reaches zero, i.e., no pills are left in the device, the monitoring process stops automatically. Overall, the software has a front-end process and a back-end process. The front-end process is responsible for taking the user information and acquiring the template image. The back-end process is responsible for determining the pill count and monitoring the medication adherence of the patient.

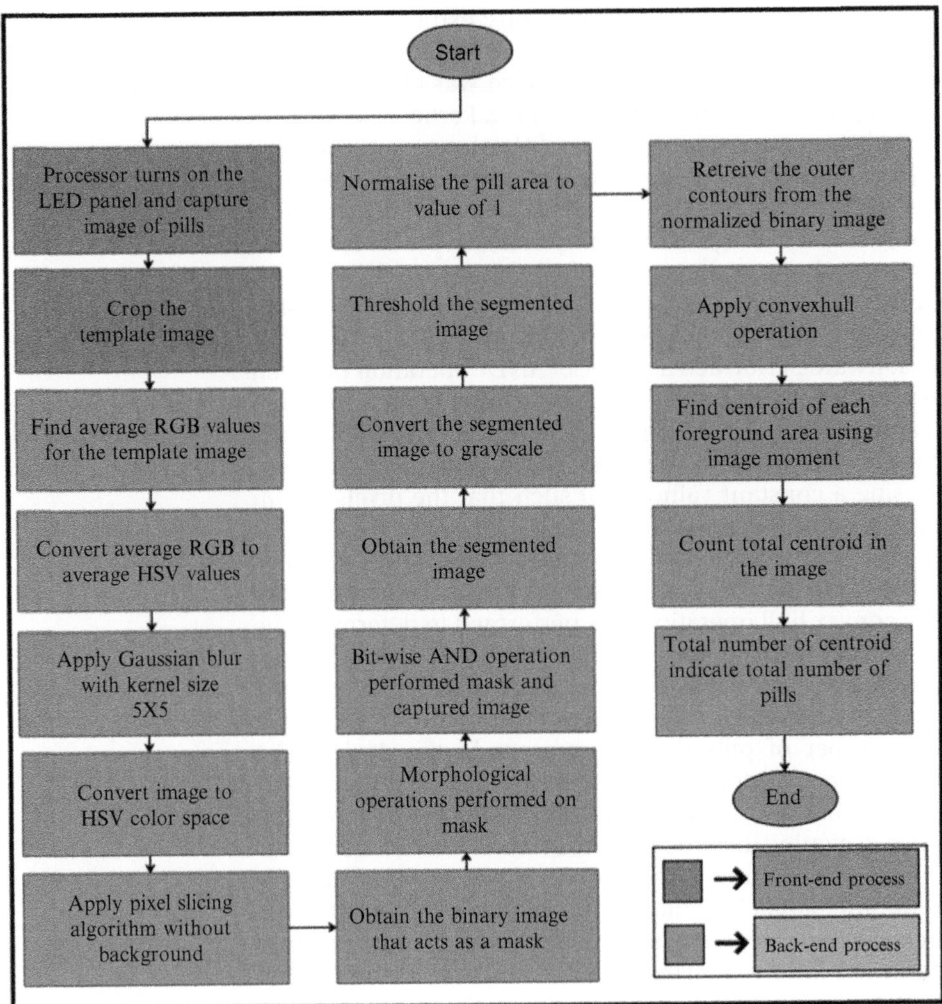

Fig. 6 The process flowchart for pill counting.

4. Results and discussions

4.1 Developing the medication monitoring system

The proposed pill monitoring system is the integration of hardware and software components. Among the hardware components, the IS is used for the proper lighting of the imaging scene. The brightness of the IS could be manipulated using a potentiometer. The PCB layout for the IS was designed in EAGLE software and served as a blueprint for laying out the copper traces

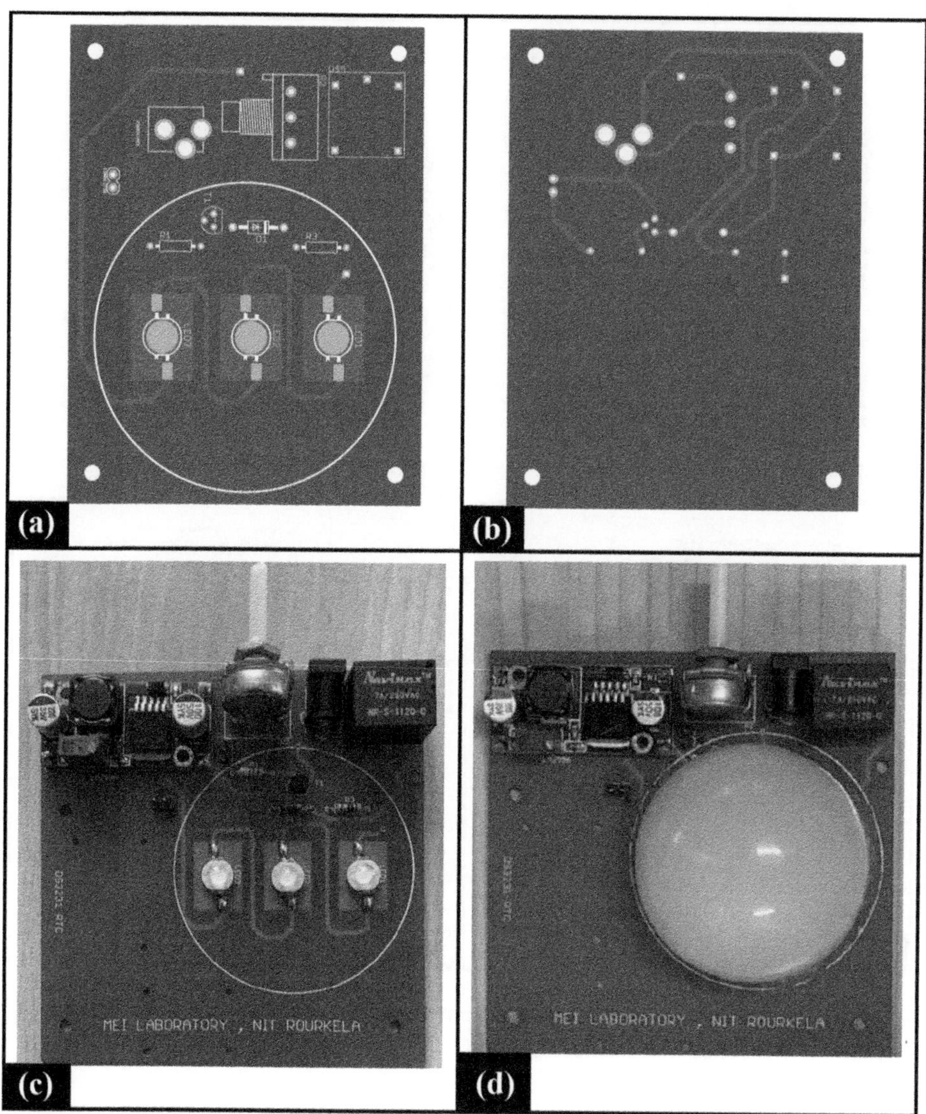

Fig. 7 PCB design of the IS. (A) Top view of the footprint, (B) bottom view of the footprint, (C) PCB with the mounted components, and (D) PCB with the mounted components and the light diffuser.

and placing the components on the PCB. The footprints of components and wiring are shown in Fig. 7A and B. The circuit components were then mounted on the top of the PCB manually (Fig. 7C). Subsequently, a light diffuser was attached to the LEDs (Fig. 7D). The image of the pills kept in the tray is captured using

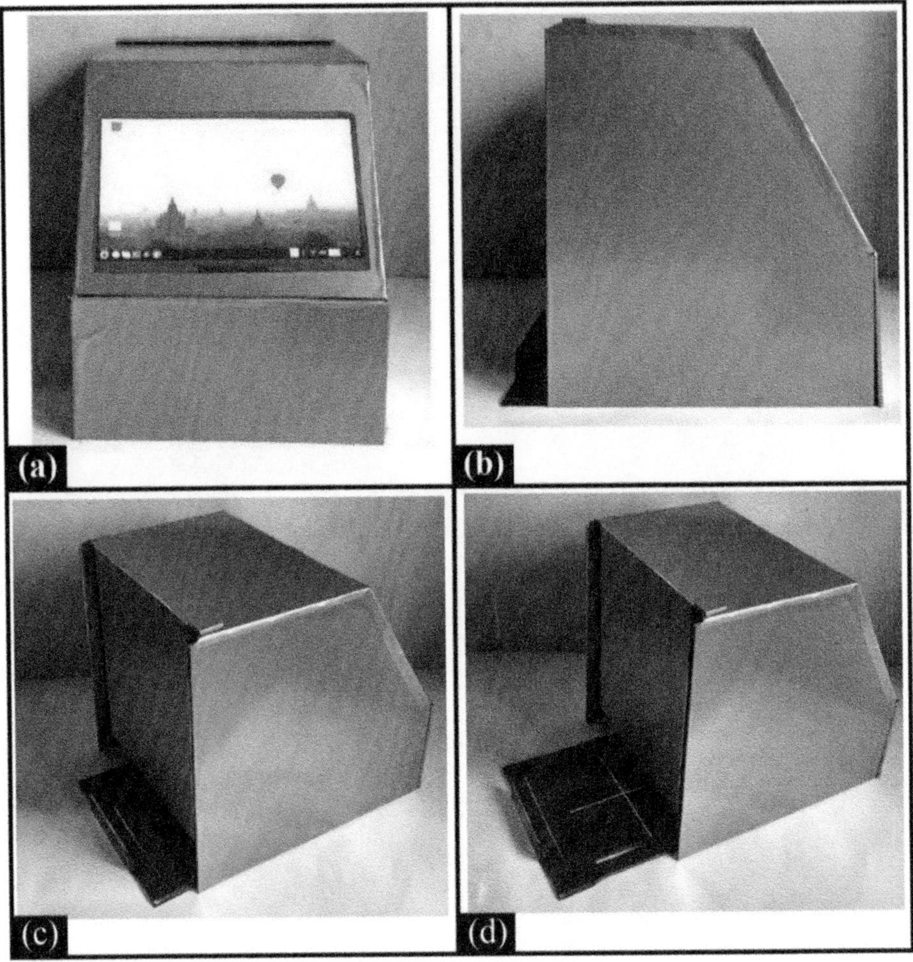

Fig. 8 Pictograph of the proposed device. (A) Front view, (B) side view, (C) trimetric view of the backside, and (D) trimetric view of the backside with extended pill tray.

the IS, controlled by the PCP. The PCP executes the developed software. In our case, the casing of the prototype device was made using a polyvinyl chloride (PVC) sheet as per the specification in the virtual 3D model (Fig. 8). The inner side of the casing was painted black to reduce the stray light on the ImS. The software component acquires the data from the ImS and computes the pill count at a definite time as per the user input to monitor the dosage adherence by the patient.

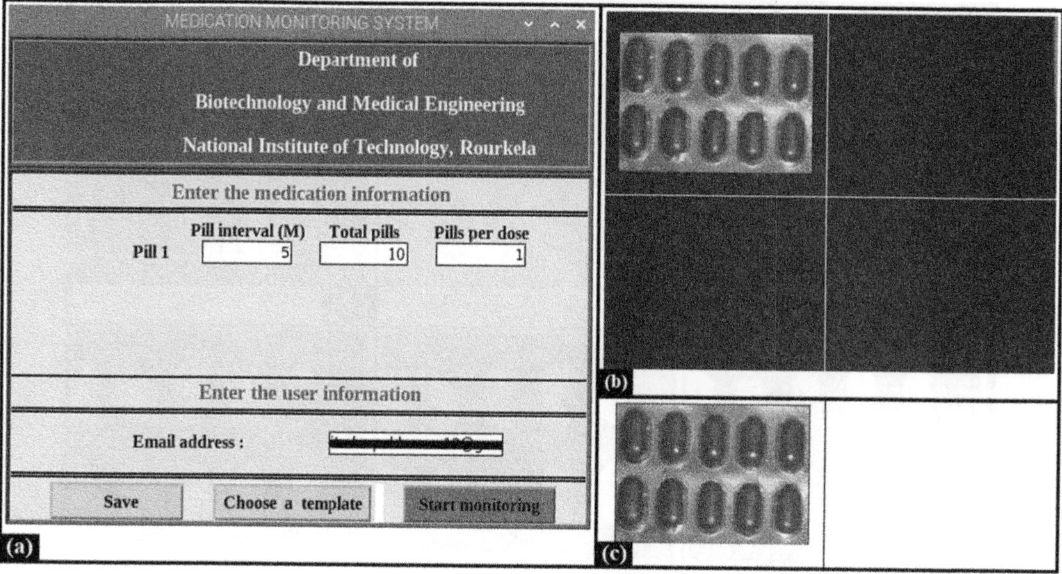

Fig. 9 Testing the medication monitoring system. (A) Dose information input GUI screen, (B) image of the pill tray, and cropping of the pill tray image into one section: (C) pill 1.

4.2 Testing the medication monitoring system

The device was tested by keeping either one, two, three, or four different types of pills in the separate pill compartments of the pill tray. The results for each pill type are presented as supplementary information (one pill: Figs. 9 and 10, two pills: Figs. 11 and 12, three pills: Figs. 13 and 14). Herein, the results with four types of pills are presented. In the main window of the GUI, the "Four pills" option was selected. This process resulted in the opening up of a second window. Thereafter, the corresponding pill dosage information (time interval between two consecutive pills, total pills loaded into pill tray, and pills to be taken per dose) was entered (Fig. 15A). The brightness of the IS of the device was adjusted, and the preview image of the camera was captured. The region of the pill tray was then automatically cropped from the image captured by the camera (Fig. 15B). Four subimages were obtained using the cropped image of the pill tray. Each of the subimages corresponds to one of the pills of the pill tray (Fig. 15C: pill1, Fig. 15D: pill2, Fig. 15E: pill3, Fig. 15F: pill4). The template image for every subimage was selected, and the average color parameters (RGB and HSV values) for the template

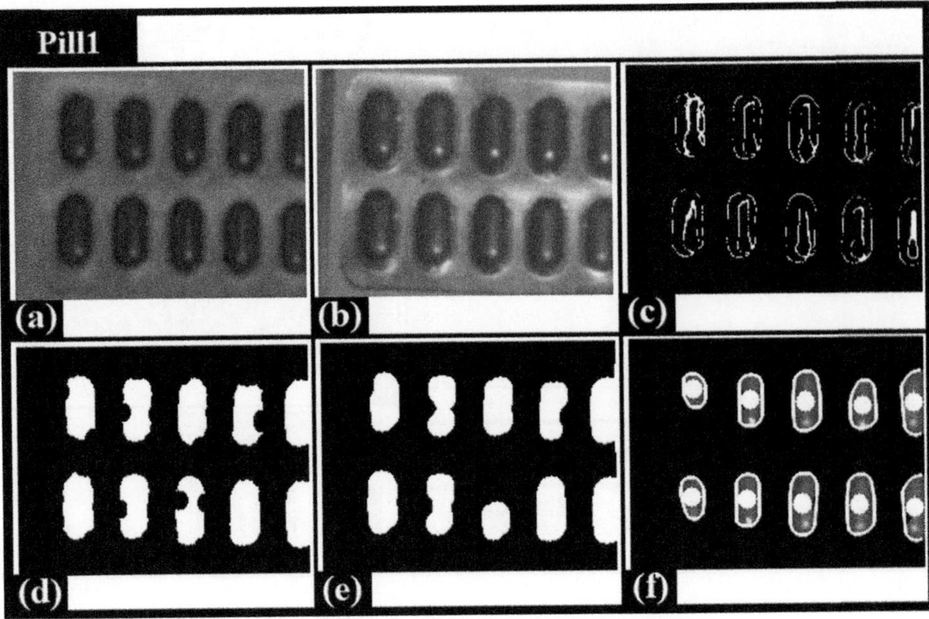

Fig. 10 The output of the image processing algorithm while monitoring one pill. (A) Image in HSV color space, (B) smoothened image, (C) image after performing "pixel slicing without background" within the computed range of HSV values (mask), (D) image obtained after the morphological closing operation on the mask, (E) image obtained after the morphological opening operation on the mask, and (F) pill areas segmented by performing bit-wise AND operation between the mask and original image with the contours and the centroid of the pills highlighted.

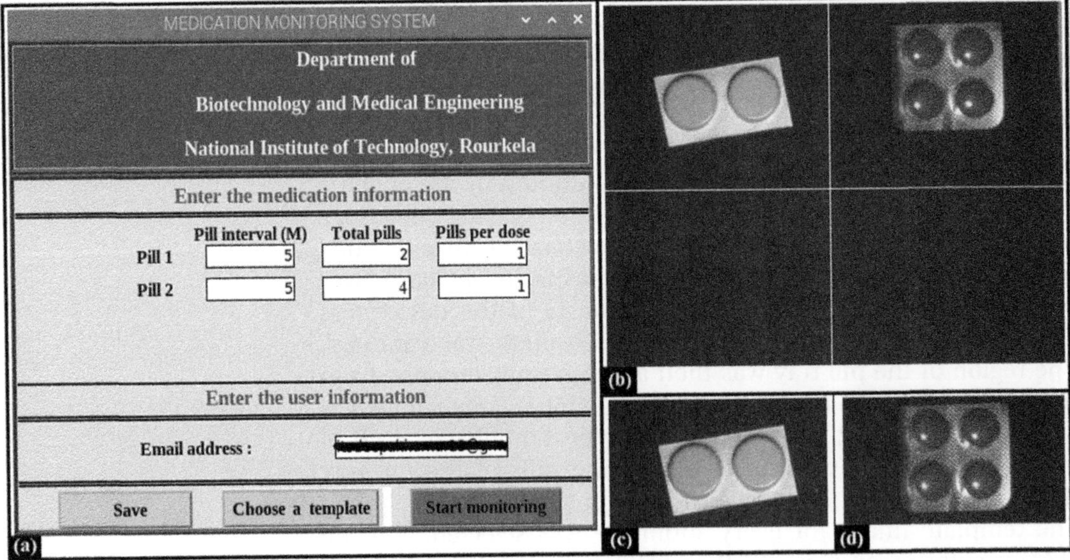

Fig. 11 Testing the medication monitoring system. (A) Dose information input GUI screen, (B) image of the pill tray, and cropping of the pill tray image into two sections: (C) pill 1 and (D) pill 2.

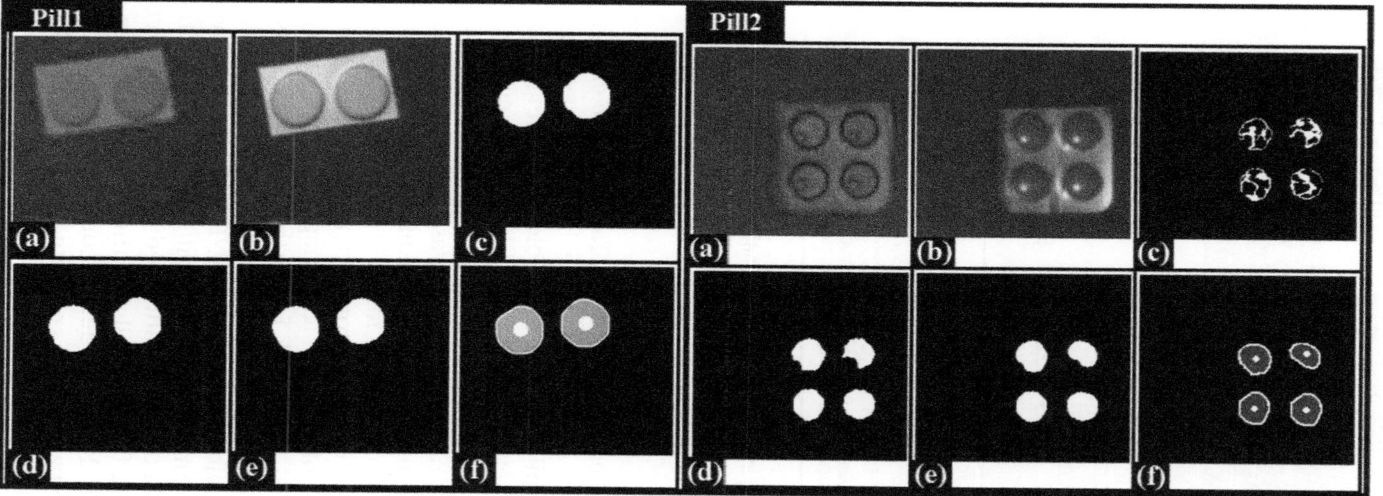

Fig. 12 The output of the image processing algorithm while monitoring two pills. (A) Image in HSV color space, (B) smoothened image, (C) image after performing "pixel slicing without background" within the computed range of HSV values (mask), (D) image obtained after the morphological closing operation on the mask, (E) image obtained after the morphological opening operation on the mask, and (F) pill areas segmented by performing bit-wise AND operation between the mask and original image with the contours and the centroid of the pills highlighted.

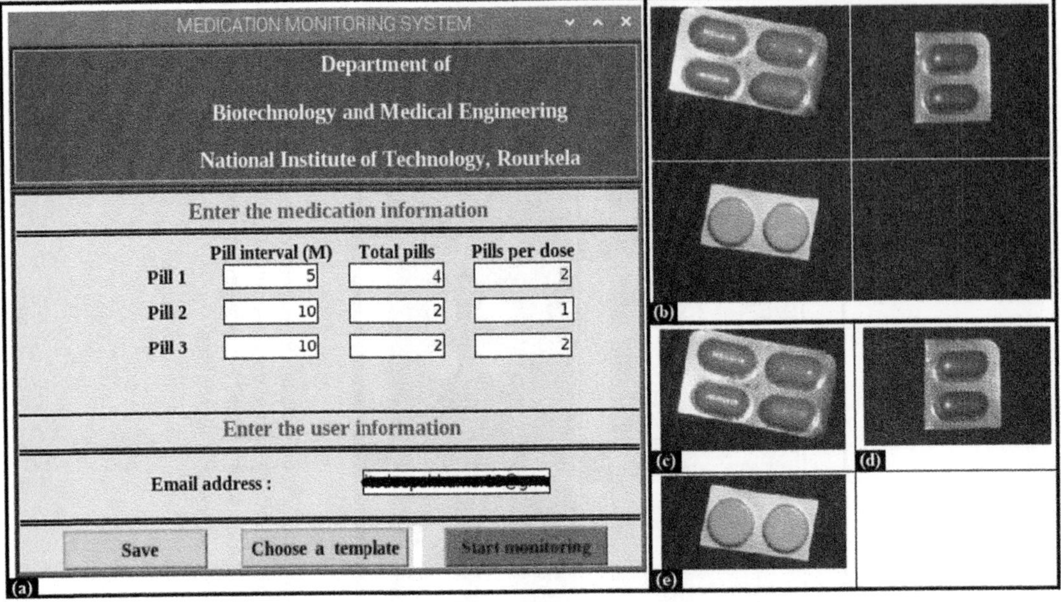

Fig. 13 Testing the medication monitoring system. (A) Dose information input GUI screen, (B) image of the pill tray, and cropping of the pill tray image into three sections: (C) pill 1, (D) pill 2, and (E) pill 3.

images were obtained (Table 1). The captured image was in RGB color space; hence the image processing algorithm converted the pill image to HSV color space (Fig. 16A). The high-frequency content (e.g., noise, edge) was removed from the captured image using the "Gaussian blur" function (Fig. 16B). The pixel region of the pills was extracted by applying the "slicing without background" algorithm (Fig. 16C). In this image, "morphological closing" (Fig. 16D) and "morphological opening" (Fig. 16E) operations, respectively, were performed using a kernel size of 15×15. The image after the morphological operations acted as a mask for further image processing applications. The shape and size of the pills in the RGB image were extracted by performing the bit-wise "AND" operation between the mask and the captured image of the pill. The contours of the pills were retrieved from the image and used to calculate the "convex hull." The centroid for each pill was then obtained using the image moments (Fig. 16F). The device continuously monitored the pill intake of the patient and generated the pill report for each pill (Fig. 17A). In a missed dosage scenario, the device sent an e-mail to the user (Fig. 17B).

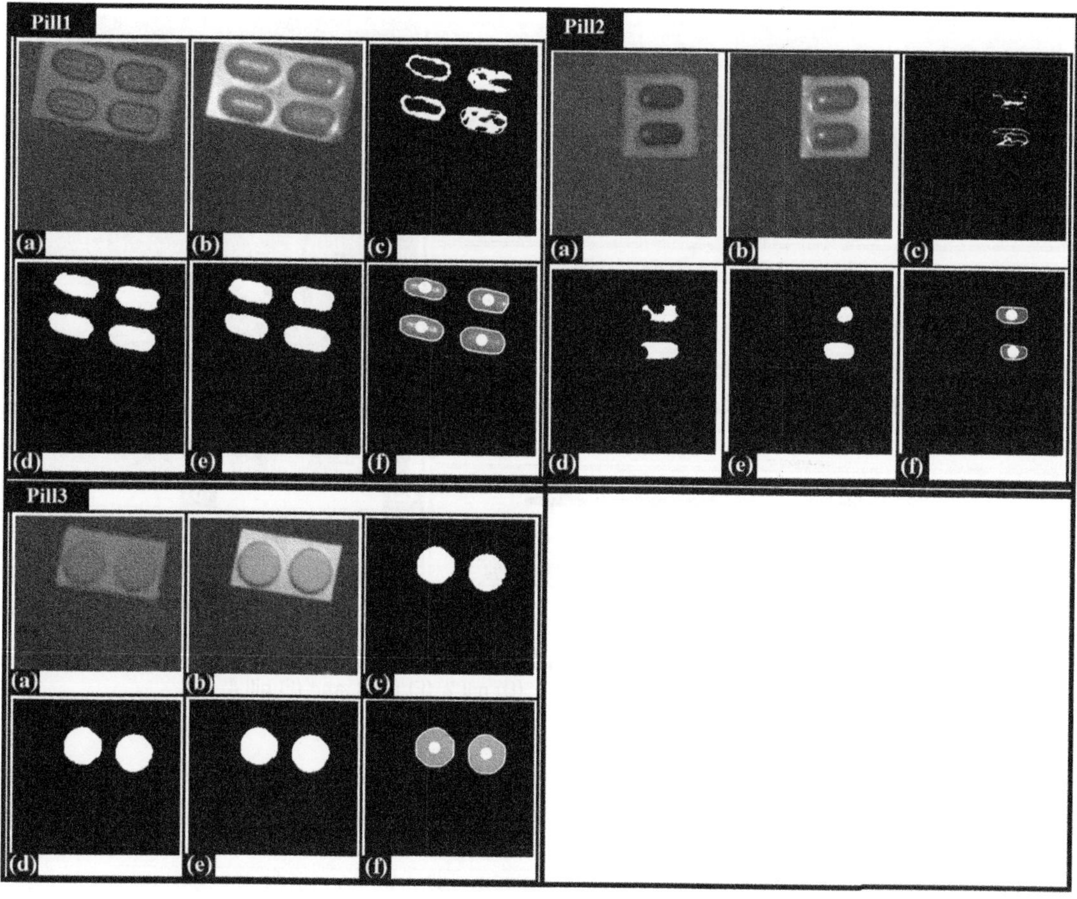

Fig. 14 The output of the image processing algorithm while monitoring three pills. (A) Image in HSV color space, (B) smoothened image, (C) image after performing "pixel slicing without background" within the computed range of HSV values (mask), (D) image obtained after the morphological closing operation on the mask, (E) image obtained after the morphological opening operation on the mask, and (F) pill areas segmented by performing bit-wise AND operation between the mask and original image with the contours and the centroid of the pills highlighted.

4.3 Discussions

In this study, an IoT-based pill monitoring device for geriatric patients has been designed using an image processing-based algorithm. The rationale for employing an IoT-based system is its advantages in the healthcare industries, including its ability for easy information exchange and decreasing the hospital stay duration and healthcare cost. The IoT is a network of things that connects different objects with a central server [34]. It has given a common platform where different medical devices, healthcare

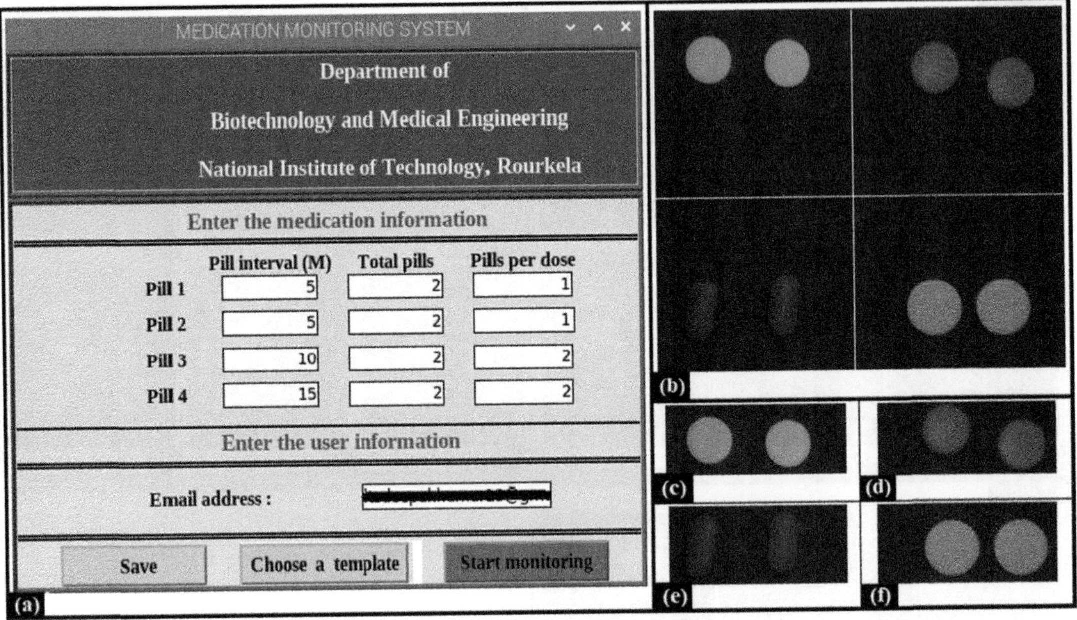

Fig. 15 Testing the medication monitoring system. (A) Dose information input GUI screen, (B) image of the pill tray, and cropping of the pill tray image into four sections: (C) pill 1, (D) pill 2, (E) pill 3, and (F) pill 4.

Table 1 The color parameters of the template image.

PILL	TEMPLATE SELECTION	AVERAGE RGB COLOR VALUES OF THE TEMPLATE			AVERAGE HSV COLOR VALUES OF THE TEMPLATE		
		R	G	B	H	S	V
Pill 1		161	181	162	83	108	181
Pill 2		117	103	77	20	87	117
Pill 3		89	77	66	15	66	89
Pill 4		104	161	108	62	91	161

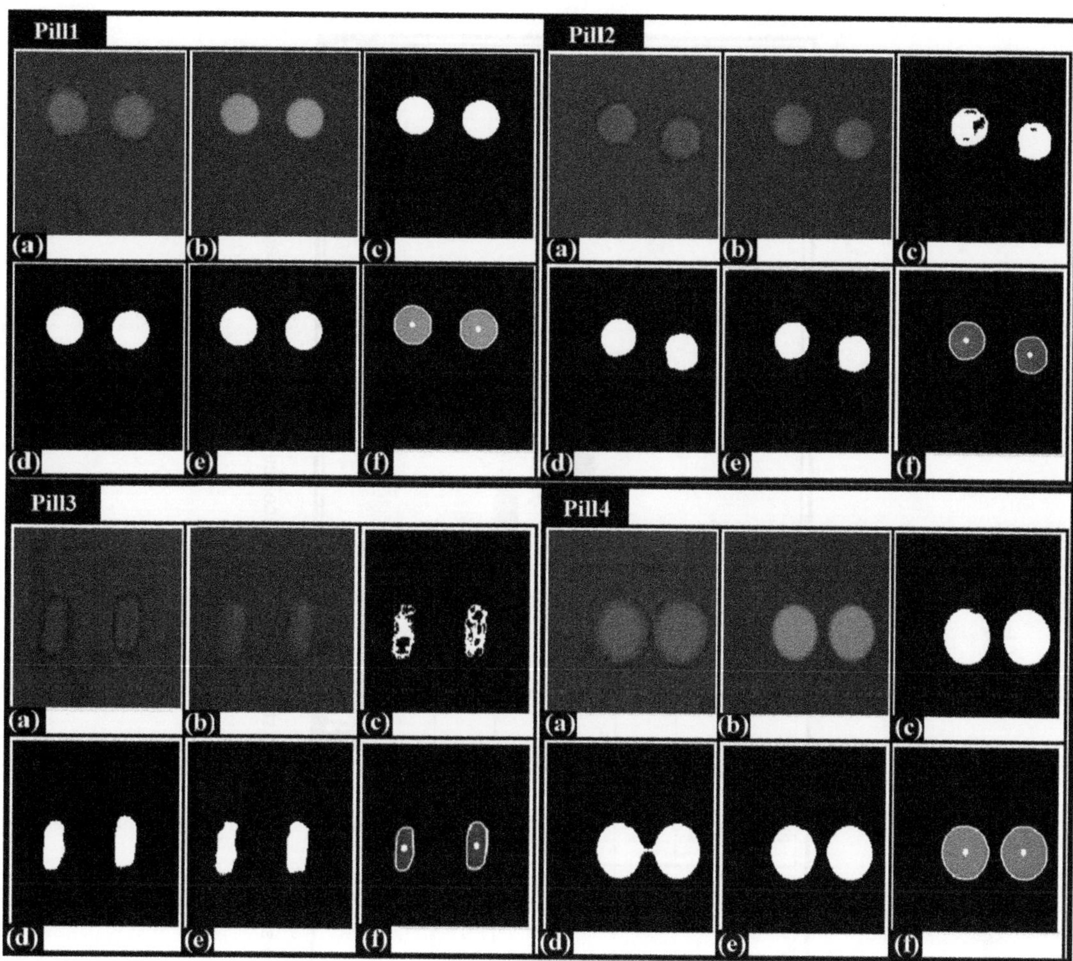

Fig. 16 The output of the image processing algorithm while monitoring four pills. (A) Image in HSV color space, (B) smoothened image, (C) image after performing "pixel slicing without background" within the computed range of HSV values (mask), (D) image obtained after the morphological closing operation on the mask, (E) image obtained after the morphological opening operation on the mask, and (F) pill areas segmented by performing bit-wise AND operation between the mask and original image with the contours and the centroid of the pills highlighted.

workers, and patients have been connected in one network. The incorporation of the IoT technology has enabled the current device to inspect and remind elderly patients to maintain their medication routine. Instead of adopting surveillance-based sensing, an image processing-based method has been employed in the proposed device. The process is to reduce the computational burden and the cost of the device. The images of the pills were processed in the HSV color space. The reason is that the HSV color model uses only one channel (Hue) to describe the color. Further,

PILL	TIME	IDEAL PILL COUNT	ACTUAL PILL COUNT	PILL STATUS
Pill 1	Tue Feb 18 09:22:24 2020	1	1	Pill is taken
	Tue Feb 18 09:27:32 2020	0	0	Pill is taken
Pill 2	Tue Feb 18 09:22:24 2020	1	1	Pill is taken
	Tue Feb 18 09:27:32 2020	0	0	Pill is taken
Pill 3	Tue Feb 18 09:27:32 2020	0	0	Pill is taken
Pill 4	Tue Feb 18 09:32:39 2020	0	1	Pill not taken*

(a)

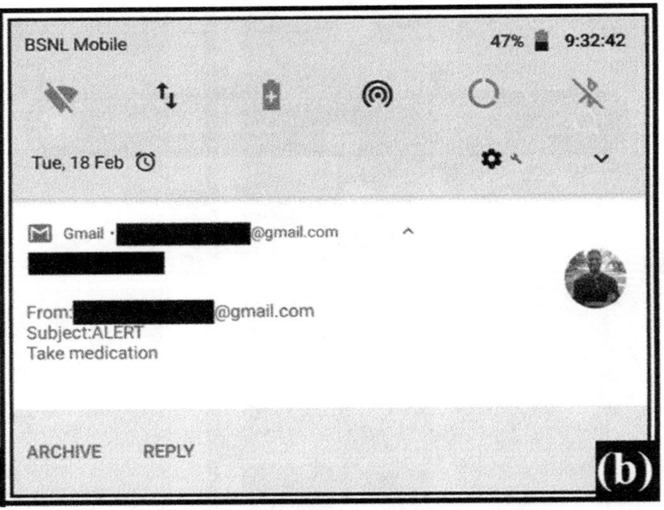

Fig. 17 (A) A sample pill intake report and (B) the screenshot of mobile showing the e-mail received in case of miss dosage.

the "hue" component is invariant of the changes in the illumination [35]. In most cases, there is uneven illumination during imaging. The lighting in our device was also inhomogeneous. Hence, the "saturation" component of the HSV color space model was considered in the processing step. However, an increase in the "saturation" component may make the colors appear to be purer. On the contrary, a decrease in the "saturation" component may generate a washed-out image. Hence, to accommodate the changes in the brightness in the image, the "value" component of the HSV color space model was considered. The "Gaussian blur" [36] filter provides gradual smoothing and preserves the edges better than any other mean filter. In our work, the edges are required for the pill counting process. So, we have used "Gaussian blur" to reduce the high-frequency components (e.g., Gaussian noise and edges) that were present in the image. The size of the Gaussian kernel depends on the noise level in the image. If the kernel size is too large, small features within the image may get suppressed, and the image may look blurred. Hence, the quality of the details of the image will be affected. If the kernel size is too small, eliminating the noises within the image will be compromised. In our experiment, we found that the "Gaussian blur" filter with the kernel size of 5×5 could effectively preserve the edges without compromising the requirement of the smoothing. So, the "Gaussian blur" filter of kernel size of 5×5 was used in our study. The effect of the kernel size of the "Gaussian blur" filter on the image has been compiled in Table 2. On the smoothened image, the "slicing algorithm without the background" was performed in the computed range of HSV values [$(H \pm 20\%\ H)$, $(S \pm 40\%\ S)$, $(V \pm 40\%\ V)$]. This algorithm generated a binary image that helped in displaying the desired pill areas (mask image). The "morphological opening" operation was performed on the mask using an elliptical structuring element (kernel size: 15×15) to smoothen the contour of the pills, break narrow isthmuses that connected the pills, remove the outlier pixels, and eliminate thin protrusions from the pills [37]. The "morphological closing" operation was performed on the mask using an elliptical structuring element (kernel size: 15×15). It smoothens sections of the pill contour, eliminates small holes (background region surrounded by a connected border of foreground pixels) that are present in the pills, and fills gaps in the contour of the pills [37]. The morphological operations (opening and closing) with a kernel size of 5×5 were ineffective in smoothing the pill contours and removing the outlier pixels and small holes. By increasing the kernel size to 15×15, the pill contour was smoothened. Also, the contour was similar to that of the actual shape of the pill. Also, the outlier pixels were eliminated. Hence, the kernel size for the implementation of the morphological operations was chosen as 15×15. But with a kernel size of 17×17, the smoothening effect on the contours was increased, and thin protrusions were observed on the pill contour. A further increment in the kernel size (19×19), elongated these thin protrusions and conjoined the contours of the adjacent pills. The effect of the kernel size on the outcome of the "morphological opening" and "morphological closing" operations has been shown in Table 2. The pill area was segmented from

Table 2 The effect of kernel size on Gaussian blurring and morphological operations.

Kernel size	Grayscale processing	Morphological operations	
	Gaussian blurring	Opening	Closing
3x3		--	--
5x5			
7x7		--	--
15x15	--		
17x17	--		
19x19	--		

the background by performing a bit-wise "AND" operation between the captured image and mask (binary image obtained from the pixel slicing algorithm). Segmenting the pills was the first step in the pill counting process. The second step in the pill counting process was contour detection. The accuracy of the contour detection process can be improved by converting the image to grayscale. For this reason, a "thresholding" operation was performed on the image before finding the contour. After the "thresholding" operation, the external contours of the pills were retrieved, and the redundant points were eliminated using the "contour approximation" operation. The removal of the unnecessary points reduces the memory requirement for storing the contour points. The convexity defects (identified by the pill contour that bulges inside) were removed from the final image, and all the foreground pixels were enclosed within the smallest possible polygon by employing the "convex hull" operation. The inclusion of an e-mail-based system is useful in reminding the patients and caregivers when the patient misses a pill. Further, with the use of IoT, the message can be sent automatically to the patient's smartphone through a wireless medium. This increases the geographical range of the application of the device.

5. Conclusion

This paper proposes an IoT-based pill monitoring device that uses an image processing algorithm to count the number of pills and efficiently monitors medication adherence. The consequence of medication nonadherence has a significant impact on elderly patients, which can strain the healthcare industry. To provide a solution to this problem, we have designed a device that captures the image of the pills using a CMOS camera. The image is then processed to find the total count of pills, and provide timely reminders based on the knowledge of the pill count. Unfortunately, the proposed device fails whenever the color of the pill matches its background. However, this problem can be solved by putting a contrasting background in the pill tray. In gist, the proposed device can help the elderly persons' family members monitor the medicine intake and take a timely intervention. Healthcare professionals in hospitals can also use the proposed device. It is expected that the device may reduce the workload and stress in these healthcare professionals. A potential extension or future development of this device is to develop a combined monitoring system that will monitor both the pill tray and patient movement. The scope of the current device is limited to the pill tray. Hence, no information about the patient after removing a pill from the pill tray is available. In other words, if a patient removes a pill from the pill tray in time, but if he does not take medicine, then the proposed device will fail to identify this. Hence, the device will be extended to include another mailing system that will alert the family members by monitoring the patient's activity and the pill tray when a patient removes a pill from the tray but has not taken the medication.

Conflict of interest

The authors declare no conflict of interest.

Appendix

RGB to HSV conversion
(a) $v = \max(R, G, B)$
(b) If $v! = 0$: $s = (v - \min(R, G, B))/v$
else: $s = 0$
(c) If $v = R$: $h = 60 \times (G - B)/(v - (\min(R, G, B)))$
Else if $v = G$: $h = 120 + 60 \times (B - R)/(v - (\min(R, G, B)))$
Else if $v = B$: $h = 240 + 60 \times (R - G)/(v - (\min(R, G, B)))$. When $h < 0$, $h = h + 360$
On output $0 \leq v \leq 1$, $0 \leq s \leq 1$, $0 \leq h \leq 360$
For 8-bit images: $V = 255 \times v$, $S = 255 \times s$, $H = h/2$ (to fit to 0–255)

References

[1] R. Hadidi, J. Cao, M. Woodward, M.S. Ryoo, H.J.I.R. Kim, A. Letters, Distributed perception by collaborative robots, IEEE Robot. Autom. Lett. 3 (4) (2018) 3709–3716.

[2] R.L. Page 2nd, S.A. Linnebur, L.L. Bryant, J.M. Ruscin, Inappropriate prescribing in the hospitalized elderly patient: defining the problem, evaluation tools, and possible solutions, Clin. Interv. Aging 5 (2010) 75.

[3] J. An, J.S. Lee, L. Sharpsten, A.K. Wilson, F. Cao, J.N. Tran, Impact of pill burden on adherence to hepatitis C medication, Curr. Med. Res. Opin. 35 (11) (2019) 1937–1944.

[4] A. Lawson, et al., Non-adherence to antihypertensive medications is related to total pill Burden, J. Hum. Hypertens. 31 (10) (2017) 682–683. Nature Publishing Group MacMillan Building, 4 Crinan St, London N1 9XW, England.

[5] J.B. Nachega, et al., Lower pill burden and once-daily antiretroviral treatment regimens for HIV infection: a meta-analysis of randomized controlled trials, Clin. Infect. Dis. 58 (9) (2014) 1297–1307.

[6] A.F. Yap, T. Thirumoorthy, Y.H. Kwan, Medication adherence in the elderly, J. Clin. Gerontol. Geriatr. 7 (2) (2016) 64–67.

[7] M.T. Brown, J. Bussell, S. Dutta, K. Davis, S. Strong, S. Mathew, Medication adherence: truth and consequences, Am. J. Med. Sci. 351 (4) (2016) 387–399.

[8] D.S.A. Minaam, M. Abd-Elfattah, Smart drugs: improving healthcare using smart pill box for medicine reminder and monitoring system, Futur. Comput. Inform. J. 3 (2) (2018) 443–456.

[9] A. Biswas, N. Sinha, K. Ray, S.K. Tripathi, A study on drug use and medication management perspectives among elderly and the impact of professional oversight, J. Clin. Diagn. Res. 12 (5) (2018).

[10] H. Ahmadi, G. Arji, L. Shahmoradi, R. Safdari, M. Nilashi, M. Alizadeh, The Application of Internet of Things in Healthcare: A Systematic Literature Review and Classification, Universal Access in the Information Society, 2019, pp. 1–33.

[11] W. Sun, Z. Cai, Y. Li, F. Liu, S. Fang, G. Wang, Security and privacy in the medical internet of things: a review, Secur. Commun. Netw. 2018 (2018).

[12] M. Srinivas, P. Durgaprasadarao, V.N.P. Raj, Intelligent medicine box for medication management using IoT, in: 2018 2nd International Conference on Inventive Systems and Control (ICISC), IEEE, 2018, pp. 32–34.

[13] A. Amira, N. Agoulmine, F. Bensaali, A. Bermak, G. Dimitrakopoulos, Empowering eHealth with Smart Internet of Things (IoT) Medical Devices, Multidisciplinary Digital Publishing Institute, 2019.

[14] H.-L. Tsai, C.H. Tseng, L.-C. Wang, F.-S. Juang, Bidirectional smart pill box monitored through internet and receiving reminding message from remote relatives, in: 2017 IEEE International Conference on Consumer Electronics-Taiwan (ICCE-TW), IEEE, 2017, pp. 393–394.

[15] K. Serdaroglu, G. Uslu, S. Baydere, Medication intake adherence with real time activity recognition on IoT, in: 2015 IEEE 11th International Conference on Wireless and Mobile Computing, Networking and Communications (WiMob), IEEE, 2015, pp. 230–237.

[16] E. Costa, et al., Interventional tools to improve medication adherence: review of literature, Patient Prefer. Adherence 9 (2015) 1303.

[17] Y.R. Manjunatha, N. Lohith, R. Bhavana, S.V. Bindushree, MEDIC—The Smart-Medicine Dispenser, Proceedings of the Second International Conference on Emerging Trends in Science & Technologies for Engineering Systems (ICETSE-2019), SSRN, 2019. Available from: https://ssrn.com/abstract=3511338 or https://doi.org/10.2139/ssrn.3511338.

[18] A.R. Sousa, P.D. Gaspar, Smart modular dispenser for medication administration, in: 6th International Conference on Biomedical Engineering and Systems: 6th International Conference on Biomedical Engineering and Systems (ICBES'19), 2019.

[19] M.O. Ibitoye, A.O. Raji, S.O. Nafiu, Inexpensive automated medication dispenser for persons with neurodegenerative illnesses in low resource settings, J. Med. Eng. Technol. 43 (8) (2019) 451–456.

[20] J. Ramkumar, C. Karthikeyan, E. Vamsidhar, K.N. Dattatraya, Automated pill dispenser application based on IoT for patient medication, in: IoT and ICT for Healthcare Applications, Springer, 2020, pp. 231–253.

[21] M.R. Kinthada, M.S.R.R. Bodda, M.S.B.K. Mande, A novel design of ARM based automated medication dispenser, Int. J. Eng. Res. Technol. 5 (2016).

[22] A. Kassem, W. Antoun, M. Hamad, C. El-Moucary, A comprehensive approach for a smart medication dispenser, Int. J. Comput. Digit. Syst. 8 (02) (2019) 131–141.

[23] J.E.P. Reddy, A. Chavan, AI-IoT based smart pill expert system, in: 2020 4th International Conference on Trends in Electronics and Informatics (ICOEI) (48184), IEEE, 2020, pp. 407–414.

[24] M.V. Moise, A.-M. Niculescu, A. Dumitraşcu, Integration of internet of things technology into a pill dispenser, in: 2020 IEEE 26th International Symposium

for Design and Technology in Electronic Packaging (SIITME), IEEE, 2020, pp. 270–273.

[25] A. Rajendran, V. Vanishwari, K.R. Varshaa, S. Pavithra, IoT based health monitoring and pill dispenser system, Ann. Roman. Soc. Cell Biol. (2021) 9927–9932.

[26] B. Ayshwarya, R. Velmurugan, Intelligent and safe medication box in health IoT platform for medication monitoring system with timely remainders, in: 2021 7th International Conference on Advanced Computing and Communication Systems (ICACCS), Vol. 1, IEEE, 2021, pp. 1828–1831.

[27] J. Joy, S. Vahab, G. Vinayakan, M.V. Prasad, S. Rakesh, SIMoP box—a smart intelligent mobile pill box, Mater. Today Proc. 43 (2021) 3610–3619.

[28] P. Pawar, C.K. Park, I. Hwang, M. Singh, Architecture of an IoT and blockchain based medication adherence management system, in: International Conference on Intelligent Human Computer Interaction, Springer, 2020, pp. 208–216.

[29] E. Chavez, B. Sifuentes, R. Vidal, J. Grados, S. Rubiños, A. Cuzcano, Remote monitoring applying IoT to improve control of medication adherence in geriatric patients with a complex treatment regimen, Lima-Peru, in: Proceedings of the 2020 3rd International Conference on Electronics and Electrical Engineering Technology, 2020, pp. 49–54.

[30] A. Ahmed, M.R. Ruman, A. Barua, Home medication for elderly sick people, in: 2019 5th International Conference on Advances in Electrical Engineering (ICAEE), IEEE, 2019, pp. 369–374.

[31] H.B. Mohammed, D. Ibrahim, N. Cavus, Mobile device based smart medication reminder for older people with disabilities, Qual. Quant. 52 (2) (2018) 1329–1342.

[32] G. Suganya, M. Premalatha, S. Anushka, P. Muktak, J. Abhishek, IoT based automated medicine dispenser for online health community using cloud, Int. J. Recent Technol. Eng. 7 (2019) 1–4.

[33] G. Guerrero-Ulloa, M.J. Hornos, C. Rodríguez-Domínguez, M. Fernández-Coello, IoT-based smart medicine dispenser to control and supervise medication intake, in: Intelligent Environments 2020, IOS Press, 2020, pp. 39–48.

[34] B. Farahani, F. Firouzi, V. Chang, M. Badaroglu, N. Constant, K. Mankodiya, Towards fog-driven IoT eHealth: promises and challenges of IoT in medicine and healthcare, Futur. Gener. Comput. Syst. 78 (2018) 659–676.

[35] J. Scandaliaris, A. Sanfeliu, Discriminant and invariant color model for tracking under abrupt illumination changes, in: 2010 20th International Conference on Pattern Recognition, IEEE, 2010, pp. 1840–1843.

[36] K. De, V. Masilamani, Image sharpness measure for blurred images in frequency domain, Proc. Eng. 64 (2013) 149–158.

[37] K.A.M. Said, A.B. Jambek, N. Sulaiman, A study of image processing using morphological opening and closing processes, Int. J. Control Theor. Appl. 9 (31) (2016) 15–21.

7

Biomedical robotics

Sumit Chakravarty
Department of Electrical Engineering, Kennesaw State University, Marietta, GA, United States

1. Introduction

Research in Medical Devices and Robotics is at the forefront of technology due to the focus on automation and technology in this era. Incorporation of safe, sustainable, and intelligent robotics systems is one of the goals of modern technology-driven development. This can be the driving force of the technological revolution that we are standing on the brink of. The First Industrial Revolution used steam power to mechanize production. The Second Revolution utilized electric power to enhance production and bring living comfort to population at large. The Third Revolution used electronics and information technology to automate and create connected production. The Fourth Industrial Revolution is using biohuman connectivity to technology to enable realistic safe, sustainable, and naturalistic products. Although the revolution has been occurring since the middle of the last century, last few years have shown tremendous growth in this arena. Significant challenges do remain on enabling such revolutions and technological developments. In this survey, we highlight recent developments in various aspects of this domain including:

1. Robotics in healthcare
2. Noninvasive robotic application
3. Surgical continuum and soft robotics
4. AI inspired medical robots
5. Augmented Reality assisted Robotics
6. Robotics in covid scenario
7. Regulatory issues

To meet the goal is to "domesticate robots" for use in healthcare and household, like the cartoon shown by Ingram publishing, in Fig. 1, we do have be cognizant about both technological and

Advanced Methods in Biomedical Signal Processing and Analysis. https://doi.org/10.1016/B978-0-323-85955-4.00011-9
Copyright © 2023 Elsevier Inc. All rights reserved.

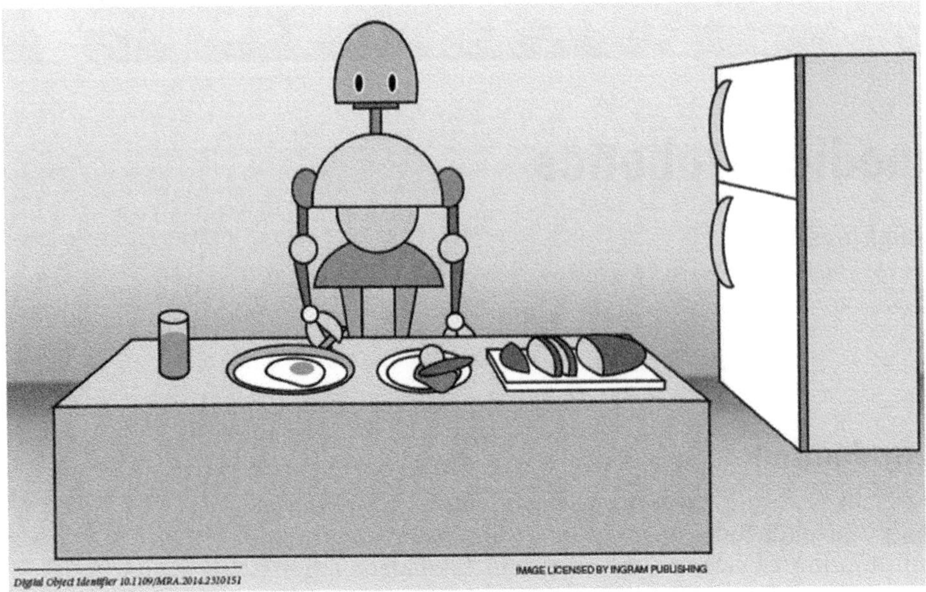

Fig. 1 The cartoon "domesticated robots" by INGRAM publishing.

societal challenges associated with the issue. For example, the economists Erik Brynjolfsson and Andrew McAfee have pointed out, the revolution could yield greater inequality, particularly in its potential to disrupt labor markets. As automation substitutes for labor across the entire economy, the net displacement of workers by machines might exacerbate the gap between returns to capital and returns to labor.

1. **Robotics in healthcare**: In medical and healthcare robotics have many different applications ranging from simple robots to those used in complicated surgeries. Having a reliable, repeatable and dedicated support in terms of robots make them a very valuable resource. They also do not have negative reactions to uncomfortable or unpleasant tasks. They can be classified as simple robots, specialized robots as well as other human–robot relationships.

   a. *Simpler robots*: Simple robots for example, giraffe portable robot or Nao humanoid robot [1]. Robots such as HELP MATE and ATHEON TUG have been used for material and supply support in healthcare industry [1]. Experts have also used robots to enable them to examine and treat patients via telehealth; for example, the University of Twente has built a robot-helped framework for adapting needles to achieve finer precision by use of a robot utilizing ultrasound imaging.

b. *Specialized robots*: The range of robotics in healthcare is massive and intricate. Robotics comes in different forms factor to serve different purposes. Instances of specialized robots are *neuromate robot* and *da Vinci robot* for stereotactic neurosurgery and laparoscopic surgery [2].

c. *Human–robot relationships*: Robots are not just restricted to advanced operations; they are also used in laboratories, nursing, and rehabilitation. The robots are utilized in pharmaceutical and telepresence, namely, recovery robots, sanitation and purification robots, and mechanical solution apportioning robots [3].

2. **Noninvasive robotic collaboration**: Various modes of interaction like elderly care, childcare and application in school and education can be considered as noninvasive robotics collaboration. Examples of interactive robots are available in [4]. A socially interactive robot HOBBIT is tailored for elderly people care for day to day operations at home like watching entertainment or making call. MOBILEROBOTS PeopleBot [5] helps people to move heavy objects. For childcare scenarios robots were used to interact with kinder-garden children to promote scientific thinking. [6] A robot system used for autistic treatment is provided [7]. The robot actors are used for mental relief as shown in [8] (Figs. 2–4).

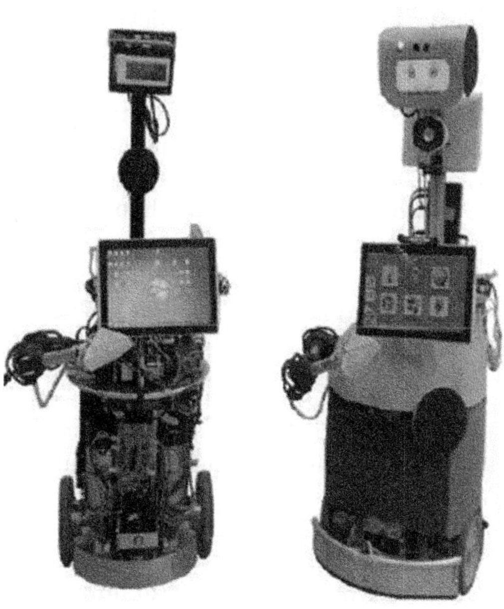
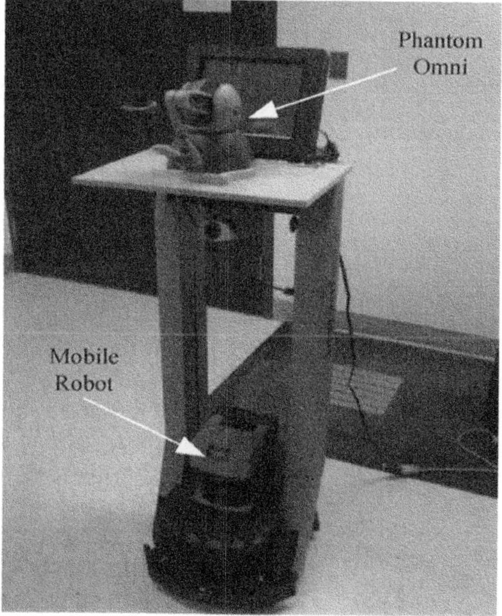

Fig. 2 Variety of robots for interacting with people [52].

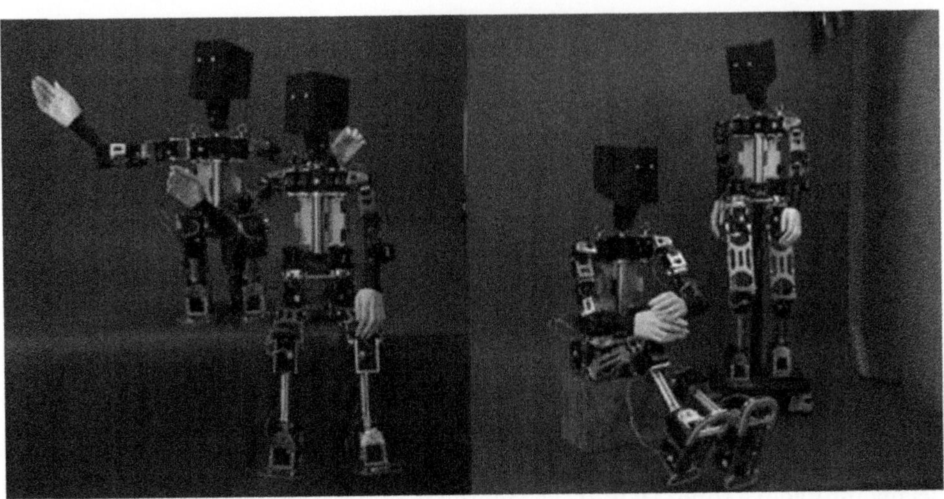

Fig. 3 Robot actors [8].

3. **Surgical and continuum robotic application**: Here is an overview of medical robot systems used in surgery. After introducing basic concepts of computer-integrated surgery, surgical CAD/CAM, and surgical assistants, we discuss the major design issues regarding medical robots. Robotics assisted Surgery aim to improve surgical precision and dexterity, to support minimally invasive procedures. Recent developments in this domain include the elements like Continuum robots and soft robots.

Continuum robots are fundamentally different due to their structure as compared to conventional manipulators, which have discrete joints and links. A robot with high degree of freedom/(DOF) can be called redundant or even hyperredundant [9]. As the number of joints approaches infinity with the link length approaching zero, it is called continuum robot [10]. The first continuum and hyperredundant robot prototypes were built in the late 1960s [11], when Hirose developed a snake inspired model. The number of researchers has increased significantly including snake-inspired hyperredundant robots [12–14], bioinspired soft robots [15,16], constant-curvature continuum robots, and concentric-tube continuum robots [17] (Fig. 5).

The application of continuum robotics has been applied to different scenarios, especially where soft tissues are involved. Neurosurgical procedures work on anatomy in human brain. This includes tasks like intracerebral drug delivery and

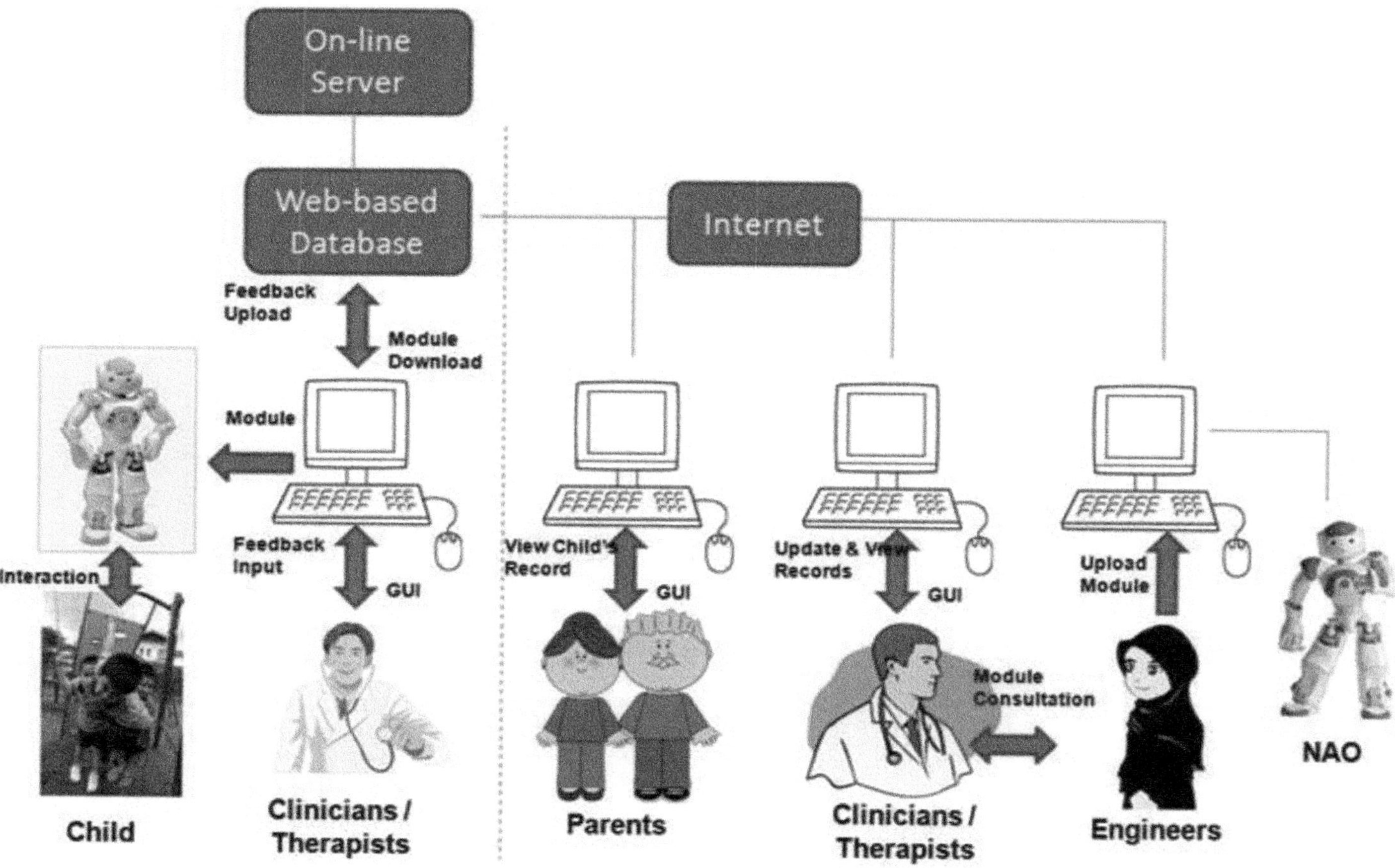

Fig. 4 Web-based system for autism [7].

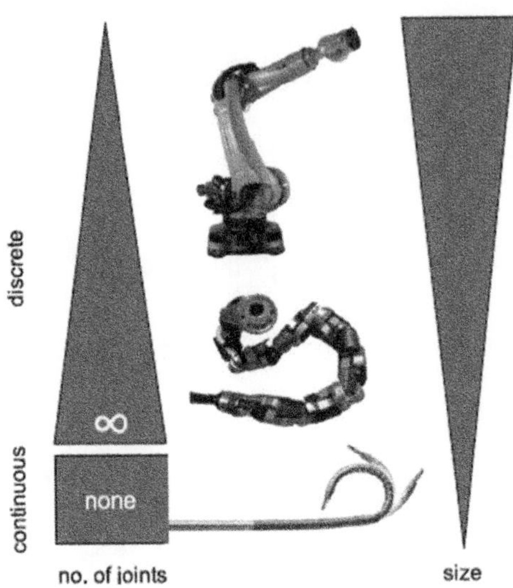

Fig. 5 Example of continuum robots showing the comparison of the number of joints and size [14].

intracerebral hemorrhage removal. Otolaryngology provides natural orifice access to regions of interest for surgical treatments. They include use of nasal or oral access for sinus surgery. Ophthalmic surgery enables precision procedures in eye with limited access. Structural heart procedures such as valve replacements/repairs can be performed on beating or nonbeating hearts, via cardiac surgery. Minimally invasive vascular surgery uses catheters and guidewires to perform injections, drain fluids, or perform procedures. Typical applications include angioplasties and aneurysms, where the key challenges include robotic guidance and steering of the catheter tips. Abdominal interventions are very popular as modes of surgery due to the quick healing and recovery via such procedures. They include ACUSITT device in collaboration with a company (Acoustic MedSystems, Savoy, IL, USA) [18,19]. Another example of use of continuum robotics is in urological applications wherein sensitive applications like prostate surgery need flexible and nimble robotic platforms.

Another aspect to such robot's set-up is soft robotics, which are made of materials that have modulus of elasticity comparable to that of biological systems' leading to several benefits like lesser trauma, simpler grip and ease of use. Recovery from trauma or other physical bodily loss requires replacement of joint, muscles, and other soft tissues via use of electroactive polymers and conductive polymers actuators [20–23]. Soft robots made of elastomers have been used in locations like are surrounding of the heart to provide ventricular assistance [24]. Elastomer actuators are flexible, thin and light, and they operate on low voltage with fast reaction times. These characteristics provide great potential for polymer actuators in medical applications. Polymer actuators due to their flexible, light and low voltage and fast operation properties, are used for catheter driving, localized drug delivery systems as well as for making the balloons that are utilized in percutaneous transluminal coronary angioplasty (PTCA) treatments. Such robots are quite challenging to manufacture as nonlinear geometry design as well as procurement of such soft materials make the fabrication techniques significantly different from that of rigid robots (Fig. 6).

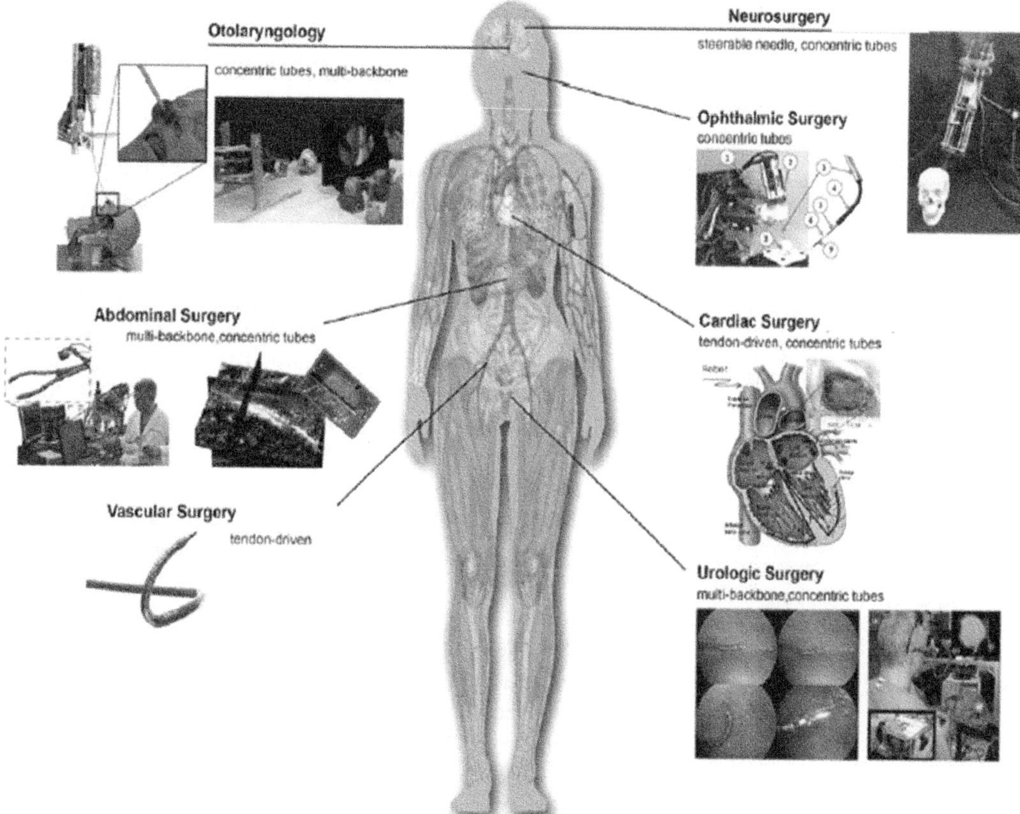

Fig. 6 Use of continuum and soft robotics [17].

4. **Augmented reality assisted robotics**: In 1968, Sutherland invented the world's first head-mounted display HMD: The Sword of Damocles [25], which tracks the user's head via either an ultrasonic position sensor or renders 3D lines. The term "Augmented Reality" (AR) was coined in 1990 by Boeing researchers, which was proposed as Knowledge-based Augmented Reality for Maintenance Assistance (KARMA) [26]. Researchers also started to use AR in the medical domain; where AR system to visualize 3D ultrasound inside the body pas proposed in [27] followed by deployment of AR in the operating room [28]. Augmented Reality in 2016 to draw the First- & Ten-Yard line in an NFL game and Is used in football broadcasting to this day. Other AR instruments including the Google Glass and the Microsoft HoloLens. In 2001, Wörn and Mühling [29] and Devernay et al. [30] utilized AR for surgical applications for example integrating KasOp, an operation planning system, with the CASPAR (Orto Maquet, Germany) orthopedic robot, for craniofacial surgery [29]. Other examples include use of AR to distinguish between coronary arteries as well as improve location awareness in robotic-assisted cardiac surgery [30]. The dimensions of AR in surgical robotics can be considered in various dimensions including:
   a. *Master–slave teleoperation robot*: The da Vinci Surgical System is a popular robotic platform with AR. During the operation, the surgeon is seated at the console to teleoperate the robot, with robotic arms holding the instruments together with a stereo laparoscope that captures the view inside the patient, which is streamed to the surgeon console.
   b. *Patient side robot*: The patient-side manipulators can autonomously execute a defined surgery plan with the surgeon still enabling some decision in the loop by use of AR tools. This includes NeuroMate, NeuroMaster [31], and ROBODOC [32].
   c. *Applications like surgical guidance and planning, port placement and sensory substitution and skill training*: AR applications include providing surgical guidance via AR as in da Vinci procedures. Such activity is done while developing surgical plan, real-time registration as well postoperative analysis. Projector based AR systems are often used with preoperative model and the ablation plan projected onto the patient body and interactively adjust the plan with hand gestures [33,34] and is a staple tool for microsurgery cases. Port placement is another critical application which simulation the placement of the virtual instruments onto the surgery area to study chances of potential collision together with the dexterity and ergonomic functionalities,

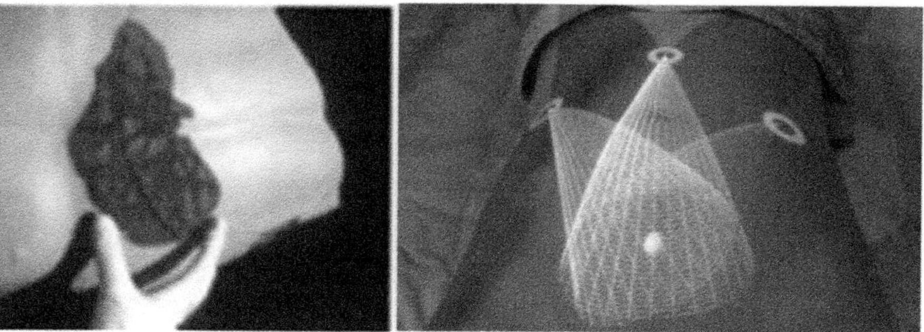

Fig. 7 Projector-camera AR system that allows hand gestures and port planning [34].

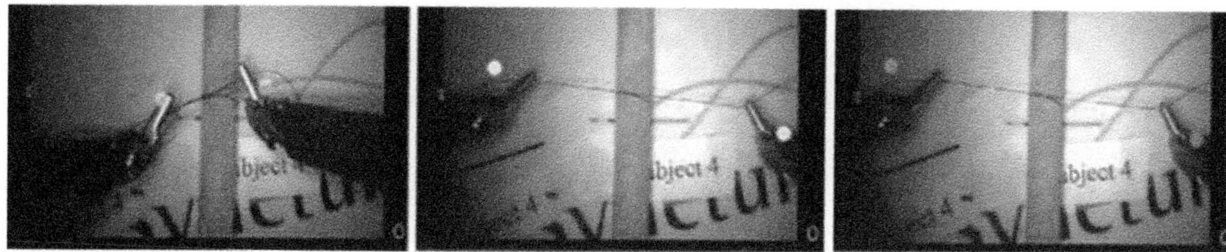

Fig. 8 Force feedback on surgical instrument, with the color indicating the amount of force [53].

as shown in Figs. 7 and 8. Another application of AR is sensory substitution, wherein the AR simulates the possible sensory feedback when operation is carried. They render a sphere, colored based on the current force category for the surgeon can be aware of. Such approach is greatly beneficial for skill training and transfer and AR based mentorship for surgery training.

5. **AI inspired medical robotics**: Machine learning (ML) and artificial intelligence (AI) is an expanding field which has shown significant applications in many domains. Use of ML and AI is becoming a game changer in the field of healthcare by providing much of the additional support so critically needed. Future systems endowed with cognitive capabilities could undertake simpler parts of a procedure and allow surgeons to focus on complex tasks. For example, systems like the Unimation Puma 200 [35], the ROBODOC [36], MINERVA [36], or Cyberknife [37] operated using AI in independent manner. However, such techniques require servo mechanisms for accurate control of instruments which may require aspects like modeling of trajectories and interactions during surgical tasks, e.g., for knot tying [38], suturing [39],stitching [40], tissue retraction [41,42], puncturing [43], and cochleostomy [44].

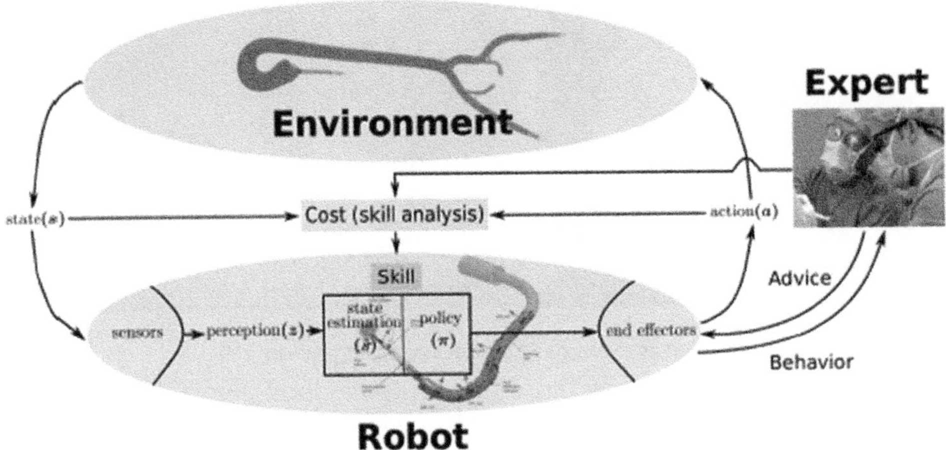

Fig. 9 Use of learning mechanism via reinforcement learning process for surgical tasks [54].

Machine learning in medical robotics can be classified into at least three aspects as detailed below:

a. *Expert based knowledge transfer*: To make the surgical system perform comparable to experienced surgeons, learning of the expert's behavior is critical. As shown in Fig. 9, the aim is to get guidance from experts in terms of reward function. The reward function is used to update the current state via undertaking action. The overarching aim is to accrue as much a reward as possible and thereby develop expertise.

b. *Analysis of surgeons' skill*: By using an expert system and comparing the performance of the expert system with that of the novice users, quantitative comparison of their difference in skill as well as required areas of improvement for learning can be recommended. Such effective training and evaluation of surgeons' skill can be very beneficial for healthcare industry in general.

c. *Workflow analysis and task segmentation*: If a surgical procedure can be broken into a set of sequential tasks then the study of a surgical procedure can be significantly simplified by studying and mastering the individual the tasks. Such identification of tasks can be made via autonomous -expert guided procedures. Such a way complex surgeries can be compartmentalized into simpler procedures, thereby enabling easier learning of the overall task. For example, in [45,46], laparoscopic cholecystectomy procedures are segmented into 14 different segments based on the presence and action of instruments in the surgical scene.

6. **Robotics in covid scenario**: As a result of the COVID-19 and its associated lockdowns, many institutions have turned to use of robots to mitigate the challenges of the pandemic. The robots have provided a continuous availability of manpower immune to the pathogen as well while significantly resisting its spread. Unfortunately, there are still significant technical hurdles for the robotics industry to overcome for the robots to excel in domains like diagnosis, screening, disinfection, telehealth, care and broader interpersonal problems unique to the effects of the pandemic.

To alleviate the spread of virus while performing diagnosis and testing, robots have been developed to automate the swabbing process. Both oropharyngeal (OP) and nasopharyngeal (NP) swab process have been robotized by developing significant degree of freedom force control. Many recently developed robots are equipped with multiple sensors such as cameras, thermal sensors, etc., to develop multifunctional robots which can perform diagnosis tasks such as temperature checking and questionnaires [47].

As shown in Fig. 10, autonomous robots are shown to be used for disinfecting hospital zones. These robots normally integrate the human detection and the building navigation

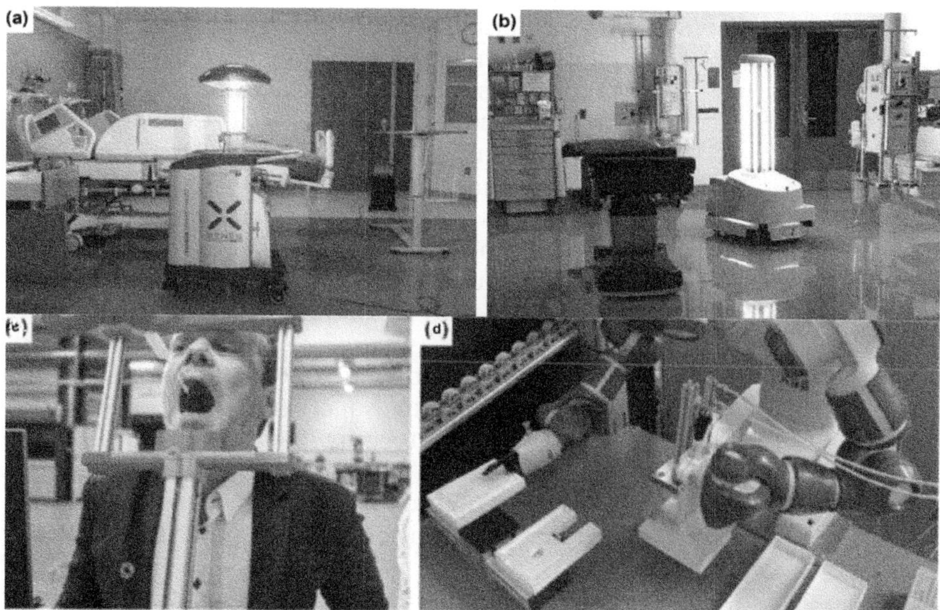

Fig. 10 Various use of medical robotics in CoVID-19 scenario [55].

process [48]. It automatically deactivates the UV in the presence of humans. This allows the medical staff to be free from this repetitive task to do more meaningful tasks such as taking care of the patients. During this pandemic, different types of disinfection robots have been developed. Some designs are mixed matches of commercially available robots with customized UV lamps, while other robots are more sophisticated with complete robotic mechanisms tailored for switching on/off UV-C lamps [49].

7. **Regulatory issues**: Regulatory and Legal/ethical barrier exist to ensure that the use of technology is not used unfathomed and without due consideration from society. [50]. The regulatory, ethical, and legal barriers imposed on medical robots dictates the levels of autonomy allowed in the robotic apparatus, especially in the medical sector. This is used to generate five autonomous levels to categorize the equipment and process as mentioned below [51]:

- *Level 0*: No autonomy. This level includes teleoperated robots or prosthetic devices which simply follows the user instructions.
- *Level 1*: Robot assistance. While the user has a continuous control, the robot just provides some mechanical assistance. Examples include prosthetic support robots or machines.
- *Level 2*: Task autonomy. The robot is autonomous for specific tasks initiated by a human, so the robot is in control for certain segments of the task which the user has discrete control over the overall process. The difference from Level 1 is that the operator has discrete, rather than continuous, control of the system. An example is surgical suturing (3) process.
- *Level 3*: Conditional autonomy. A system generates task strategies but relies on the human to select from among different strategies or to approve an autonomously selected strategy.
- *Level 4*: High autonomy. The robot can make medical decisions but under the supervision of a specialist.
- *Level 5*: Full autonomy (no human needed). This is a "robotic surgeon" that can perform an entire surgery and is currently in the realm of science fiction.

As technology typically grows in much faster rate than medical, legal, and ethical frameworks, it is critically therefore to have frequency updates in legal and ethical groundwork to keep up with the technology. On the other hand, technological improvements need to consider the societal, environmental, ethical and legal concerns to ensure they do not operate on the loopholes or work on the gray-zones in the framework. In fact, the technologists should play an active part in adding legal and ethical representatives for continuous development of the framework.

2. Challenges and opportunities

Like the revolutions that preceded it, the Fourth Industrial Revolution has the potential via the use of technology to raise global health levels and improve the quality of life around the world. In this review, we survey a variety of aspects of robotics in healthcare including general usage of robotics, like simple or specialized robots to ease the human life. Further, we study noninvasive robots like the robots which have been providing sanitation and disinfection services to our hospitals during the CovID-19 pandemic. Other aspects of use of robotics in this scenario include automated testing facilities as well as automated analysis of the tests.

Net we discuss the surgical application of robotics including highly flexible continuum robotics which can be very agile and accommodate complex surgical procedures. Augmented reality is often used in tandem with robotical systems in surgical procedures. Augmented systems are further improved via use of artificial intelligence wherein the augmented systems together with the action procedures can enable use of learning procedures like reinforcement learning which relies on learnt reward scenarios to gain expertise on robotic handling of procedures. Finally, we discuss the aspects of the regulatory nature on use of robotics by asking the key questions; how to keep up with technological advances; how to strike a balance between innovation and the protection of users' rights. At the same time, economist such as Erik Brynjolfsson and Andrew McAfee have pointed out, technological revolutions could cause further inequality in the healthcare services, due to cost, availability and lack of technological transfer of expertise to poor communities.

References

[1] T.S. Dahl, M.N. Kamel-Boulos, Robots in health and social care: a complementary technology to home care and telehealth care? Robotics 3 (1) (2013) 1–14.
[2] S. Shamsuddin, N.A. Malik, H. Yussof, S. Mohamed, F.A. Hanapiah, F. Wan Yunus, Telerehabilitation in robotic assistive therapy for children with developmental disabilities, in: 2014 IEEE Region 10 Symposium, IEEE, 2014 April, pp. 370–375.

[3] https://www.theatlantic.com/magazine/archive/2019/04/robots-human-relationships/583204/. (Accessed 7 August 2021).

[4] https://interactive.mit.edu/. (Accessed 7 August 2021).

[5] M.L. Walters, et al., Close encounters: spatial distances between people and a robot of mechanistic appearance, in: 5th IEEE-RAS International Conference on Humanoid Robots, 2005, 2005, pp. 450–455, https://doi.org/10.1109/ICHR.2005.1573608.

[6] G. Keren, A. Ben-David, M. Fridin, Kindergarten assistive robotics (KAR) as a tool for spatial cognition development in pre-school education, in: 2012 IEEE/RSJ International Conference on Intelligent Robots and Systems (IROS), 2012, October, pp. 1084–1089.

[7] E.T. Bekele, U. Lahiri, A.R. Swanson, J.A. Crittendon, Z.E. Warren, N. Sarkar, A step towards developing adaptive robot mediated intervention architecture (ARIA) for children with autism, IEEE Trans. Neural Syst. Rehabil. Eng. 21 (2) (2013) 289–299.

[8] D. Lee, S. Park, M. Hahn, N. Lee, Robot actors and authoring tools for live performance system, in: 2014 International Conference on Information Science and Applications (ICISA), 2014, May, pp. 1–3.

[9] G. Chirikjian, J. Burdick, A hyper-redundant manipulator, IEEE Robot. Autom. Mag. 1 (4) (1994) 22–29.

[10] G. Robinson, J. Davies, Continuum robots—a state of the art, in: Proceedings of the IEEE International Conference on Robotics and Automation, 1999, pp. 2849–2854.

[11] V.C. Anderson, R.C. Horn, Tensor arm manipulator design, Trans. ASME DE-57 (1967) 1–12.

[12] S. Hirose, H. Yamada, Snake-like robots [Tutorial], IEEE Robot. Autom. Mag. 16 (1) (2009) 88–98.

[13] J.K. Hopkins, B.W. Spranklin, S.K. Gupta, A survey of snake-inspired robot designs, Bioinspir. Biomim. 4 (2) (2009), 021001.

[14] A.A. Transeth, K.Y. Pettersen, P.I. Liljebäck, A survey on snake robot modeling and locomotion, Robotica 27 (7) (2009) 999.

[15] D. Trivedi, C. Rahn, W. Kier, I.D. Walker, Soft robotics: biological inspiration, state of the art, and future research, Appl. Bionics Biomech. 5 (3) (2008) 99–117.

[16] S. Kim, C. Laschi, B. Trimmer, Soft robotics: a bioinspired evolution in robotics, Trends Biotechnol. 31 (5) (2013) 287–294.

[17] H.B. Gilbert, D.C. Rucker, R.J. Webster III, Concentric tube robots: the state of the art and future directions, in: Proceedings of the International Symposium on Robotics Research, 2013, pp. 1–16.

[18] E.M. Boctor, M.A. Choti, E.C. Burdette, R.J. Webster III, Three dimensional ultrasound-guided robotic needle placement: an experimental evaluation, Int. J. Med. Robot. Comput. Assist. Surg. 4 (2) (2008) 180–191.

[19] E.C. Burdette, D.C. Rucker, P. Prakash, C.J. Diederich, J.M. Croom, C. Clarke, P. Stolka, T. Juang, E.M. Boctor, R.J. Webster III, The ACUSITT ultrasonic ablator: the first steerable needle with an integrated interventional tool, Proc. SPIE 7629 (2010) 76290V-1–76290V-10.

[20] I.A. Anderson, T.A. Gisby, T.G. McKay, B.M. O'Brien, E.P. Calius, Multifunctional dielectric elastomer artificial muscles for soft and smart machines, J. Appl. Phys. 112 (4) (2012), 041101, https://doi.org/10.1063/1.4740023.

[21] T. Tanaka, I. Nishio, S.-T. Sun, S. Ueno-Nishio, Collapse of gels in an electric field, Science 218 (4571) (1982) 467–469, https://doi.org/10.1126/science.218.4571.467.

[22] N. Ogawa, M. Hashimoto, M. Takasaki, T. Hirai, Characteristics evaluation of PVC gel actuators, in: 2009 IEEE/RSJ International Conference on Intelligent Robots and Systems, St. Louis, MO, USA, 2009, pp. 2898–2903, https://doi.org/10.1109/iros.2009.53544.17.

[23] K. Wales, S. Frederick, Surgical instrument having fluid actuated opposing jaws. US 7,559,452, 2009.

[24] E.T. Roche, et al., Soft robotic sleeve supports heart function, Sci. Transl. Med. 9 (373) (2017), eaaf392, https://doi.org/10.1126/scitranslmed.aaf3925.

[25] I.E. Sutherland, A head-mounted three-dimensional display, in: Proceedings of ACM Fall Joint Computer Conference I, 1968, pp. 757–764.

[26] S. Feiner, B. Macintyre, D. Seligmann, Knowledge-based augmented reality, Commun. ACM 36 (7) (1993) 53–62.

[27] M. Bajura, H. Fuchs, R. Ohbuchi, Merging virtual objects with the real world: seeing ultrasound imagery within the patient, ACM SIGGRAPH Comput. Graph. 26 (2) (1992) 203–210.

[28] N. Navab, T. Blum, L. Wang, A. Okur, T. Wendler, First deployments of augmented reality in operating rooms, Computer 45 (7) (2012) 48–55.

[29] H. Wörn, J. Mühling, Computer- and robot-based operation theatre of the future in cranio-facial surgery, in: Proceedings of the International Congress Series, vol. 1230, 2001, pp. 753–759.

[30] F. Devernay, F. Mourgues, È. Coste-Manière, Towards endoscopic augmented reality for robotically assisted minimally invasive cardiac surgery, in: Proceedings of the IEEE MIAR, 2001, pp. 16–20.

[31] W. Chou, T. Wang, Y. Zhang, Augmented reality based preoperative planning for robot assisted tele-neurosurgery, in: Proceedings of the IEEE International Conference on Systems, Man and Cybernetics, 3, 2004, pp. 2901–2906.

[32] J.M. Sackier, Y. Wang, Robotically assisted laparoscopic surgery, Surg. Endosc. 8 (1) (1994) 63–66.

[33] J. Leven, et al., DaVinci canvas: a telerobotic surgical system with integrated, robot-assisted, laparoscopic ultrasound capability, in: Proceedings of MICCAI, 2005, pp. 811–818.

[34] T. Akinbiyi, et al., Dynamic augmented reality for sensory substitution in robot-assisted surgical systems, in: Proceedings of IEEE EMBS, 2006, pp. 567–570.

[35] H. Paul, W. Bargar, B. Mittlestadt, B. Musits, R. Taylor, P. Kazanzides, J. Zuhars, B. Williamson, W. Hanson, Development of a surgical robot for cementless total hiparthroplasty, Clin. Orthop. Relat. Res. 285 (1992) 57–66.

[36] C.W. Burckhardt, P. Flury, D. Glauser, Stereotacticbrain surgery, IEEE Eng. Med. Biol. Mag. 14 (3) (1995) 314–317.

[37] J. Adler, S. Chang, M. Murphy, J. Doty, P. Geis, S. Hancock, The Cyberknife: a frameless robotic system for radiosurgery, Stereotact. Funct. Neurosurg. 69 (1–4) (1997) 124–128.

[38] H. Kang, Robotic assisted suturing in minimally invasive surgery, PhD thesis, Rensselaer Polytechnic Institute, Troy, New York, 2002.

[39] R. Jackson, M. Cavusoglu, Needle path planning for autonomous robotic surgical suturing, in: IEEE International Conference on Robotics and Automation (ICRA), 2013, pp. 1669–1675.

[40] F. Nageotte, P. Zanne, C. Doignon, M. de Mathelin, Stitching planning in laparoscopic surgery: towards robot-assisted suturing, Int. J. Robot. Res. 28 (2009) 1303–1321.

[41] R. Jansen, K. Hauser, N. Chentanez, F. van der Stappen, K. Goldberg, Surgical retraction of non-uniform deformable layers of tissue: 2d robot grasping and path planning, in: IEEE/RSJ International Conference on Intelligent Robots and Systems (IROS), October 2009, pp. 4092–4097.

[42] S. Patil, R. Alterovitz, Toward automated tissue retraction in robot-assisted surgery, in: IEEE International Conference on Robotics and Automation (ICRA), May 2010, pp. 2088–2094.

[43] R. Muradore, D. Bresolin, L. Geretti, P. Fiorini, T. Villa, Robotic surgery—formal verification of plans, IEEE Robot. Autom. Mag. 18 (3) (2011) 24–32.

[44] P. Brett, R. Taylor, D. Proops, C. Coulson, A. Reid, M. Griths, A surgical robot for ochleostomy, in: Proceedings of 29th Annual International Conference of the IEEE Engineering in Medicine and Biology Society (EMBS), 2007, pp. 1229–1232.

[45] N. Padoy, T. Blum, I. Essa, H. Feussner, M.-O. Berger, N. Navab, A boosted segmentation method for surgical workow analysis, in: Medical Image Computing and Computer-Assisted Intervention (MICCAI), Volume 4791 of Lecture Notes in Computer Science, Springer, Berlin Heidelberg, 2007, pp. 102–109.

[46] S.-A. Ahmadi, T. Sielhorst, R. Stauder, M. Horn, H. Feussner, N. Navab, Recovery of surgical workow without explicit models, in: Medical Image Computing and Computer-Assisted Intervention (MICCAI), vol. 4190, Springer, 2006, pp. 420–428.

[47] B. Varadarajan, C. Reiley, H. Lin, S. Khudanpur, G. Hager, Data-derived models for segmentation with application to surgical assessment and training, in: Medical Image Computing and Computer-Assisted Intervention (MICCAI), 5761, Springer, 2009, pp. 426–434.

[48] C. Reiley, G. Hager, Task versus subtask surgical skill evaluation of robotic minimally invasive surgery, in: Medical Image Computing and Computer-Assisted Intervention (MICCAI), 5761, Springer, 2009, pp. 435–442.

[49] . https://www.therobotreport.com/ava-robotics-uv-light-disinfection robot/. (Accessed 7 August 2021).

[50] . https://www.theregreview.org/2020/01/08/kunwar-robotic-surgeries-need-regulatory-attention/. (Accessed 7 August 2021).

[51] G.-Z. Yang, J. Cambias, K. Cleary, E. Daimler, J. Drake, P.E. Dupont, N. Hata, P. Kazanzides, S. Martel, R.V. Patel, V.J. Santos, R.H. Taylor, Medical robotics—regulatory, ethical, and legal considerations for increasing levels of autonomy, Sci. Robot. 2 (2017), eaam8638.

[52] http://www.mobilerobots.com/Libraries/Downloads/PeopleBot-PPLB-RevA.sflb.ashx. (Accessed 7 August 2021).

[53] http://biorobotics.harvard.edu/research/ff_surgery.html. (Accessed 7 July 2021).

[54] B. Thananjeyan, A. Garg, S. Krishnan, C. Chen, L. Miller, K. Goldberg, Multilateral surgical pattern cutting in 2D orthotropic gauze with deep reinforcement learning policies for tensioning, in: 2017 IEEE International Conference on Robotics and Automation (ICRA), 2017, pp. 2371–2378, https://doi.org/10.1109/ICRA.2017.7989275.

[55] Y. Shen, et al., Robots under COVID-19 pandemic: a comprehensive survey, IEEE Access 9 (2021) 1590–1615, https://doi.org/10.1109/ACCESS.2020.3045792.

8

Combating COVID-19 by employing machine learning predictions and projections

Anvita Gupta Malhotra[a], Pranjali Borkar[a], Rashmi Chowdhary[b], and Sarman Singh[a]

[a]Molecular Medicine Laboratory, Department of Microbiology, AIIMS, Bhopal, India. [b]Department of Biochemistry, AIIMS, Bhopal, India

"Machine learning can't get something from nothing…What it does is get more from less."

~Dr. Pedro Domingo, University of Washington

1. Introduction

COVID-19 was declared a global pandemic on March 20, 2020, by the World Health Organization (WHO). There have already been 20,78,34,266 documented infected cases, causing 43,71,025 fatalities through August 17, 2021 [1]. The transmission of the disease was so rapid that the doubling time of the first million cases reported was one-seventh of the time required to report them [2]. Almost the entire world has undergone a difficult period of lockdown with desolation. It calls for an urgent requirement of competent and cutting-edge science technology solutions to combat pandemics like these before they become an unmanageable crisis.

The coronavirus outbreaks turned out to be a major cause of infection to humans in the form of fatal pneumonia. Severe Acute Respiratory Syndrome CoronaVirus-2 (SARS-CoV-2), the causative pathogen for this disease, is a novel and highly pathogenic coronavirus exhibiting rapid transmission and extreme mortality. There is no definite antiviral therapy available to date against this virus. Initially, the only possible resolution of this pandemic was patient management by containment and mitigation [3], which has now been replaced by an extensive vaccination drive.

Advanced Methods in Biomedical Signal Processing and Analysis. https://doi.org/10.1016/B978-0-323-85955-4.00003-X
Copyright © 2023 Elsevier Inc. All rights reserved.

This has been described as the worst catastrophe for mankind since World War II and has put healthcare systems across the globe in a crisis situation [4]. Looking back to 2003, major morbidity was caused by the coronaviruses SARS-CoV and Middle East Respiratory Syndrome CoronaVirus (MERS-CoV), which have their origins from animal reservoirs that led to global epidemics [5]. However, COVID-19 has surpassed SARS and MERS in its topographical transmissibility and mortality.

During this pandemic, global administrative authorities were unsuccessful in predicting the scale of the problem and thus were not prepared in advance. They were out of time to use additional resources and deploy the latest technologies. However, for the first time ever, this pandemic generated a critical need for developing resources that would integrate emerging predictive technologies like machine learning (ML) and artificial intelligence (AI) to aid in combating a disease like COVID-19. These technologies can be employed in various arenas like screening and tracking of disease and development of effective treatment or vaccination [6,7].

In India, the outbreak of COVID-19 intruded into the routine functioning of everyone. People were forced to stay indoors to safeguard themselves, and more caution was advised for senior citizens and immune-compromised individuals [8]. We have faced several outbreaks caused by microbes before, but to confront a situation like this, a planned predictive strategy was required—an approach that managed and analyzed data pertaining to daily reported cases, patient details, and transmission dynamics, and integrated it with clinical trials, vaccination, and whole genome sequencing data to deliver meaningful predictions using ML and AI [9]. These forecasts might determine the epidemiological correlations for the origin and spread of disease and alert regions to make necessary arrangements and precautions [10]. The best example for this is a cloud and AI solution developed by Alibaba for China to predict the peak, size, and duration of the outbreak. This model claimed 98% accuracy when compared to real world data from various regions of China [11]. Also, ML can be used for the diagnosis of different types of pneumonia by using CT scan images [12]. These ML techniques can also be used to fast track the development of vaccines for COVID-19 by high throughput genome analysis and molecular docking [13]. Additionally, this technology is the most reliable technique for pattern recognition and therefore is widely employed to predict the systematic classification of individuals with COVID-19. In this chapter, the focus is on the COVID-19 pandemic and implementation of ML technology to aid in tackling this dreadful disease. The chapter also discusses types of ML algorithms along with the advantages and disadvantages of this existing prediction technique [14].

2. COVID-19: The 2020 pandemic

2.1 Origin and classification

There are various studies that presume or project the origin of COVID-19 from Bat-CoV-RaTG13 or Pangolin-CoV-2019 [15–17] than previously anticipated [18]. To prove this, virus genome sequencing revealed a 96.2% overall genome sequence identity of SARS-CoV-2 with Bat-CoV-RaTG13 [19] suggesting that both genomes might share the same ancestor. Furthermore, there is the strong possibility of alternative intermediate hosts, such as pangolins, bats, civet cats, pig, camel, cow, snakes, and non-human primates as revealed by protein sequence alignment and phylogenetic analysis [20] (Fig. 1). Human-to-human SARS-CoV-2 transmission mainly occurs when there is intimate contact of a person with patients or incubation carriers.

The taxonomic classification of the SARS-CoV-2 genome is the family Coronaviridae and genus Betacoronavirus [3]. Human coronavirus infections are caused by α- and β-CoVs. These alpha-coronaviruses (229E and NL63) and Betacoronaviruses (OC43 and HKU1) circulate in humans and cause the common cold.

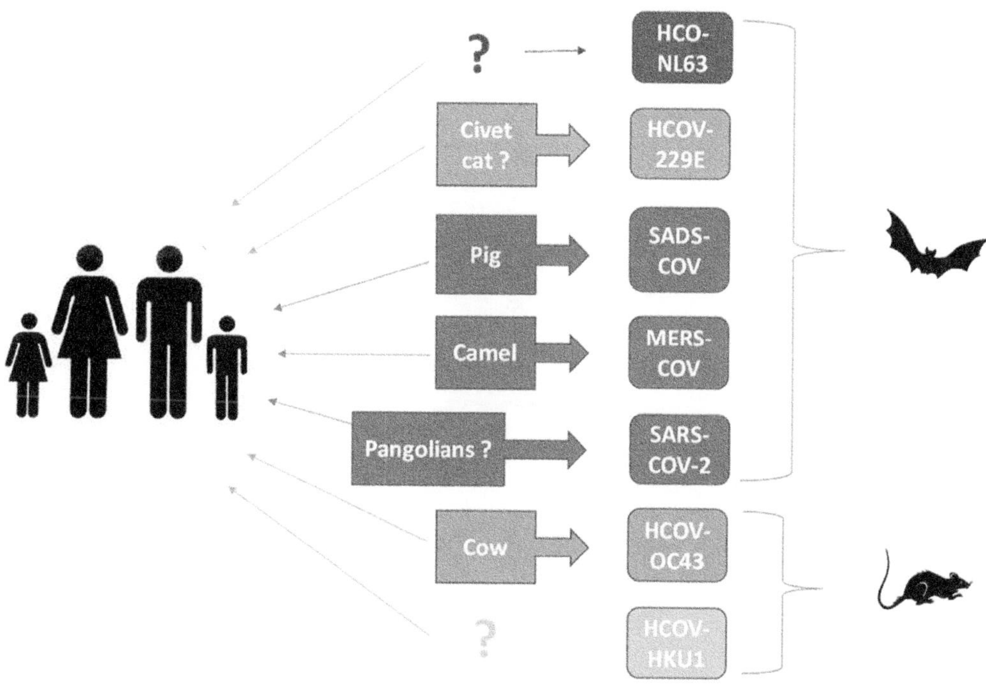

Fig. 1 Transmission of coronavirus infection from animal to humans.

Betacoronaviruses are supposed to be more pathogenic for humans. These include SARS-CoV, MERS-CoV, and now SARS-CoV-2 [21]. The phylogenetic analysis at the genomic level indicates that this novel SARS-CoV-2 shares 79.5% and 50% sequence identity to SARS-CoV and MERS-CoV, respectively [22].

2.2 The genome

SARS-CoV-2 from the Betacoronavirus family are enveloped, positive-sense, single-stranded RNA viruses which is 50–200 nm in diameter [23] with a genome size of ~30,000 bases. There are 14 open reading frames (ORFs) in the genome, which codes for 27 proteins. Of them, four are major structural proteins (spike [S], nucleocapsid [N], membrane [M], and envelope [E]), which are required to make a complete virus particle, and 16 nonstructural proteins (nsp1–nsp16), which assist in viral RNA replication and transcription (Fig. 2).

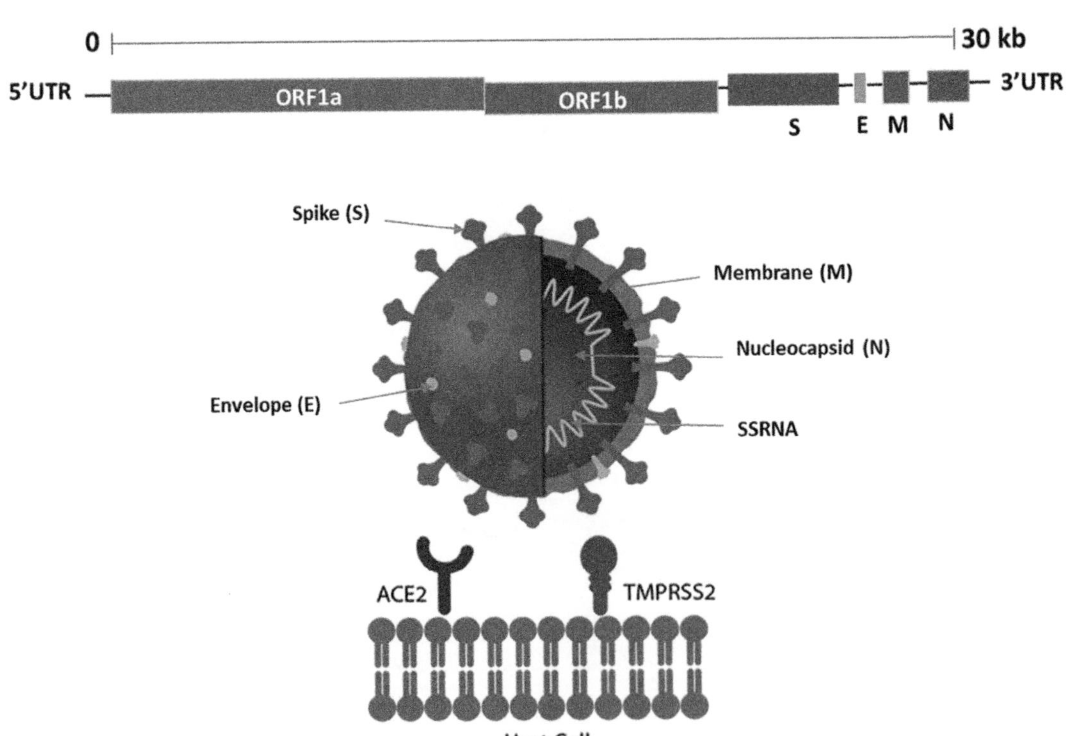

Fig. 2 Genome organization of SARS-CoV-19.

2.3 Epidemiology

SARS-CoV-2 has resulted in a distressing effect on public health across the globe. The number of globally confirmed cases has reached several million by September 2020 and doubled by April 2021. The least-affected population is children, and maximum death rates is observed in people with comorbidities. The effect of this pandemic is clearly visible by the percentage of population infected, its forest fire-like transmissibility, and the severity of clinical infection. Accordingly, the world needed to enlarge its health facilities and social and economic planning to reduce the consequences on the social, medical, and financial well-being of its people.

During the first wave, the global peak was observed during late September and early October 2020, when there were 35,109,317 cases, of which 1,035,341 died [24]. Researchers illustrated the probable estimate of COVID-19 severity as 2–2.5 [25], which means that each COVID-19-positive person can spread it to two to three new people at minimum. In the second surge, the condition was more grave with the daily number of daily cases being as high as 194,105 in April 2021. Countries with the highest number of cases reported are United States, India, United Kingdom, and Brazil [26].

2.3.1 *Source and spectrum of infection*

Since last 2 decades, three viral infections have led to an epidemic. This includes H5N1 in 1997, SAR-CoV in 2003, and MERS-CoV in 2012 [27]. The 2019–20 viral upsurge caused by SARS-CoV-2 turned into a pandemic by March 2020. This coronavirus was first identified in Wuhan, the capital city of the Hubei province of China, in December 2020 and has spread widely since then. The genome analysis of SARS-CoV-2 revealed its zoonotic origin from the strain found in bats (betaCoV-RaTG13). Similar to SARS and MERS, it has been predicted that transmission of the virus from bats to humans occurred via intermediate hosts such as pangolins and minks [28]. The worldwide spread of this disease is now believed to be transmitted through human-to-human transmission via droplets spread from an infected person by coughing or sneezing [29,30].

2.3.2 *Disease etiology*

Viruses including SARS-CoV-2 require the host's cell machinery for successful integration into the host genome. Viral entry inside the host cell happens via interaction between a virus spike protein and angiotensin converting enzyme 2 (ACE2) receptor of the host protein [20]. The ACE2 protein of the host present in the lower respiratory tract acts as a cell receptor for SARS-CoV-2. This protein also regulates within- and cross-species transmission. The first step of infection is the binding of the S-glycoprotein (spike) of SARS-CoV-2 to the human ACE2 receptor. The spike protein contains two subunits, S1 and S2. S1 subunit with receptor binding domain (RBD) determines the viral host range and cell adhesion. On the other hand, the S2 unit involves viral and host cell membrane fusion by two tandem domains, heptad repeats 1 and 2 [31,32]. Thereafter, the RNA (viral genome) is released into the cytoplasm of the host cell where it translates two polyproteins, pp1a and pp1ab. These protein codes for nonstructural proteins (NSP) and form replication-transcription complex (RTC).

2.3.3 Pathogenesis

COVID-19 patients exhibit symptoms of high leukocyte count, abnormal lung radiology report, respiratory distress, and increased levels of plasma proinflammatory cytokines. These are responsible for disease severity. The positive real-time polymerase chain reaction results for patient's nasopharyngeal swab confirms COVID-19 infection. The pathological analysis of the patient's blood also reveals leucopenia with high C-reactive protein (CRP), erythrocyte sedimentation rate (ESR), and D-dimer [33]. The primary symptom of COVID-19 infection linked to the respiratory system is severe pneumonia, RNAaemia, along with the incidence of ground-glass opacities and acute cardiac injury [11].

2.4 Treatments

The SARS-CoV-2 pandemic has spread very quickly all over the world. The detection of the SARS-CoV-2 infection can be done by several serological, pathological, and molecular tests. However, the confirmatory test to date is the molecular RT-PCR-based diagnosis test (Fig. 3). Currently, the research community is focusing on effective vaccinations for all. The next-generation sequencing has paved a way for the identification of emerging new variants. The treatment regime per Indian Council of Medical Research (ICMR) guidelines is to start oxygen therapy at $5\,L/min$ to achieve target $SpO_2 \geq 90\%$ in nonpregnant adults and $SpO_2 \geq 92\%$–95% in pregnant women. Empirical antibiotic administration should be in alignment with the treatment guidelines and based on the clinical symptoms and resident epidemiology and susceptibility

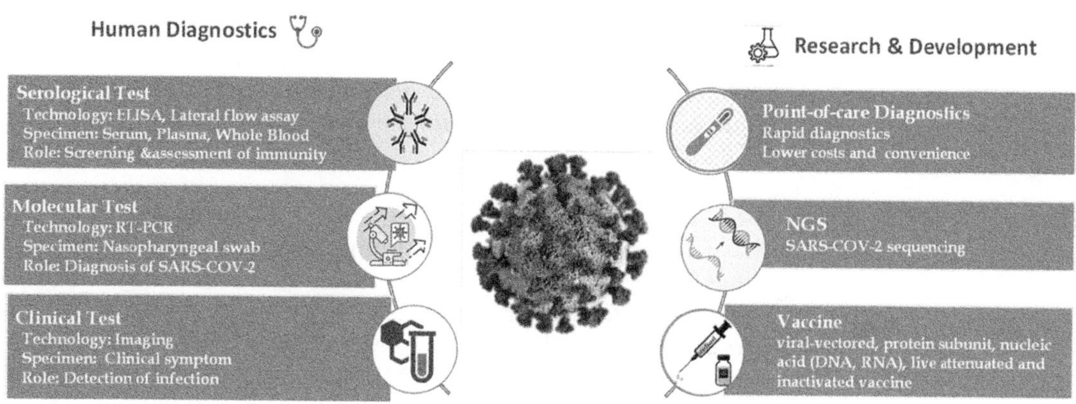

Fig. 3 The current diagnostic tools for COVID-19 detection along with recent research and development for prevention, diagnosis, and treatment.

information. The COVID-19-associated clinical manifestation can be identified by the altered values of biological markers like CRP, IL-6, white cell count (WCC), lactate dehydrogenase (LDH), D-dimers, platelet count, cardiac troponin, and renal markers [34]. In the case of critically ill patients, convalescent plasma can also be used. Since this plasma is taken from COVID-19-recovered patients, it contains corresponding antibodies that can suppress viremia.

The treatment of COVID-19 can target the following aspects of infection. It can prevent RNA replication by either targeting the viral RNA or inhibiting the key enzymes involved in replication. It can also block the virus and host cell interaction by blocking the ACE receptors. The treatment can interact with the viral structural protein and inhibit its self-assembly process. Some repurposed drugs that can be used immediately include a few broad-spectrum antiviral drugs against RNA viruses, like Remdesivir (GS-5734), a 1′-cyano-substituted adenosine nucleotide analog prodrug. Also, chloroquine (antimalarial) or hydroxychloroquine (used for rheumatoid arthritis or systemic lupus erythematosus) were earlier thought to be very effective for COVID-19 treatment and controlled its spread [35].

3. What is machine learning (ML)?

In a very simple way, ML can be defined as a process of enabling computers to make accurate predictions based on provided information. However, it uses the competence of AI that enables the system to self-learn from the given knowledge and improve upon it gradually without being hardcoded. ML was defined by computer scientist and ML pioneer Tom M. Mitchell as "…*The study of computer algorithms that allow computer programs to automatically improve through experience.*"

3.1 What does ML do?

The main difference of ML from traditional coding languages is that its algorithm does not specifically give a set of instructions to the computer to perform a task, but the system instead learns from the given data and makes informed predictions just like the humans do. Moreover, an ML algorithm learns and improvises itself as and when it is exposed to new data or information. Thus, it also evolves with time.

ML is comprised of algorithms and statistical models used by machines to perform tasks and learn in a self-sufficient manner. It also provides us with statistical tools to explore and analyze the data.

3.2 What is data in ML?

Recently, data have become very readily accessible due to the availability of enormous amounts of open-source data. Data is the first and most important aspect of ML, as this is where the system will learn from. So, these data are called the training dataset. Compiling and inputting these data comprise 80% of the time and effort involved in this process, as the concept of "garbage in, garbage out," i.e., quality of the output entirely depends on the input provided (Fig. 4).

Data is the information or knowledge that we already have for the topic under consideration. However, determining knowledge of the data is the most importance challenge. Thus, the data needs to be properly prepared and processed to be used for learning by the system.

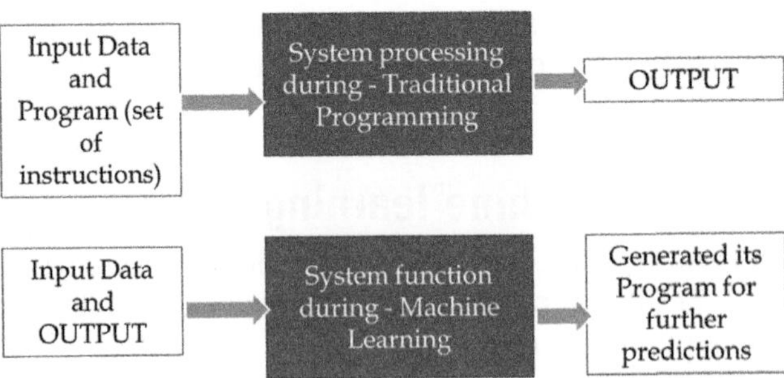

Fig. 4 Difference between traditional programming and machine learning.

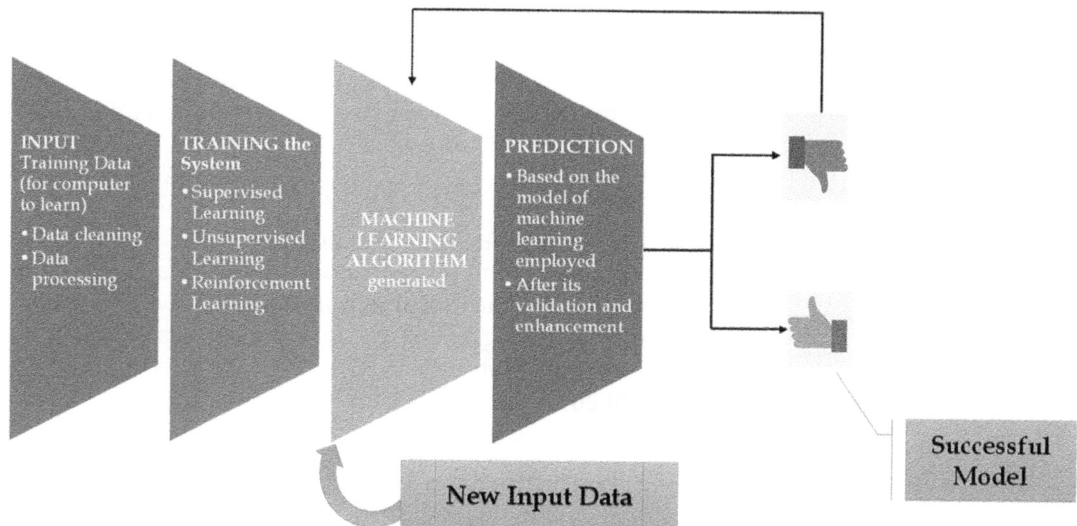

Fig. 5 Framework of machine learning.

3.3 Framework of ML-based prediction and projections

There are numerous algorithms of ML known and being made, but the basis of all of them includes the same four key aspects (Fig. 5):

1. **Representation of the training data:** It involves the illustration of the data or knowledge about the subject under study. It must focus on the key differentiating factors and should be filtered and processed.
2. **Hypothesis building:** The computer generates a candidate program, also known as a search process, for making predictions, which means when the system is given loads of raw data, it discovers patterns and rules to describe it on its own. This is further used to make predictions in the same line.
3. **Evaluation of the hypothesis:** Several statistical parameters are employed to validate the learning program generated by the computer. These includes accuracy, prediction and recall, squared error, likelihood, posterior probability, cost, margin, entropy, k-L divergence, and others.
4. **Optimization of the program generated:** The training program generated is constantly improved by input of any new data or information. On arrival of new data, the program recognizes and categorizes it into the patterns and rules already created by the computer program. Eventually, as more data

is received, it adds to the computer's "intelligence" by mathematical approaches like combinatorial optimization, convex optimization, and constrained optimization. Finally, it makes the patterns and rules ever more refined and reliable.

3.4 Demystifying machine learning

We give the machine input data and the results we need, then the machine figures out how that result can be obtained from the input data. Basically, the machine is trying to learn a way to come to the result by putting in or forming certain rules, e.g., Input is $x=1$ and $x=2$, and output is $y=6$ and $y=12$, then the rule that machine will come up with is $y=x \times 6$.

3.5 Machine learning: The process

The field of ML evolved from the arena of pattern recognition and computational learning theory. ML learns from the data without human intervention via indulging the concepts of computer science and AI. The process of learning involves the following steps:

1. **Data Collection:** Data as input comes from varied sources and includes observations, examples, direct learning, or instructions. The ML algorithm will learn from the data, therefore cleaner data leads to good model building, which will in turn give better predictions. For example: Hospital, emergency response unit, commercial flights, satellite data, government, army, and news media data to establish a network to track the contagion and how it has spread.
2. **Data Preparation:** Data is a raw entity; it needs to be worked on for the next steps to follow. We need to setup or concoct the data in the desired format to ensure it is consistent and accurate.
3. **Training:** Learning of the system is done on the training dataset via techniques based on data mining and statistical analysis. The system is trained to emulate the human brain, which has properties like reasoning and decision making alongside the features of learning and adapting.
4. **Evaluation:** Done on the test dataset to test how well the model has learned to generate reliable and repeated results [36].
5. **Fine Tuning:** The adaptability of the model to implement new input is very essential as it ensures the development and improvement of the smart system. Also, it leads maximization of the detection performance to attain 100% prediction efficiency.

3.6 Types of machine learning

ML is an arena of computer science that involves learning from input data without explicitly being instructed how to do so. This is a continuous process from the analyzed data and new input data. These iterations of learning lead to the identification of hidden perceptions and patterns in the system and will aid in adaption of this system when exposed to new data [37].

There exists a wide variety of ML applications in the field of commercial products analysis, healthcare sectors, transportation to weather predictions, and many other applications [38]. The four main techniques of ML are Supervised Learning, Unsupervised Learning, Semi-supervised Learning, and Reinforcement Learning. Fig. 6 illustrates the types of ML, and the related algorithms will be discussed hereon.

3.6.1 Supervised learning

In this type of ML, the data entered to train the learning algorithm is labeled in pairs, i.e., there will an input (represented as an vector) and the corresponding desired output (supervisionary signal). This learning process is termed "supervised" since the desired output is known and the algorithm iteratively tries to predict the output so there is a minimal difference between the predicted and the actual output [39,40]. Based on the type of output, the learning algorithm generates the functions. Classifier function is produced if the output is discreate and regression function if the

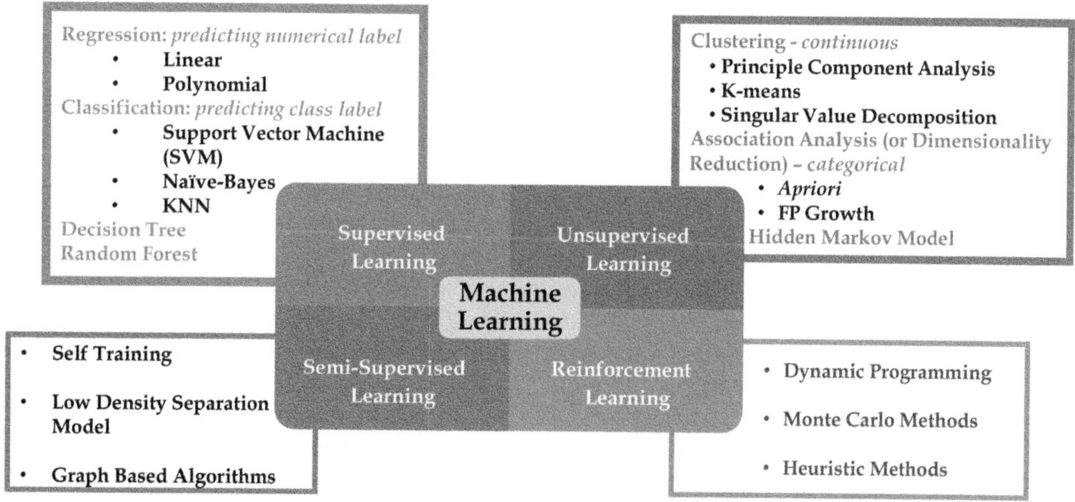

Fig. 6 Types of machine learning.

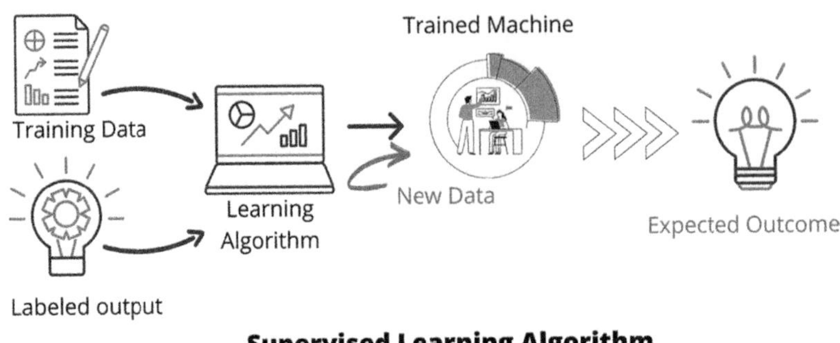

Fig. 7 Illustration of a supervised learning algorithm.

output is continuous. The algorithm detects the generalized features or patterns from the input data, generates revised input data, and produces the desired given output from it (similar to the provided output) (Fig. 7). The main categories of supervised ML are:

1. **Regression Algorithms (continuous output)**: It tries to unfold the best function that fits the points of the input training dataset. Linear, multiple, and polynomial regressions are the main types of the regression employed.
2. **Classification Algorithms (discreate output)**: It aims to assign the best fit class to the input data. In this type, the output is the discreate form, and its value is one of the different classes available [41]. It includes the algorithms like decision trees, random forest, support vector machines (SVM), Naïve Bayes, Logistic Regression, and K nearest neighbor (KNN).

3.6.2 Unsupervised learning

In contrast to supervised learning, this method employs the input dataset without the desired labeled output to train the algorithm. Once the input data is given the algorithm, it figures out the most suited distribution pattern or fundamental structure. It follows a "learning by self" principle by which it creates clusters. These clusters are unlabeled but based on features identified from the input data [42]. Fig. 8 suggests different stages of unsupervised learning.

Though unsupervised learning cannot assign specific names or labels to the clusters, it can still form different clusters based on the input features. The success of the algorithm solely relies on the quality and quantity of the input data. It discovers a similar group of data and then assigns new members to the existing group

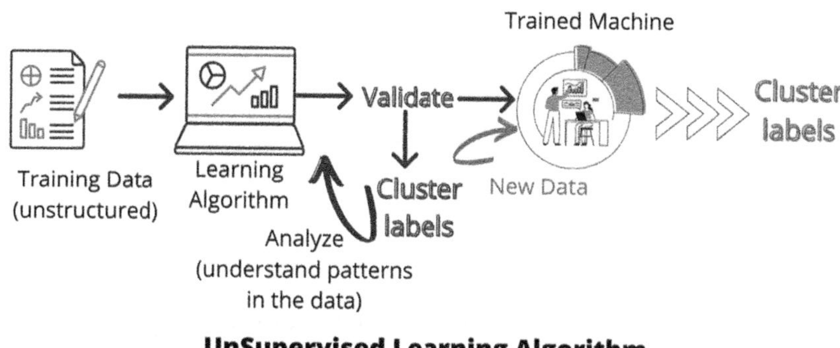

UnSupervised Learning Algorithm
("Self Learning Mode")

Fig. 8 The algorithm behind unsupervised learning.

based on their characteristics. Algorithms under this group can be broadly classify as:

- Clustering (based on similarity of data, it will cluster the data, i.e., Euclidian distance)
  - K-means clustering
  - Hierarchical clustering
  - DB scan clustering
  - Dimensionality reduction

3.6.3 Semi-supervised learning

As the name suggests, this method lies between the two previous methods wherein some data is labeled output and some is not. Its prime advantage of this method is that it uses less labeled data and a large number of unlabeled data [43] and hence is governed by minimal human involvement. It utilizes the skills of both the learning algorithms: unsupervised learning techniques can be used to identify patterns and structures in the data, and supervised learning can aid in the labeling of the formed clusters. The supervised learning techniques can also aid to make predictions on the unlabeled data, feed the data back to the learning algorithm as training data, and use gained knowledge to make predictions on new sets of data. In other words, the unlabeled or new data is used to enhance prediction by modifying or reprioritizing hypothesis made by labeled data (Fig. 9).

3.6.4 Reinforcement learning

Reinforcement involves learning from interaction with the environment to determine the best solution of the problem. The learning algorithm is trained from its own actions and is not

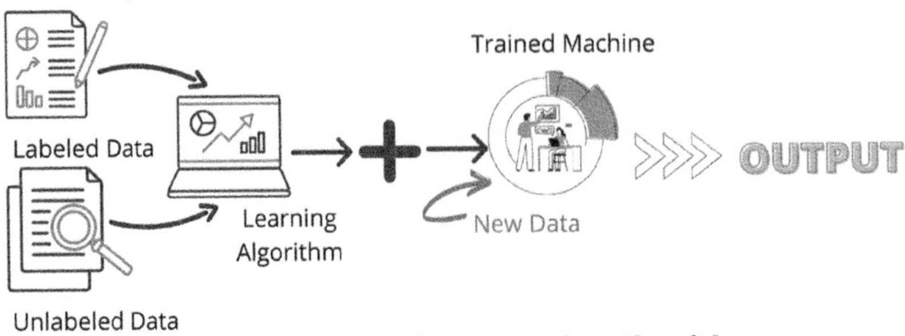

Fig. 9 Details of the semi-supervised learning algorithm.

instructed in any way (Hit and Trial Method). It selects its present action based on learning from past experiences and also exploration of new choices. Thus, it is best described as a trial-and-error-based learning process. The model is rewarded or penalized for each correct or wrong prediction. On this basis, it is trained and then creates a prediction of new data presented to it [44]. The learning models here have a set of goals and can understand the environment it is in; thus, it takes actions that bring it closer to the goal. It differs from supervised learning by the fact that, in supervised learning, the model learns from the input given, whereas the reinforcement learning model uses interaction with the problem environment to gain knowledge [45]. It includes methods like Monte-Carlo, dynamic programing, and heuristic methods.

4. Key application of machine learning with illustrative examples: Fighting COVID-19

COVID-19 has affected almost all countries, and its incident rate is increasing at an alarming rate. However, prediction techniques involving ML can be inculcated in the present healthcare scenario for better planning and implementation of government strategies to restrain the spread of COVID-19. These forecasting approaches can aid in the containment of the contamination. There are various aspects of the pandemic cycle in which ML can help with its predictions and projections (Fig. 10). A few of them are described as follows:

4.1 Pandemic preparedness

(a) **Predictive maintenance (*predicting the disease outbreak*):** Taking time and risky manual inspections are tedious jobs to do in the field of infectious diseases. In COVID times, even

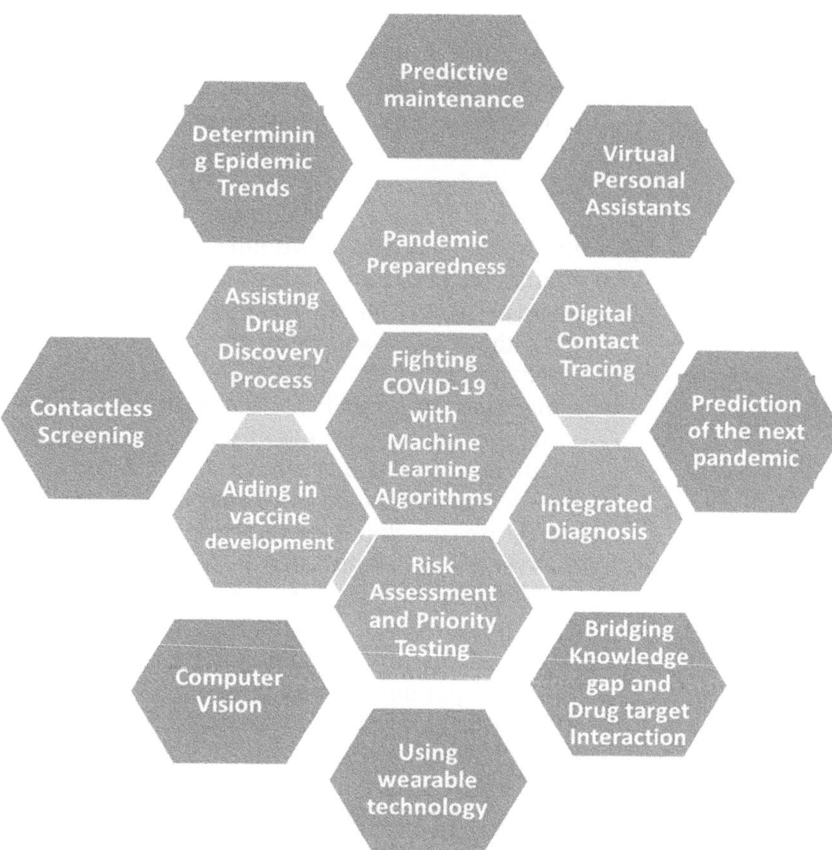

Fig. 10 Application of machine learning for combating COVID-19.

before any medical predictions, we had models based on deep learning, ML, and natural language processing to indicate the outbreak of this mysterious virus. This is a kind of insight that the world of medicine can use for tracing these anomalies and take necessary precautions in advance.

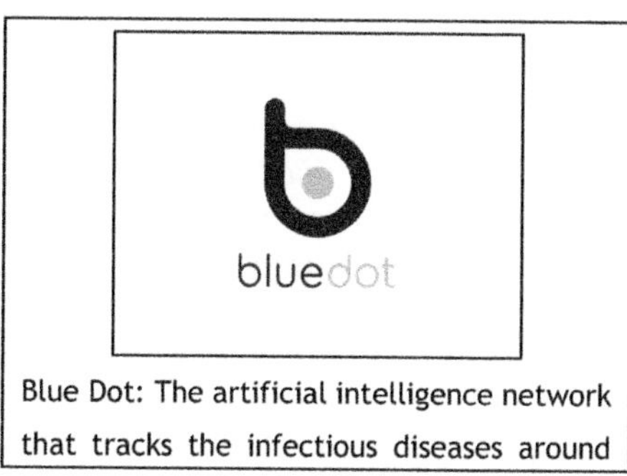

Blue Dot: The artificial intelligence network that tracks the infectious diseases around

Bluedot is an ML- and AI-based infectious disease surveillance system that can be used for early prediction. It has a successful record for prediction of ZIKA (2016) and EBOLA (2014) infections in the past. Also, for SARS-CoV-2, it predicted a cluster of "unusual pneumonia" near the Wuhan market 9 days prior to release of a WHO statement regarding the discovery of a novel coronavirus in a patient with pneumonia hospitalized in Wuhan.

(b) **Virtual personal assistants:** ML is such a brilliant part of personal assistants. On the basis of previous interaction with the data, they collect and refine information that is employed to fetch preferential results. Popular examples of virtual personal assistants are Siri, Alexa, and Google Now. These assistants can act as a source of data to learning algorithms for predictions and projections of the disease.

(c) **Prediction of the next pandemic:** Based on the data of infectious diseases globally, predictions can be anticipated about a novel disease occurrence. Like the ML algorithms, they can also help in the prediction of a zoonotic dive (transmission from one species to another) of a strain of influenza. Doctors and medical professionals can get help with anticipating potential pandemics and prepare accordingly.

(d) **Determining epidemic trends:** COVID-19 has taken a grip on the world with millions of people infected worldwide. Global efforts have been taken to stop the spread of the virus. However, it's difficult to forecast when the epidemic will end all over the world. Therefore, predicting the trend of COVID-19 is the need of the hour. "Epidemic prediction technology" developed by Alibaba Cloud is an ML-based technology for epidemic prediction and calculations of epidemic characteristics with 98% prediction accuracy. Also, a time series prediction model based on ML was developed by Wang et al. to determine the epidemic curve for some countries like Brazil, Russia, India, Peru, and Indonesia, and to also predict the trend of the global epidemic. It predicted in an analysis that the global outbreak would peak in late October, with an estimated 14.12 million people infected worldwide. However, recent confirmed cases have even exceeded the prediction. So, these models can be used by policy makers to decide on mitigation and reopening strategies [46].

There are a few other studies that use ML algorithms to predict the timeframe for the decrease in cases of COVID-19 and also estimate pandemic endpoints in some countries. T. Chakraborty and I. Ghosh (2020) [47] and Xu et al. [48] proposed a short-term trend of the SARS-CoV-2 for various countries like United Kingdom, Canada, South Korea, and France, including India, to assist policy makers and healthcare professionals to make necessary arrangements in the target country. In another study, Yang et al. [49] introduced an excellent model for forestalling the COVID-19 pandemic apices and extents. They applied an AI model prepared with past SARS to predict the epidemic curve to determine its peak and gradual decline in China.

4.2 Risk assessment and priority testing

This involves the screening of the population to identify who is most at risk of infection by the SARS-CoV-2 virus. These predictions can be based on factors like geographic location, age, medical record, etc. To achieve the maximum screening in a population, priority testing can be done. This ML technique can be used to increase the number of tests per million in less time. Collecting data on a larger scale, which might not be very accurate, would be better and faster in comparison to waiting a long time for an expensive lab report. Also, these data could be used for initial scrutiny and patient prioritization.

Contactless Screening (Remote patient monitoring): There are applications for healthcare personnel to remotely screen patients that use *machine learning-enabled chatbots* for interaction with patients for screening of COVID-19 symptoms, and it can also be used to address public queries related to the disease. Since SARS-CoV-2 is highly contagious, it is recommended for the medical community to guard themselves; therefore, several robotic systems are in use. For this, unmanned aerial vehicles (UAVs) are used for medical samples and to quarantine material transport. Exchange of COVID-19 information might be easier by some applications like *chatbot* by Clevy.io, a French company that uses Amazon Web Services (AWS). These chatbots will assist doctors to screen patients based on symptoms reported by the patients. Many other nations have now developed "self-triage" systems, like *Arogyasetu* in India, wherein the patient needs to answer a questionnaire about their symptoms and medical history, and then doctors will instruct further action to be taken such as staying home, calling a doctor, or visiting a hospital. Companies like Microsoft have also released their chatbots to assist the public in identifying their symptoms and taking necessary action.

(a) **Computer Vision:** This is a camera-aided technology that monitors the temperature and the body language of a person. If it finds any abnormality, it will be reported to the authorities. This is being implemented in some organizations to trace fever via thermal camera (with infrared sensors) for accurate reading of body temperature by creating people's temperature profiles. Another method for temperature screening is by using face scans.

(b) **Using wearable technology:** Smart watches can be employed to look into the patients' vitals. For example, Apple Watch detects common heart concerns with ML. Fitbit watch data can also detect changes in resting heart rate and can aid in identification of "influenza-like illness" or "ILI" in patients. Certainly, this research is in a budding stage, and it is far from diagnosing COVID-19 precisely. Additionally, OURA, an activity tracking device, employs body temperature, heart rate, and breathing rate for identification of onset, progression, and recovery of COVID-19.

By these screening methods, we can forecast the rate and spread of infection and also patient prognosis. The ML methods can figure out a quick rise in the infection rate or micro-outbreak in any part of the city for better planning of resources redirection and planning of healthcare workers.

4.3 Digital contact tracing

If a person is confirmed to have COVID-19, then contact tracing is the next important step in widespread prevention of the disease. According to WHO, the major mode of infection spread is through human-to-human contact by saliva droplets or nasal discharges [50]. To prevent the spread of SARS-CoV-2, the contact chain needs to be identified and blocked. Contact tracing involves identification and screening of people concurrent with the immediate COVID-19 exposure and managing them to stop further transmission. Here, the process pinpoints the infected person with an exposure from 14 days. If employed systematically, the outbreak could be suppressed by discontinuing the transmission chain of SARS-CoV-2 and taking control of the recent pandemic. To tackle with this, many countries with higher infection rates have employed digital contact tracing processes. This involves the use of mobile technology, Bluetooth, Global Positioning System (GPS), Social graph, contact details, mobile tracking data, card transaction data, and system physical address. All these data are analyzed by ML and AI tools to predict the most vulnerable person. This virtual process is in real-time and very quick as compared to physical tracing. Some examples of contact tracing applications include Arogya Setu (India), CORONA-WARN (Germany), Smart City (South Korea), Stopp Corona (Austria), Immuni (Italy), Trace Together (Singapore), Swiss COVID (Switzerland), Covid

Tracker (Ireland), and many more. However, for these applications to work with perfection, at least 60% of the population should install it. But concerns with the tracing app lies in the fact that it could breach the personal privacy.

4.4   Integrated diagnosis

Early detection is a critically important task for any disease, be it infectious or noninfectious, to save more lives. Radiodiagnostic tools like X-ray and CT scans can be useful to test the identified patient. These tools can be assisted with statistical and computational intervention. Medical features that are a combination of clinical and laboratory features, and demographic information integrated with thermal imaging, medical imaging, ML, computer vision, and cloud computing, can help in early diagnosis of COVID-19 and will further bring down detection time to minutes. They also aid to reduce the frequency of exposure to a hazardous environment of infectious disease surrounding hospitals and analyzing the data through ML.

These pandemics have resulted in several psychological problems as well. The ML and AI techniques along with predicting the virus conduct can be implied to monitor human behavior and response assessment.

Radiological images have helped in the diagnosis of many diseases like breast cancer diagnosis; it has delivered 53% of insight. So, radiological images (CT/MRI/X-ray) analysis can predict the onset of pneumonia in the case of COVID-19. It also saves time of medical professionals for detection and diagnosis. There are several studies to illustrate the effectivity of deep learning models in early screening of COVID-19 patients. It can therefore act as a supplementary diagnostic method for frontline health workers. AI and ML technologies can be applied to CT images for screening COVID-19 patients. A multicentric study based on fully automatic deep learning models revealed diagnostic precision 86.7% for COVID-19, Influenza-A viral pneumonia, and healthy cases groups [48].

A support vector machine (SVM)-based classification model was used by researchers to identify key features (age, GSH, CD3, and total protein), which can estimate the disease severity as early, mild, and severe in COVID-19 cases. The empirical statistical analysis results confirm that this four-feature combination results in an Area Under Receiving Operating Curve (AUROC) of 0.9996 and 0.9757 in training and testing datasets, respectively [51].

A study was designed to develop a supplementary tool to enhance the accuracy of COVID-19 diagnosis based on a deep learning algorithm [52]. This model was developed based on chest X-ray images of 127 infected patients compared with 500 healthy cases and 500 pneumonia patients. The model performed remarkably well for binary class with 98.08% accuracy and multiclass with 87.02%. However, the multiclass was later found to be a more appropriate expert system to assist the radiological findings in screening process quickly and precisely.

Similarly, another ML- and AI-based model, Deep Convolutional Network Model was developed based on 1020 CT images of 108 COVID-19 patients and 86 viral pneumonia patients. This tool showed accuracy and specificity of 86.27% and 83.33%, respectively [53].

4.5 Assisting drug discovery process

COVID-19 made drug discovery and repurposing a prerequisite that helps to devise a better strategy to tackle this emergency across the globe. Given the magnitude of the coronavirus pandemic and its spread across the world, investment in biomedical and pharmaceutical research and development has increased significantly to combat this disaster. Development of a potential molecule is a possible choice to tackle COVID-19. Here, taking into consideration the time and cost of developing new treatments would require quick drug screening and ML constitutes to be a beguiling way through. For example, during discovery of small potent molecules for the treatment of the Ebola virus, it was found that Bayesian ML models could be trained with two assay data; first, the viral pseudotype entry assay and, second, the Ebola virus replication assay, which aided to accelerate the scoring process of the small molecules as potent drugs [54]. This speeded process led to the identification of three potential candidate drug molecules. Likewise, it was revealed during an H7N9 study that accuracy of the scores could be improved substantially with ML-assisted (random forest algorithm) virtual screening and scoring [55]. In the current situation of the COVID-19 pandemic, wherein there is a rapid transmission of virus, it is advisable to employ techniques that can give quick and accurate scores to help in early drug discovery. In another study, researchers from the United States and Korea jointly proposed a novel model to address the requirement of an effective antiviral drug for COVID-19 treatment [56]. Here, they compared AutoDock Vina (an in silico virtual screening/molecular docking application) with the deep learning-based model on a 3C-like proteinase of COVID-19 and 3410 pre-existing FDA-approved drugs. They found that Antazanavir, a antiretroviral drug used for HIV treatment, is the best repurposed drug for COVID-19, followed by Remdisivir.

Drug Repurposing: When finding existing drugs that can help, ML can serve as the fastest drug decoder by automatically:

(a) **Building knowledge graphs**: Research articles provide us with plethora of information about drugs, viruses, their mechanism, and mode of action. Biomedical knowledge graphs could be built with language processing (ML applied to text), which reads and interprets a large number of research literature working as well-thought-out grids and meaningfully connecting these different entities, such as drugs and targets [57]. Researchers have tailored an ML-built information quest to discover the link between SARS-CoV-2 and the Baricitinib drug for the treatment of COVID-19 [58].

(b) **Identifying Drug-target interactions (DTIs)**: The virus-host protein interactome can act as a communication model and tell us the mechanism of virus infestation in our body. For a complex network like this, a neural network algorithm was applied to understand and decode them [56,59]. Further, the large DTI databases are used to train these networks to assemble a list of promising candidate drugs that can bind and inhibit the action of the viral protein. Another noteworthy study found Baricitinib as a candidate drug by applying a neural network algorithm [60].

For the rapid drug design and discovery of SARS-CoV-2 antivirals, SUMMIT, the world's most powerful supercomputer, is in game now, which is performing high throughput virtual screening for the identification of small molecules that bind to the SARS-CoV-2 S-protein or the S protein-human ACE2 interface. It is assumed that the selected small molecules will inhibit the host-virus interactions and/or limit viral recognition [61].

4.6 Aiding in vaccine development

Vaccine development is a time-consuming process that can be boosted by ML and AI by applying an integrative approach. There are a couple of studies that have shown the utility of ML in the prediction of a suitable target group for vaccine administration [62]. Moreover, these deep learning algorithms can be used to predict suitable vaccine candidates [63,64]. We now have a variety of vaccines in the market, and the vaccination drive is in full swing globally. Therefore, based on the post-vaccination data across the world, a desirable ML-based model can be built that can effectively predict the best vaccine for a given population based on their geographic location.

Another major concern with vaccination is to reassure the adequate uptake of the vaccine, since more than one dose of a vaccine is required or a booster dosage is needed to ensure long-term immunity against the virus. It was learned from the past that the dropout rate of vaccinations in low and medium income countries (LMICs) is 34.6% [65]; therefore, ML can be used to identify the target population who is unlikely to take the complete dose of vaccination and can focus efforts to that region. As far as herd immunity is concerned, ML algorithms can be used to prioritize those geographic locations to start vaccinations where it is needed the most. In India, the rural areas are around 66%, which are difficult to trace and explore; here, ML-based maps can be optimally utilized for better distribution of vaccines to a susceptible population that may be missed otherwise.

5. Concerns

There have been great advances in the field of computing with each passing year. However, there are certain limitations associated with it as well. It is still very difficult to handle computers in a logical perspective. The major factor that affects use of ML is lack of expertise, which is a key factor in data analysis. Human intervention is extremely crucial in any computational approach to incur the essential information. Hence the analysis and predictions are biased toward the person performing it. Also, in the case of viruses, we do lot of work and then the virus mutates, wasting all the efforts and eventually all the setup has to be redone. Whenever it will be, if we develop a ML algorithm in the future that is robust enough to handle mutations and recombinations to detect COVID-19 quickly with that much accuracy, it will be a "holy grail."

6. Final thoughts

There were and there will be outbreaks of infections before and after COVID-19. This prompts an immediate need for a system to succumb it. Researchers around the globe are trying hard to find a cure for the novel SARS-CoV-2 virus. Computational-assisted methods like ML and AI, when employed with the medical data, can deliver quick and useful predictions. This chapter describes the ML methods and their applications for early diagnosis and prevention of COVID-19 for assisting medical experts and healthcare providers in real-world problems.

The use of prominent technology like ML presents an ability to assist and improve screening processes, early prediction/diagnosis, digital contact tracing, and drug/vaccine development with high consistency and precision. Deep learning, support vector machine, and random forest-like algorithms of ML are favored among all the other learning algorithms. However, the recent scenario demands more advanced models to analyze the clinical, geographical, and demographical data of the suspected and infected patients for better predictions and screening. Furthermore, it is clear and concluded that learning by machine can tremendously help in screening and treatment of COVID-19 patients, thus lightening the workload of medical experts. The use of computational algorithms, along with existing docking applications, result in a faster drug development process by reducing the cost and manpower. Today, the need of the hour is data sharing and global collaboration to fight against this heath emergency and the battle against the pandemic.

Several computer-based, state-of-the-art, and up-to-date technologies are required to assist in the fight against this pandemic. Current advances in computational research have established that these technologies have immense utility, and they along with medical knowledge laid the foundation for the upcoming Medical Informatics Industry [66]. Therefore, there is an important role of the ML technologies to manage the existing global emergency related to public health. COVID-19 management and cure can be achieved by increasing the horizon of the medical industry by joining hands with these emerging and promising technologies.

The limitations with this technology lie in the fact that the SARS CoV-2 virus is unraveling itself continuously, and the data presented here is solely based on current information, which is limited. However, it can be modified as more information becomes available, and the published literature can direct the management of COVID-19.

But one of the biggest challenges lies in the optimum utilization of limited resources available with LMICs. ML can help in the reasonable and effectual distribution of spare funds. The volatile and asymptomatic transmission of COVID-19 can be handled by computational algorithms that employ real-time data that improves with time to provide an accurate prediction for COVID-19 management mitigation.

Finally, training, orientation, and technology enhancement should be a role for world health organizations (CDC, WHO, UN health), so that nations will be ready to handle these types of pandemics or will be careful not to repeat the same.

7. Takeaway points

ML is proven to be an essential aid in combating the current pandemic. For this, a collection of medical and sociodemographic data should be done, followed by pooling of expertise and skills to make decisive predictions, projections, and implementation. By doing so, we can help to save lives. A few top points of this technology include:

1. The outbreak of a pandemic has created an **urgent need** for managing resources, healthcare, and essential services.
2. Given the current situation, the screening and treatment of diseases need to be done **quick and fast**.
3. ML can help medical experts with a substitutive method of quick and contactless screening, contact tracing, and drug repurposing.
4. It is well proven that the **accuracy and reliability** of this technology is acceptable.
5. Learning algorithms can assist healthcare providers and researchers in multiple dimensions to **address the challenges** of the current pandemic scenario.
6. Applications based on ML can help in COVID-19 screening with **minimal human intervention**.
7. **Globalization of data sharing** with regard to research, scientific, diagnosis, and medical data is highly essential for the appropriate implementation of ML for COVID-19.

Key terms

(1) **Data**: Data is a digital collection of information. It is the quantities, characters, or symbols on which operations are performed by a computer, which may be stored and transmitted in the form of electrical signals and recorded on magnetic, optical, or mechanical recording media.

(2) **Data Sources**: A data source is the location where data that is being used originates from. A data source may be the initial location where data is born or where physical information is first digitized; however, even the most refined data may serve as a source, as long as another process accesses and utilizes it.

(3) **Data Mining**: Data mining is defined as a process used to extract usable data from a larger set of any raw data. It implies analyzing data patterns in large batches of data using one or more software.

(4) **Natural language processing**: It is a collective term referring to automatic computational processing of human languages. This includes both algorithms that take human-produced text as input and algorithms that produce natural-looking text as outputs.

(5) **Machine learning**: It refers to the practice of using algorithms to parse large volumes of data, learn from it, detect patterns, and make decisions or predictions based on these patterns.

(6) **Deep learning**: It is a subset of machine learning. It is based on neural networks and is a technique for implementing machine learning that has recently proved highly successful. Again, it is dependent on massive datasets to "train" itself.

(7) **Neural Network**: A neural network is a series of algorithms that endeavors to recognize underlying relationships in a set of data through a process that mimics the way the human brain operates. It involves an interconnected group of natural or artificial neurons that uses a mathematical or computational model for information processing based on a connectionistic approach to computation.

(8) **SVM**: A support vector machine (*SVM*) is a supervised machine learning model that uses classification algorithms for two-group classification problems. SVM are a set of supervised learning methods used for classification, regression, and outliers detection.

(9) **Random forest algorithm**: Random forest is a robust machine learning algorithm that can be used for a variety of tasks including regression and classification. It is an ensemble method made up of a large number of small decision trees, called estimators, which each produce their own predictions. The random forest model combines the predictions of the estimators to produce a more accurate prediction.

(10) **Artificial intelligence**: It is the broadest term, having been coined as early as 1955. It is wide-ranging branch of computer science concerned with building smart machines capable of performing tasks that typically require human intelligence.

References

[1] Coronavirus—Worldometer, Worldometer, 2020. 20th April.

[2] Covid-19 Outbreak: It Took the World 13 Days to Get Its Second Million, Hindustan Times, 2020. 16th April.

[3] N. Zhu, et al., A novel coronavirus from patients with pneumonia in China, 2019, N. Engl. J. Med. 382 (8) (2020) 727–733, https://doi.org/10.1056/NEJMoa2001017.

[4] J.H. Tanne, E. Hayasaki, M. Zastrow, P. Pulla, P. Smith, A.G. Rada, Covid-19: how doctors and healthcare systems are tackling coronavirus worldwide, BMJ (2020) m1090, https://doi.org/10.1136/bmj.m1090.

[5] C.I. Paules, H.D. Marston, A.S. Fauci, Coronavirus infections-more than just the common cold, JAMA 323 (8) (2020) 707, https://doi.org/10.1001/jama.2020.0757.

[6] A. Haleem, M. Javaid, R. Vaishya, S.G. Deshmukh, Areas of academic research with the impact of COVID-19, Am. J. Emerg. Med. 38 (7) (2020) 1524–1526, https://doi.org/10.1016/j.ajem.2020.04.022.

[7] C.J. Wang, C.Y. Ng, R.H. Brook, Response to COVID-19 in Taiwan, JAMA 323 (14) (2020) 1341, https://doi.org/10.1001/jama.2020.3151.

[8] R. Sujath, J.M. Chatterjee, A.E. Hassanien, A machine learning forecasting model for COVID-19 pandemic in India, Stochastic Environ. Res. Risk Assess. (2020), https://doi.org/10.1007/s00477-020-01827-8.

[9] S. Zhao, et al., Preliminary estimation of the basic reproduction number of novel coronavirus (2019-nCoV) in China, from 2019 to 2020: a data-driven

analysis in the early phase of the outbreak, Int. J. Infect. Dis. 92 (2020) 214–217, https://doi.org/10.1016/j.ijid.2020.01.050.

[10] S. Tuli, et al., Next generation technologies for smart healthcare: challenges, vision, model, trends and future directions, Internet Technol. Lett. (2020), https://doi.org/10.1002/itl2.145.

[11] C. Huang, et al., Clinical features of patients infected with 2019 novel coronavirus in Wuhan, China, Lancet 395 (10223) (2020) 497–506, https://doi.org/10.1016/S0140-6736(20)30183-5.

[12] A. Depeursinge, et al., Automated classification of usual interstitial pneumonia using regional volumetric texture analysis in high-resolution computed tomography, Invest. Radiol. 50 (4) (2015) 261–267, https://doi.org/10.1097/RLI.0000000000000127.

[13] M.W. Libbrecht, W.S. Noble, Machine learning applications in genetics and genomics, Nat. Rev. Genet. 16 (6) (2015) 321–332, https://doi.org/10.1038/nrg3920.

[14] S. Lalmuanawma, J. Hussain, L. Chhakchhuak, Applications of machine learning and artificial intelligence for Covid-19 (SARS-CoV-2) pandemic: a review, Chaos Solitons Fractals 139 (2020), https://doi.org/10.1016/j.chaos.2020.110059, 110059.

[15] T.T.-Y. Lam, et al., Identifying SARS-CoV-2-related coronaviruses in Malayan pangolins, Nature 583 (7815) (2020) 282–285, https://doi.org/10.1038/s41586-020-2169-0.

[16] A. Banerjee, K. Kulcsar, V. Misra, M. Frieman, K. Mossman, Bats and coronaviruses, Viruses 11 (1) (2019) 41, https://doi.org/10.3390/v11010041.

[17] W. Li, Bats are natural reservoirs of SARS-like coronaviruses, Science 310 (5748) (2005) 676–679, https://doi.org/10.1126/science.1118391.

[18] X. Tang, et al., On the origin and continuing evolution of SARS-CoV-2, Natl. Sci. Rev. 7 (6) (2020) 1012–1023, https://doi.org/10.1093/nsr/nwaa036.

[19] P. Zhou, et al., A pneumonia outbreak associated with a new coronavirus of probable bat origin, Nature 579 (7798) (2020) 270–273, https://doi.org/10.1038/s41586-020-2012-7.

[20] Z. Liu, et al., Composition and divergence of coronavirus spike proteins and host ACE2 receptors predict potential intermediate hosts of SARS-CoV-2, J. Med. Virol. 92 (6) (2020) 595–601, https://doi.org/10.1002/jmv.25726.

[21] S. Su, et al., Epidemiology, genetic recombination, and pathogenesis of coronaviruses, Trends Microbiol. 24 (6) (2016) 490–502, https://doi.org/10.1016/j.tim.2016.03.003.

[22] R. Lu, et al., Genomic characterisation and epidemiology of 2019 novel coronavirus: implications for virus origins and receptor binding, Lancet 395 (10224) (2020) 565–574, https://doi.org/10.1016/S0140-6736(20)30251-8.

[23] X. Xu, et al., Evolution of the novel coronavirus from the ongoing Wuhan outbreak and modeling of its spike protein for risk of human transmission, Sci. China Life Sci. 63 (3) (2020) 457–460, https://doi.org/10.1007/s11427-020-1637-5.

[24] WHO "Novel Coronavirus (COVID-19) Situation", WHO Coronavirus (COVID-19) Dashboard, 7 October 2020, Available from: https://covid19.who.int/?gclid=CjwKCAjwq_D7BRADEiwAVMDdHhgF8UuMrGwDVxV3P00vye5RJih7d_cmPY-xWzxppxsJMqdujdB0PBoCczkQAvD_BwE.

[25] J.T. Wu, et al., Estimating clinical severity of COVID-19 from the transmission dynamics in Wuhan, China, Nat. Med. 26 (4) (2020) 506–510, https://doi.org/10.1038/s41591-020-0822-7.

[26] World Health Organization, Clinical management of severe acute respiratory infection when COVID-19 is suspected: interim guidance V1.2, 2020, Available from: https://www.who.int/publications/i/item/clinical-management-of-covid-19.

[27] J.M. Abduljalil, B.M. Abduljalil, Epidemiology, genome, and clinical features of the pandemic SARS-CoV-2: a recent view, New Microbes New Infect. 35 (2020), https://doi.org/10.1016/j.nmni.2020.100672, 100672.

[28] T. Zhang, Q. Wu, Z. Zhang, Probable pangolin origin of SARS-CoV-2 associated with the COVID-19 outbreak, Curr. Biol. (2020), https://doi.org/10.1016/j.cub.2020.03.022.

[29] J. Riou, C.L. Althaus, Pattern of early human-to-human transmission of Wuhan 2019 novel coronavirus (2019-nCoV), December 2019 to January 2020, Euro Surveill. 25 (4) (2020), https://doi.org/10.2807/1560-7917.ES.2020.25.4.2000058.

[30] Y.-R. Guo, et al., The origin, transmission and clinical therapies on coronavirus disease 2019 (COVID-19) outbreak—an update on the status, Mil. Med. Res. 7 (1) (2020) 11, https://doi.org/10.1186/s40779-020-00240-0.

[31] S. Xia, et al., Fusion mechanism of 2019-nCoV and fusion inhibitors targeting HR1 domain in spike protein, Cell. Mol. Immunol. 17 (7) (2020) 765–767, https://doi.org/10.1038/s41423-020-0374-2.

[32] F. Yu, L. Du, D.M. Ojcius, C. Pan, S. Jiang, Measures for diagnosing and treating infections by a novel coronavirus responsible for a pneumonia outbreak originating in Wuhan, China, Microbes Infect. 22 (2) (2020) 74–79, https://doi.org/10.1016/j.micinf.2020.01.003.

[33] J. Lei, J. Li, X. Li, X. Qi, CT imaging of the 2019 novel coronavirus (2019-nCoV) pneumonia, Radiology 295 (1) (2020) 18, https://doi.org/10.1148/radiol.2020200236.

[34] M. Kermali, R.K. Khalsa, K. Pillai, Z. Ismail, A. Harky, The role of biomarkers in diagnosis of COVID-19—a systematic review, Life Sci. 254 (2020), https://doi.org/10.1016/j.lfs.2020.117788, 117788.

[35] C. Harrison, Coronavirus puts drug repurposing on the fast track, Nat. Biotechnol. 38 (4) (2020) 379–381, https://doi.org/10.1038/d41587-020-00003-1.

[36] P. Domingos, A few useful things to know about machine learning, Commun. ACM (2012), https://doi.org/10.1145/2347736.2347755.

[37] R. Schapire, COS 511: Theoretical Machine Learning, Princeton University, Computer Science Department, 2008.

[38] A. Mukherjee, A. Pal, P. Misra, Data analytics in ubiquitous sensor-based health information systems, in: 2012 Sixth International Conference on Next Generation Mobile Applications, Services and Technologies, Sep. 2012, pp. 193–198, https://doi.org/10.1109/NGMAST.2012.39.

[39] J.T. Senders, et al., An introduction and overview of machine learning in neurosurgical care, Acta Neurochir. (Wien) 160 (1) (2018) 29–38, https://doi.org/10.1007/s00701-017-3385-8.

[40] E. Alpaydin, Introduction to Machine Learning, third ed., The MIT Press, 2014.

[41] L.C. Resende, L.A.F. Manso, W.D. Dutra, A.M. Leite da Silva, Support vector machine application in composite reliability assessment, in: 2015 18th International Conference on Intelligent System Application to Power Systems (ISAP), Sep. 2015, pp. 1–6, https://doi.org/10.1109/ISAP.2015.7325580.

[42] R. Rojas, Unsupervised learning and clustering algorithms, in: Neural Networks, Springer Berlin Heidelberg, Berlin, Heidelberg, 1996, pp. 99–121.

[43] X. Zhu, Semi-Supervised Learning Literature Survey, Eur. Sp. Agency, (Special Publ.), 2006. ESA SP.

[44] P.R. Montague, Reinforcement learning: an introduction, in: R.S. Sutton, A.G. Barto (Eds.), Trends Cogn. Sci, 1999, https://doi.org/10.1016/s1364-6613(99)01331-5.

[45] R.S. Sutton, A.G. Barto, Reinforcement learning: an introduction, IEEE Trans. Neural Netw. (1998), https://doi.org/10.1109/tnn.1998.712192.

[46] P. Wang, X. Zheng, J. Li, B. Zhu, Prediction of epidemic trends in COVID-19 with logistic model and machine learning technics, Chaos Solitons Fractals 139 (2020), https://doi.org/10.1016/j.chaos.2020.110058, 110058.

[47] T. Chakraborty, I. Ghosh, Real-time forecasts and risk assessment of novel coronavirus (COVID-19) cases: a data-driven analysis, Chaos Solitons Fractals 135 (2020) 109850, https://doi.org/10.1016/j.chaos.2020.109850.

[48] X. Xu, et al., A deep learning system to screen novel coronavirus disease 2019 pneumonia, Engineering (2020), https://doi.org/10.1016/j.eng.2020.04.010.

[49] Z. Yang, et al., Modified SEIR and AI prediction of the epidemics trend of COVID-19 in China under public health interventions, J. Thorac. Dis. (2020), https://doi.org/10.21037/jtd.2020.02.64.

[50] World Health Organization, Modes of transmission of virus causing COVID-19: implications for IPC precaution recommendations, 29 March 2020, World Health Organization, Geneva, 2020. Available from: https://www.who.int/news-room/commentaries/detail/modes-of-transmission-of-virus-causing-covid-19-implications-for-ipc-precaution-recommendations.

[51] L. Sun, et al., Combination of four clinical indicators predicts the severe/critical symptom of patients infected COVID-19, J. Clin. Virol. 128 (2020), https://doi.org/10.1016/j.jcv.2020.104431, 104431.

[52] T. Ozturk, M. Talo, E.A. Yildirim, U.B. Baloglu, O. Yildirim, U. Rajendra Acharya, Automated detection of COVID-19 cases using deep neural networks with X-ray images, Comput. Biol. Med. 121 (2020) 103792, https://doi.org/10.1016/j.compbiomed.2020.103792.

[53] A.A. Ardakani, A.R. Kanafi, U.R. Acharya, N. Khadem, A. Mohammadi, Application of deep learning technique to manage COVID-19 in routine clinical practice using CT images: results of 10 convolutional neural networks, Comput. Biol. Med. 121 (2020), https://doi.org/10.1016/j.compbiomed.2020.103795, 103795.

[54] M. Anantpadma, et al., Ebola virus Bayesian machine learning models enable new in vitro leads, ACS Omega 4 (1) (2019) 2353–2361, https://doi.org/10.1021/acsomega.8b02948.

[55] L. Zhang, et al., Virtual screening approach to identifying influenza virus neuraminidase inhibitors using molecular docking combined with machine-learning-based scoring function, Oncotarget 8 (47) (2017) 83142–83154, https://doi.org/10.18632/oncotarget.20915.

[56] B.R. Beck, B. Shin, Y. Choi, S. Park, K. Kang, Predicting commercially available antiviral drugs that may act on the novel coronavirus (SARS-CoV-2) through a drug-target interaction deep learning model, Comput. Struct. Biotechnol. J. (2020), https://doi.org/10.1016/j.csbj.2020.03.025.

[57] J. Fauqueur, A. Thillaisundaram, T. Togia, Constructing large scale biomedical knowledge bases from scratch with rapid annotation of interpretable patterns, in: Proceedings of the 18th BioNLP Workshop and Shared Task, Jul. 2019, pp. 142–151, https://doi.org/10.18653/v1/W19-5016.

[58] P. Richardson, et al., Baricitinib as potential treatment for 2019-nCoV acute respiratory disease, Lancet 395 (10223) (2020) e30–e31, https://doi.org/10.1016/S0140-6736(20)30304-4.

[59] H. Zhang, et al., Deep learning based drug screening for novel coronavirus 2019-nCov, Interdiscip. Sci. Comput. Life Sci. 12 (3) (2020) 368–376, https://doi.org/10.1007/s12539-020-00376-6.

[60] F. Wan, L. Hong, A. Xiao, T. Jiang, J. Zeng, NeoDTI: neural integration of neighbor information from a heterogeneous network for discovering new drug-target interactions, Bioinformatics (2019), https://doi.org/10.1093/bioinformatics/bty543.

[61] M. Smith, J. Smith, Repurposing therapeutics for COVID-19: supercomputer-based docking to the SARS-CoV-2 viral spike protein and viral spike protein-human ACE2 interface, ChemRxiv (2020), https://doi.org/10.26434/chemrxiv.11871402.

[62] G. Liu, et al., Computationally optimized SARS-CoV-2 MHC class I and II vaccine formulations predicted to target human haplotype distributions, Cell Syst. 11 (2) (2020) 131–144.e6, https://doi.org/10.1016/j.cels.2020.06.009.

[63] E. Ong, H. Wang, M.U. Wong, M. Seetharaman, N. Valdez, Y. He, Vaxign-ML: supervised machine learning reverse vaccinology model for improved prediction of bacterial protective antigens, Bioinformatics 36 (10) (2020) 3185–3191, https://doi.org/10.1093/bioinformatics/btaa119.

[64] E. Ong, M.U. Wong, A. Huffman, Y. He, COVID-19 coronavirus vaccine design using reverse vaccinology and machine learning, Front. Immunol. 11 (2020) 1581, https://doi.org/10.3389/fimmu.2020.01581.

[65] S. Chandir, et al., Using predictive analytics to identify children at high risk of defaulting from a routine immunization program: feasibility study, JMIR Public Health Surveill. 4 (3) (2018), https://doi.org/10.2196/publichealth.9681, e63.

[66] J.J. Reeves, H.M. Hollandsworth, F.J. Torriani, R. Taplitz, S. Abeles, M. Tai-Seale, M. Millen, B.J. Clay, C.A. Longhurst, Rapid response to COVID-19: health informatics support for outbreak management in an academic health system, J. Am. Med. Inform. Assoc. 27 (6) (2020) 853–859, https://doi.org/10.1093/jamia/ocaa037.

9

Deep learning methods for analysis of neural signals: From conventional neural network to graph neural network

Chen Liu[a], Haider Raza[b], and Saugat Bhattacharyya[c]
[a]Sun Yat-Sen University, Guangzhou, China. [b]University of Essex, Colchester, United Kingdom. [c]Ulster University, Londonderry, United Kingdom

1. Introduction

Neural signal processing plays an essential role in the field of neuroscience and neuroengineering. Researchers use advanced neural signal recording techniques to extract information for understanding and exploiting the behaviors of neurons [1]. Information within the brain is transmitted as electrical neuronal impulses generated by the membrane potentials that lead to the formation of signature neural signals for all activities. Currently, various invasive and noninvasive recordings are capable of extracting such electrical signals, and they differ among each other in terms of accuracy and transferability. Invasive methods have more resistance to artifacts; however, their applications are normally restricted to certain clinical research where surgery and electrodes implantation is a requisite. Alternatively, noninvasive techniques including electroencephalography (EEG), magnetoencephalography (MEG), and functional magnetic resonance imaging (fMRI) are popularly adopted for human brain research. Numerous computing algorithms are explored to facilitate the processing of signals collected by these recordings mainly dedicated to dealing with noises coming from: (1) the transmission obstacles caused by layers of cortex and (2) brain scalp artifacts from facial muscle movements. By using more state-of-the-art methods, the signal-to-noise ratio is improved, which accelerates progress in the field of neurotechnology. Spatial recording techniques such as fMRI indirectly measures the change in the oxygen level contained within the blood during the activation of neurons,

Advanced Methods in Biomedical Signal Processing and Analysis. https://doi.org/10.1016/B978-0-323-85955-4.00010-7
Copyright © 2023 Elsevier Inc. All rights reserved.

giving us an understanding of the activation of different brain regions during mental tasks. Nevertheless, fMRIs are not chosen for brain-computer interface (BCI) studies because of relevant low temporal resolution and bulkiness. Therefore, fMRI studies are mainly adopted by cognitive and neuroscience scholars working on developing the representation of some activities in the brain. Convenient and cheaper recording modalities exist, mostly EEG, which is largely adopted by the scientific community, and numerous literatures exists that aims at designing robust processing techniques for neural engineering applications. Table 1 lists some popular neural recording techniques so far as we know.

Common neural signal processing methods are usually applied during preprocessing, analyzing, and prediction stages of the mental state detection pipeline. Now we focus mainly on feature extraction and prediction parts. In fact, after the advent of deep learning methods, the use of intricate preprocessing has been reduced to only those methods that are necessary, such as band-pass filtering the raw EEG signal to remove environmental noise. The boundaries among preprocessing and data analyzing have become blurry. Normally, analysis of characteristic features can be categorized into (1) temporal-spatial, (2) spectral, and (3) combination of both aforementioned domains. To extract features from temporal and feature domains, some methods are applied to

Table 1 GNN methods applied to neural data.

Electrical recordings	Single-unit recordings (spikes)	Microelectrodes insert into neurons or placed between adjacent neurons	Invasive
	Local field potential (LFP) recordings	Multielectrode arrays placed inside the brain	Invasive
	Electrocorticography (ECoG)	Implanted electrodes placed on the upper layers ofcerebral cortex	Invasive
	Electroencephalography (EEG)	Electrodes placed on the surface of the scalp	Noninvasive
Magnetic recordings	Magnetoencephalography (MEG)	Measures the magnetic field produced by electrical activity in the brain	Noninvasive
	Functional magnetic resonance imaging (fMRI)	Multielectrode arrays placed inside the brain	Invasive
	Positron emission tomography (PET)	Detects the radioactive compound as a result of metabolic activity caused by brain activity	Invasive

signals collected from multielectrodes, by which interchannel connectivity of neuron activities can be detected and aggregated. Moreover, neural signals can also be considered as a form of time-series data where groups of neurons shift their behaviors dynamically in real time. Therefore, useful features can also be extracted by computational models aimed at operating on the time domain. However, for some signals (such as EEG signals) that are low in time-spatial resolution, frequency analysis is more likely to reveal more information about the oscillatory activities. Usually signals can be decomposed within short-time windows by Fast Fourier transform (FFT) or wavelet transformation into various spectral bands (which are delta, theta, alpha, beta, and gamma). Last but not least, by taking advantage of all three perspectives of time-, frequency-, and spatial domain, researchers can also conduct time-frequency analysis and spatial-frequency analysis on brain signals (see surveys [2–7]). Signals are usually sliced into short-time windows to generate the amount of samples needed. Machine learning methods are implemented to detect feature patterns and predict the mental tasks, usually in the form of unsupervised/self-supervised or supervised learning. As for unsupervised learning, clustering methods like principal component analysis [8] and independent component analysis [9] are mostly used to reduce the dimensions of the feature while also finding the underlying structures of recorded neural data. Generalized linear models [10], support vector machines (SVMs) [11], linear discriminant analysis (LDA) [12], and artificial neural networks (ANNs) [13] are commonly implemented in supervised learning for training feature representation and building predictive relationships between features with their corresponding labels. By using machine learning frameworks, neuroengineers and engineers are capable of training and testing batches of large data collected from recording techniques, letting the data speak for themselves with predictive power.

We have introduced popular neural signal recording techniques and traditional statistical methods to deal with the data collected from them. In this chapter, we are going to introduce deep learning, which is a subset of machine learning methods based on ANNs. Algorithms belonging to machine learning are typically trained with samples and automatically learned for making decisions. Attributed to its strong capability of capturing features and learning representations from those features, it has been broadly adopted to substitute the traditional methods in many fields, including neural signal processing. Furthermore, in recent years, graph neural networks (GNNs) have attracted lots of attention in research communities. Since big data, especially brain signals, are naturally structured as a complex and dynamic graph with multiple attributes, graphs integrated into neural networks have been reasonably adopted to embed both attribute and structural features. Therefore, we continue our journey to GNNs after an overview of basic deep learning frameworks and mechanisms, as a promising trend of methods toward better understanding and utilization of neural signals. Finally, we discuss both the pros and cons of deep learning, emphasizing the importance for developing explainable and reproducible infrastructures for brain data processing in the future.

2. Deep learning methods

Deep learning is a family of algorithms within the bigger family of machine learning. In recent times, deep learning is the most commonly used machine learning tool for numerous prediction-related problems. This branch of machine learning was clarified by LeCun et al. [14] in their co-authored paper "deep learning." Based on the assumption that the world around us is compositional and hierarchically represented, this field has changed the trend of traditional machine learning that required feature engineering and specialist knowledge into parallelized feature parameters learning. Deep learning is broadly used in the fields of computer vision, natural language processing, robotics, and scientific research. When it comes to supervised learning, traditional machine learning methods need to calibrate the design of intricate feature extractors. Classifiers based on general linear models simply partition the input features by a hyperplane, which could not distinguish relevant features from irrelevant ones (such as position, backgrounds, orientation, etc.) for pattern recognition on images and speech. Kernel methods draw raw inputs from a low-dimension to a high-dimension space where the data become more separable as the partition plane number increases, but it lacks the robust generalization between the training and testing samples [15]. In contrast, a key advantage of deep learning as compared to traditional machine learning methods is that it allows automatic feature learning from raw data, progressively from the basic features to assembled patterns within a general-purpose framework [14].

In fact, the concept of deep learning is inspired by the brain. The history of deep learning can be traced back to the 1940s with McCulloch and Pitts, who came up with the idea of threshold binary neurons as a logical inference machine, and expanded by Norbert Wiener with cybernetics, which is the prototype idea of an ANN [16]. In 1957, Frank Rosenblatt proposed the Perceptron concept, which learns through modifying weights of simple neural networks [17]. However, deep learning had been abandoned periodically by many researchers during the 1960s and early 2000s for decades because the idea of continuous neuron back-propagation was not considered. Before this, the traditionally used discrete neurons left the problem of how information flowed mathematically unresolved until the continuous neuron backpropagation mechanism was proposed, when it was possible for a neural network to transmit information back and forth through updating the weight parameters, as there was also no sufficient hardware to carry out parallel computation and limited big data resources. The revival of deep learning began around 2003 under the efforts of LeCun, Hinton and Bengio et al. [14, 18–22], with a series of research projects and workshops aimed at encouraging the use of neural networks among the machine learning scientists. Together with the low-cost general-purpose TFLOPS-class graphic processing units, consumable and practical language frameworks (Torch, Tensorflow, Keras, etc.), and open-source resources have contributed to the new surge in deep learning. This field has been experiencing a flourish of models and mechanisms ever since 2013, evidenced via record-breaking results on numbers of pattern recognition tasks, such as semantic segmentation and target detection, which then spread from computer vision to other research communities. All frameworks emerging in succession are based on the early developed fundamental frameworks following three essential points of deep learning: (1) complex feature representation learning can be divided into simple parameterized linear and nonlinear transform blocks, (2) learning processes can be conducted by gradient-descent methods on parameters to minimize the objective function, and (3) the gradient is calculated by a back-propagation algorithm following chain-rule, which is then computed as the partial derivative of an objective with respect to all parameters and updated throughout the network [23]. These fundamental frameworks are mainly feedforward neural networks (FNNs), convolutional neural networks (CNNs), recurrent neural networks (RNNs), and neural network with attention. Specifically, CNNs are more appropriate to deal with spatially structured data formats, while RNNs are designed mainly for time-sequential ones. Attention mechanisms play an important role in memorizing the important parts of long sequence information by assigning more weights to them. The most impressive model inspired from this idea is called a

Transformer, which applies multihead attention mechanisms and results in state-of-the-art performance in language translations.

In this chapter, we will provide a detailed introduction to their basic structures and their recent adaptation to neural signal processing. Moreover, these models are intended and designed to deal with data format collected from brain activity signals; therefore, explainability and interpretability of the models are also an important point of consideration when designing a deep learning-based model. Despite its sufficient representation ability and effective practical results, deep learning results are still met with suspicion because of its black model, and improving the explainability/interpretability of these models is still an open area of research. Rather than drawing inference from a data-driven perspective, neuroscientists and bioengineers are searching for tools that are theoretically explainable and data efficient, and hence, are two central considerations for many scientific uses [14]. Through deep learning, we are still exploring what the learned features from various neural signal data represent and how to draw a significant understanding/learning from networks when it comes to concrete study cases. Meanwhile, neuroscience researches on human and animal brain signals are also inexhaustible fountains for new deep learning ideas. Current deep learning methods are quite efficient in learning from bottom-to-up representations but less capable to formulate up-to-bottom concepts and regulate further representation learning as humans consciously. New findings using deep learning methods as tools can be reciprocal to the artificial intelligence research communities as well. Therefore, it is mutually beneficial to bring deep learning methods for data processing with neural signals. We are going to elaborate on the mainstream methods used in this field and the papers mainly published within 5 years. Since neural signal encoding and decoding are mainly studied for brain functional exploration and engineering settings, there is little differences between those two branches of studies: the latter one needs more careful model design considering transferability and timeliness. It means that good algorithms are robust so that they allow neural control devices across subjects and sessions and predict outputs rapidly with every sequence of incoming online signals.

2.1 Some discussion on CNNs and RNNs

CNNs were inspired by the discovery of information hierarchically processed in the ventral visual cortex pathway. Neurophysiologists Hubel and Wiesel [24] experimented on a cat's brain using different types of visual stimuli. They found that "simple cells" in the primary visual cortex are only responsive to edges in certain receptive fields. But "complex cells" detect edges despite their variation of orientation and locations. The former cell types are local detectors of specific edge features while the latter can be viewed as position-permutable aggregation of the local information. It was Yann LeCun who brought up the ConvNet framework (1998) that is the foundation of modern CNN structures. There are two key components in CNN: convolutional layers and pooling layers, respectively. In convolutional layers, filters are adopted to scan over the data array by dot-product and summation, before which usually padding with zero is added around the edges to keep the dimension unchanged. Those filters can be regarded as a matrix representing different local pattern detectors with a set of weights. This process is ideally similar to the functional activities of simple and complex neurons mentioned earlier. Usually feature maps are acquired for filters accordingly and set into a nonlinear activation (usually a ReLU transformation) as input of the next layer (see Fig. 1). The next component is the pooling layer, which is simply an aggregation operation (sum, average, max, and more) of small pooling filters conducted on the feature map out of computation complexity and translation invariance consideration. A typical ConvNet is constructed by sequential input-hidden-output structured layers combined by a convolutional layer (including nonlinearity activation), a pooling layer, and fully connected layer, resulting in a learned representation (see Fig. 2). Normally the sigmoid or softmax function is utilized following a fully connected layer for label prediction. Popular CNN architectures are LeNet [25], ResNet [26], AlexNet [27].

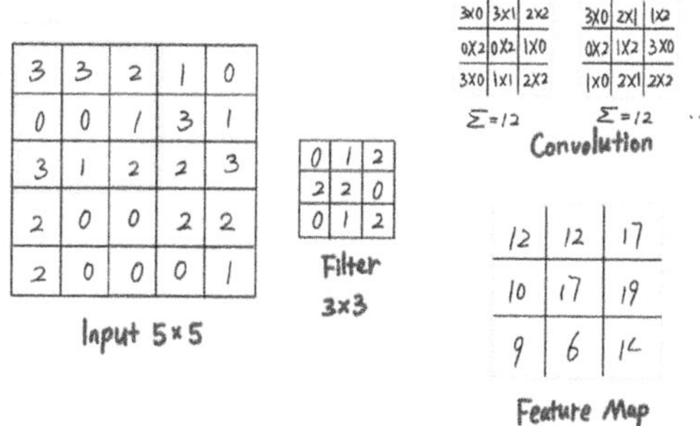

Fig. 1 Convolution operations: A 3 × 3 filter is going to slide on the 5 × 5 input feature matrix with one stride, from upper left to right bottom. The process generates several pieces of element-wise multiplicated and summed values that form the feature map.

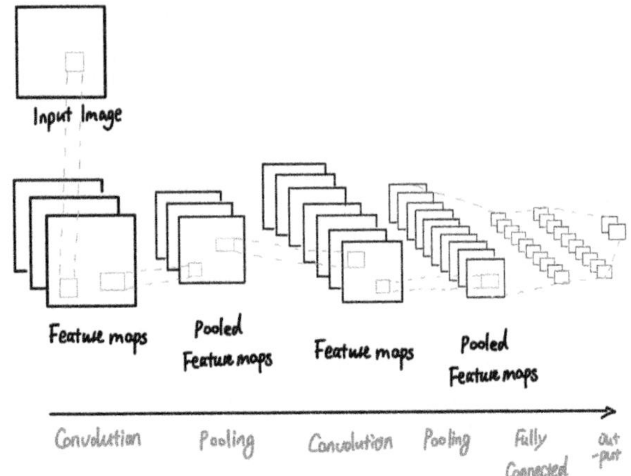

Fig. 2 A framework case of convolutional neural networks.

Local connection and shared weights allow CNNs to be more computationally efficient than a fully connected neural network.

Another framework, RNNs, is a class of self-connected neural networks that allow previous outputs to iteratively combine with hidden states as inputs for next time steps. They are designed to deal with sequential data. A simple RNN's structure is composed of the following: (1) a time step t, (2) hidden states in which h^t is the nonlinear activation of weighted current inputs x^t adding weighted hidden states h^{t-1} resulted from step $t-1$, and (3) outputs y^t, which is the nonlinear transformation of weighted h^t (see Fig. 3).

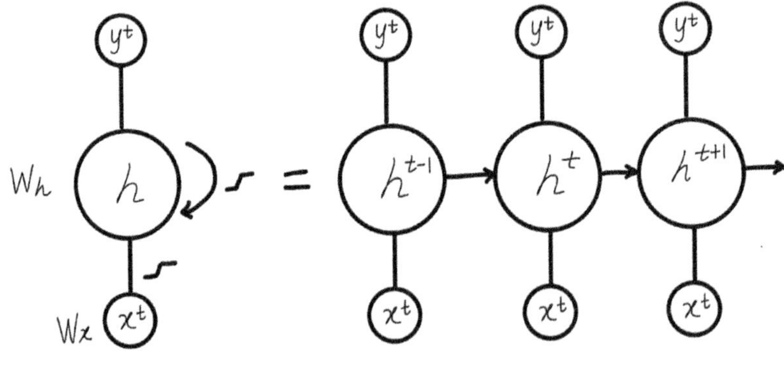

Fig. 3 A simple RNN framework. A hidden state h^t is the nonlinear activation of weighted current input x^t adding weighted hidden state h_{t-1} from step $t-1$.

Bi-directory RNN (BRNN) is another architecture [28] that has two hidden layers learned from the forward and backward sequences separately and combined to calculate outputs. Early research on RNNs took place in the 1980s [29–31], which are the basis for long-short-term memory neural networks (LSTMs) proposed by Hochreiter and Schmidhuber [32]. Vanilla RNNs (Rumelhart & Hinton et al., 1986) with backpropagation through time (BPTT) [33] suffer from the problem of gradient vanishing, which means information is usually lost as it travels through long sequences. LSTM has introduced a state cell C_t to control the information passing through the network through different gates. Specifically, those gates are forget (which is indeed do not forget), input and output gates represented by a scalar between [0, 1] and calculated using a sigmoid activation of a weighted combination (W_f, W_i, W_o, respectively) of concatenated inputs of vector $x^{(t)}$, and hidden state $h_{(t-1)}$ separately. The larger the value of the scalar, the more the information it allows to flow through. In simpler terms, the LSTM works as follows: First, the forget layer decides what information to throw away from the state cell. Second, new information is stored in the cell state by the input gate. Then a tanh layer computes a new candidate $\widetilde{C}_t$ on weighted (W_C) concatenated inputs. Then we add a forget gate of $f_t * C_{t-1}$ and gated candidate $i_t * \widetilde{C}_t$. Finally, the hidden state h_t is decided by multiplication of the output gate o_t with tanh-activated C_t (see Fig. 4). Ever since LSTMs, many studies have redesigned the memory gates, in which Cho et al. [34] proposed a gated recurrent unit (GRU). It is more computationally efficient and popularly used because it combines forget and input gates into a single

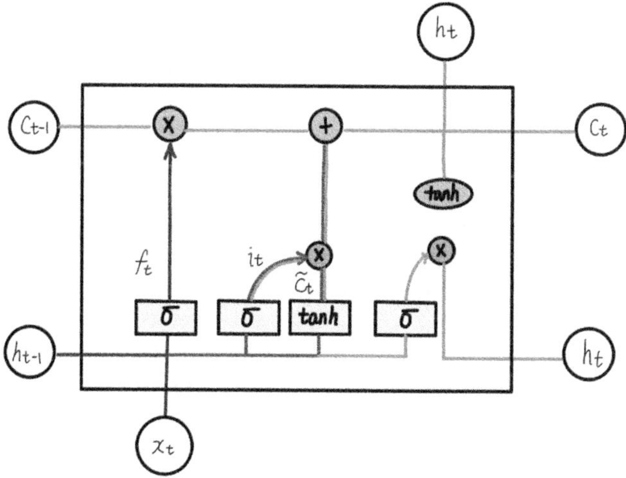

Fig. 4 LSTM frameworks. *Different colors/shapes* denote different gates and operations. Forget gate: *blue line with arrow* f_t; input gate: *red line* i_t; update information: *green line connecting* h_{t-1}; and output: *orange line connecting to x and* h_t. *Pink circle* indicates element-wise operations, and *yellow box* represents neural network layer.

"update gate" for merged units of state-hidden cells. Similar to RNN, LSTM-based methods can also be bi-directional.

fMRI data can be analyzed to recognize brain disorder diagnosis within CNN frameworks. Preprocessed 4D volume (3D brain plus time dimension) data can be considered as a sequence of continuous 2D or 3D functional activation images. Sarraf and Tofighi [35] proposed a DL (deep learning) pipeline to recognize Alzheimer's disease (AD) from normal brains. They adjusted LeNet-5 [25] as two Conv layers with a pooling layer following, and two fully connected layers with sigmoid activation for final binary output, which achieved 96.85% accuracy. Furthermore, by inspecting multidegree neurodegenerative process of AD with ResNet, Ramazan et al. [36] improved the results of their fine-tuned model for multiprogress AD stages with an accuracy of 100%, 96.85%, 97.38%, 97.43%, and 97.40%, respectively, which were also supported by other performance metrics such as Recall and F1 score. Intuitively, ResNet [26] introduced a block of residuals that divides the inputs as identity and residual parts, then lets the identity part skip to the next layer and only "learn" from the residual part. It allows the network to go deeper without losing efficiency. With a Deep Network Optimizer designed, Aradhya and Ashfahani [37] were able to decide the optimal number of fully connected layers and nodes of CNN architecture for predicting attention deficit hyperactivity disorder (ADHD). They adopted evolutionary strategies for the last fully connected layer, which controls the node and layer's growth with T randomly initialized nodes and layers interpolated before it. The growth of the nodes and layers is regulated by the network's minimum observed network bias and variance, and node pruning was decided by the $|mean - sd|$ of expected outputs. The accuracy of the ADHD200 dataset was significantly higher (80.39%) as compared to that of 3D-CNN (69.15%), in which volumetric hidden layers are settled between input and output layers. It was popularly adopted by researchers [38–45] on other neural diseases. A recent work by Kam et al. [46] derived brain functional networks (BFNs) from MRI (rs-fMRI). They combined the multiple paired static and dynamic BFNs for individuals through two 3D conv-pool structures before concatenating them to a fully connected layer, resulting in a 10% improvement of diagnostic performance for early-stage mild cognitive impairment.

EEG data can be formatted and illustrated as time-frequency sequences. Signals collected are characterized by increase or decrease of amplitude in the temporal domain, which can be observed as a power increase and decrease of a particular frequency band in the spectral domain. Specifically, according to

Zhang et al. [47], the EEG signal classification problem can be elaborated as: "Each trial is T-second long, each channel representing an electrode is a node, so an EEG recording can be interpreted as $\gamma_{i \in [1,n]} = [s_1^i, s_i^i, ..., S_k^i] \in R^k$ through $k = T \times f$ time points, where f is the sampling frequency and s is the measurement at time point t. The raw EEG features of a trial T is $X_T = [r_1, r_2, ... r_n] \in R^{n \times k}$." CNN architectures are leveraged for classification in different settings such as Brain-Computer Interface (BCI) [2, 48–55], mental disease of clinical environment [56–65], and cognitive monitoring [3, 66–71]. Movement-related imagery or motor imagery (MI) is heavily explored in the field of BCI. Schirrmeister and colleagues found that a shallow CNN architecture with techniques of a cropped training strategy reached a comparable accuracy (84.0%) to the widely used filter bank common spatial patterns (FBCSP) algorithm, for the purpose of decoding imagined or executed tasks. They also visualized the learned features and found components in different frequency bands contributing to classification. A compact CNN (EEGNet) inspired by the Filter-Bank Common Spatial Pattern (FSCSP) was introduced by Lawren and colleagues (2018) for EEG-based paradigms. This architecture applies a temporal filter with length half of the sampling rate and a spatial filter with a depth of the channels separately. Then a depth-wise and point-wise convolution was applied together to extract movement-related cortical potential (MRCP) and other types of EEG signals. Another way is to construct images with time-frequency spectra of EEG signals [72]. By combining the entire theta and alpha band as well as beta band to STFT plots, motor-related ERD and ERS signals are identified.

RNNs are also attempted by some researches to decode EEG recordings. LSTM was attempted [73] on DEAP dataset for extracting emotional features, and a fully connected layer classifies these into low/high arousal, valence, and liking, resulting in an average accuracy of 85%, 85.45%, and 87.99%, respectively, compared with the traditional methods. Tsiouris et al. [74] selected a two-layer LSTM network to predict seizure happenings in 185 samples, with low false prediction rates (FPR) of 0.11–0.02 false alarms per hour. Similarly using fMRI recordings, Dvornek et al. [75] proposed the use of LSTMs to predict individuals with autism and typical controls from multisourced (Autism Brain Imaging Data Exchange) resting-state fMRI time series, achieving an accuracy of 68.9%. One recent study [76] showed that speech can be decoded from human brain signals directly and accurately at the word level. Through encoding ECoG using RNNs and then decoding it word by word, their model reached an average word error rate as low as 3%. Another study [77] conducted spike recording level on rats and using neural activity recorded from a bunch of hippocampal place cells compared between the performance of point process filter and LSTMs in decoding 2D movement trajectory of a rate. Results showed that LSTM is more computationally efficient than point-process filter and deals with raw inputs directly. It was also adopted by Yoo et al. [78] as a classifier to predict three mental tasks and showed it superior (83.3% accuracy) over traditional SVM (37.50%) and LDA methods (37.96%).

As for other recording techniques, Hasasneh et al. [79] applied CNN structure to identify cardiac and ocular artifacts from MEG data and revealed a medium accuracy of 94.4% with augmented samples, which indicated high reliability of their proposed DCNN model. Dash et al. [80] applied CNNs on the spatial, spectral, and temporal features extracted from the imagined and spoken speech MEG data collected. The results indicated the possibility of decoding speech phase activity directly from MEG signals. There are more studies based on CNNs, RNNs, or both. But their purposes are more or less the same: extracting the spatial-temporal information extensively by whatever means appropriate from neural recordings for representation learning. We are going to introduce them in the next section.

2.2 Hybrid models

A survey by Craik et al. [4] has shown that only 10% of the EEG researches employs a stand-alone RNN architecture. It is usually combined with CNN to capture both temporal and spatial information, because a stand-alone RNN is time-consuming, but EEG signals are generally formed as a long sequence [47] based on the topology of brain. Also for fMRI datasets, hybrid structures are more likely to be adopted. Prosperous hybrid methods based on CNNs and RNNs have been adopted to process neural signals in recent years. Since deep learning itself is a toolbox of representative learning, other combined methods such as generative structures, dimension-reducing approaches, and transfer methods mainly deal with the shortage of data and high variance inter-/intra-subjects. Compared with communities such as computer vision (CV) and natural language processing (NLP), benchmark datasets are still highly demanded, and data collected from various studies are restricted by the available subjects. Moreover, neural activities vary between individuals and times. So, it is necessary that algorithms can be generalized across sessions or even subjects. Therefore, generating more samples and transferring models adaptively are important for neural activity analysis. We are going to introduce hybrid models as (1) CNNs + LSTMs and

(2) generative models such as Autoencoders. But in practice, there are more hybrid possibilities with diverse available methods.

Li et al. [81] combined a series of 3D CNN filters to extract features from individual 3D images in fMRI image sequences of AD. Then the output feature maps were fed into an LSTM network, and their C3d-LSTM model was able to directly tangle the 4D volumes and showed better results than using functional connectivity, 2D, or 3D fMRI data. Another ConvRNN pipeline was proposed [82] to identify individuals with resting-state fMRI data, which achieved better results than RNN alone. The results showed better extraction of local features between neighboring regions of interest (ROIs). A study by Spampinato et al. [83] applied RNNs to capture EEG features when viewing different categories of pictures, and then projected the images onto the learned feature dimensions through CNNs, which allowed the machine learning process to leverage neural signal features. It reached a competitive performance and generalization compared with solely CNN classification on images. Another study [84] detected epileptiform discharge with various combinations of CNN and RNN, resulting in the area under the ROC curve (AUC) for the test of 0.94, 47.4% sensitivity, and 98.0% specificity.

Autoencoder is an unsupervised neural network that transforms inputs into latent spaces and then tries to reconstruct the original inputs from those embeddings. The smaller the distance between original inputs and constructed outputs, the better the hidden layers have learned the latent attributes. Suk et al. [85] focused on time-varying patterns of functional networks (such as inherent in rs-fMRI et al.) and proposed a novel architecture to recognize mild cognitive impairment (MCI) disease. They adopted a deep autoencoder to transform the original inputs to low embedding spaces, then used a Hidden Markov Model (HMM) to catch the dynamic characteristics to estimate the likelihood of rs-fMRI signals with MCI and normal labels. This method outperformed the other mentioned comparative models on two datasets (ADNI2 cohort, In-house cohort) consistently. A study [86] resorted to using autoencoders to denoise EEG artifacts noises and learned representation, then was fed into an XGBoost classifier with K trees for estimating intersubjects movement. Comprehensive exploring was conducted on different normalization methods, training data size, as well as hidden neuron size. Said et al. [87] presented a joint learning approach of EEG and EMG signals by a multimodal stacked autoencoder architecture by projecting EEG and MEG signals to a combined latent representation, which contributed to the accuracy stage of emotion classification.

There are models that combine preprocessed neural signal data with DL structures. However since the power of DL comes from its strong representative learning in end-to-end style, we indeed want to minimize such kinds of preprocessing. In fact, how to tailor DL methods into a specific domain with their end-to-end advantage retained is of significant importance, which will be discussed in Section 5.

2.3 Attention mechanism in deep learning

The attention mechanism is motivated by biology that eye fovea only focuses on patches of objective within the receptive field. Such a mechanism in animals is reasonable because it allows only relevant information to be processed and manipulates the environment in the same way. Attention mechanism in deep learning can be viewed as a vector of importance weights: to predict one element of inputs, we need to estimate the attention vector correlated to other elements and sum their weighted values for a final prediction. In fact, it is a mechanism of soft address searching, during which a task-related query vector Q is given to calculate the attention distribution with a key (K as a vector) and then added to the value (V as a vector). It takes the form of an attention pooling as:

$$f(X) = \rho\left(\sum_{x \in X} \alpha(x, w)\phi(x)\right)$$

where $\phi(x)$ is an embedding of x. There are numerous attention functions $\alpha(x, w)$. The popular ones are weighted dot products and sum of nonlinear transformations of weighted products. Seq2Seq model is a popular model in machine translation. It has an encoder-decoder architecture with two parts: (1) the encoder takes the input sequence and outputs a context state of the sequence as distribution of attention. (2) The decoder takes this context vector with new input to the network to get a prediction for the next input. Both decoder and encoder are usually LSTM or GRU. But it has difficulties in memorizing long sequences and therefore loses information at the beginning of a sequence after processing the whole sentence. Attention mechanism [88] is hence the most appropriate way to deal with this problem (see Fig. 5). Suppose we have an encoder structure that has a hidden state $(h_1, h_2, ..., h_T)$ and a decoder with hidden state of s_{t-1}. Correlation of each input position j and the current output position is calculated as $e_{tj} = a(s_{t-1}, h_j)$ for which a is an operation of correlation: weighted dot product $e_t = s_{t-1}^T h$, then using softmax to get a normalized distribution of α_{tj}. After this,

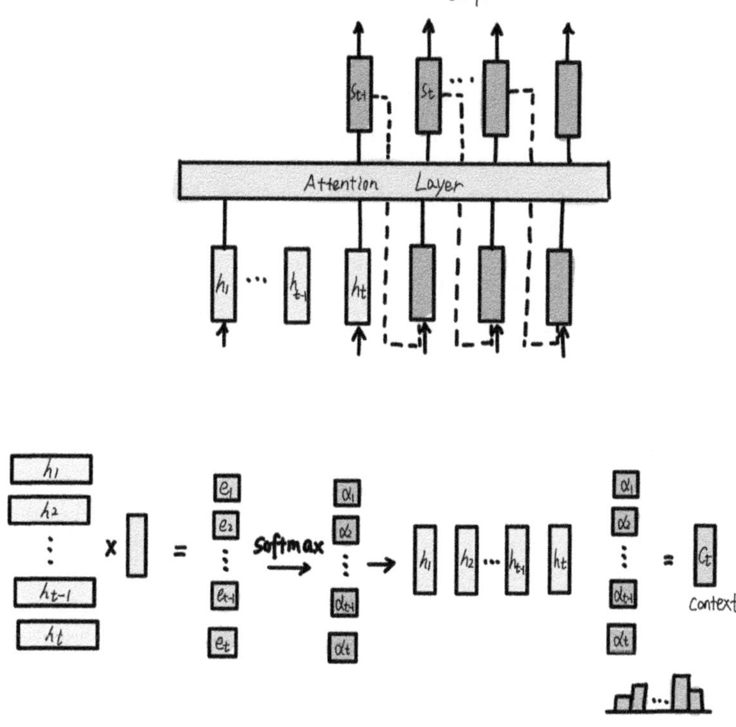

Fig. 5 Seq2Seq with attention model.

corresponding context vector is calculated as $c_t = \sum_{j=1}^{T}\alpha_{tj}h_j$. Based on all this, the next hidden state and outputs as $s_t = f(s_{t-1}, y_{t-1}, c_t)$ and $p(y_t|y_1, ..., y_{t-1}, x) = g(y_{i-1}, s_i, c_i)$, respectively (see Fig. 5). Moreover, multiheads attention proposed by Vaswani et al. [89] has been popular in recent studies. It projects the injury key and value array into multiple subspaces before concatenating them together. Specifically given the N inputs as $X = [x_1, x_2, ..., x_n]$, three initial vectors as K, Q, V are calculated by weighted matrix, respectively. Then scaled dot-product attention z_i is calculated by the formula:

$$\text{Attention}(Q, KV) = \text{softmax}\left(\frac{QK^T}{\sqrt{d_k}}\right)V$$

Multihead is the operation that segments the inputs into several parts and calculates the attention scores accordingly. Finally a concatenation of z_i applied with a linear transformation W_o gets the final output vector of attention for inputs X. We will mention attention again when introducing graph attention networks (GATs).

3. Graph neural network

3.1 Transition from basic models to graph-based models

When it comes to graphs, representing node i takes not only its attributes but also the features of its neighbors into consideration. Different mechanisms are designed to aggregate the embeddings of node i's neighbors to strengthen the representation of the central node. Therefore, models based on graphs are expressive at learning both structural and attributes information at the same time. In nature and society, data are easily found or can be organized as graphs. For example, it is reasonable to represent molecules as graphs with atoms as nodes, bonds as edges, and features could be a type of atom or their charge. It is also common to study social network connection by a graph with individuals as nodes and connections as edges, while node features could be attributes (such as ages, genders, etc.) of the individual and the connections. As for the case of neural processing, viewing them as complicated connectivity and adopting graph-based models for analyzing brain connectomes is a prior and appropriate choice. Research communities have been traditionally applying methods of connectivity for studying neural cells, usually with many predefined measurements and filters to diminish noises and amplify ROIs. Also as in the introduction of Section 2, deep learning methods based on CNNs and RNNs have provided researchers with more flexible approaches to deal with raw signals. In recent years, graph-based methods were integrated into deep learning that led to many longitudinal researches and applications. One advantage of graph-based deep learning is its encoding effectiveness in non-Euclidean spaces.

3.2 GNN: Convolutional, attention, and message passing flavors

GNNs used to be categorized into spectral-based and spatial-based. In fact, the boundary between them is blurry because the true spectral operators are computationally intricate. After being approximated by polynomial function, it can be considered similar to spatial convolution essentially, which is more obvious after our following elaboration.

We are going to introduce them based on how messages are passing on the graph into three "flavors" of GNN layers: (1) convolutional layers, (2) attentional layers, and (3) message-passing layers [90]. Their way of representing the input node x_i into a hidden embedding are formularized as follows: (1) $\mathbf{h}_i = \phi(\mathbf{x}_i, \oplus_{j \in \mathcal{N}_i} c_{ij} \psi(\mathbf{x}_j))$ where features of neighbors are aggregated with fixed weights c_{ij}, (2) $\mathbf{h}_i = \phi(\mathbf{x}_i, \oplus_{j \in \mathcal{N}_i} \psi(\mathbf{x}_i, \mathbf{x}_j))$ where features of neighbors are aggregated with implicit weights via attention, and (3) $\mathbf{h}_i = \phi(\mathbf{x}_i, \oplus_{j \in \mathcal{N}_i} a(\mathbf{x}_i, \mathbf{x}_j) \psi(\mathbf{x}_j))$ where arbitrary vectors ("messages") are computed to be sent across edges. Here x_i and x_j denote node i and its neighboring nodes j, ϕ, and ψ indicate any function conducted on nodes, while $\oplus$ represents any aggregation function (such as sum, average, or max functions) that are permutation invariant.

First, let us consider convolution on graphs. We have already mentioned convolution operation in Section 2.1 while discussing CNN structures. Convolution is straightforward as Euclidean structure as dot-wise multiplication, because at grid-level, the relationship between pixels are invariant. When it comes from grid to graph case, convolution needs to be shifted from spatial-temporal domain to spectral domain. Based on spectral graph theory, Bruna et al. [91] developed a graph convolution. Several improved models have been proposed ever since, such as ChebyNet by Defferrard et al. [92], GCN by Kipf and Welling [93], and SGC by Wu et al. [94]. Spectral graph theory is the study of graph attributes by using eigenvalues and eigenvectors of the Laplacian matrix. Here, we take Kipf and colleagues' work to clarify graph convolution in detail. Given an undirected graph containing n nodes, the normalized graph Laplacian matrix is a mathematical representation of such a graph. This matrix is defined by $L = D - A$, where A is the adjacency matrix and D is the diagonal matrix of node degrees. It is characterized by the following properties: (1) Nonzero elements are only in the position of central vertex (degree numbers) and one-hop neighbors (negative 1), respectively. (2) It is a real symmetric positive semidefinite. With the second property, it can be decomposed as $L = U \Lambda U^T$, where $U = [u_0, u_1, ..., u_{n-1}] \in R^{n*n}$ is the matrix eigenvector, U^T is the conjugate transpose of U, and Λ is the diagonal matrix of eigenvalues. The elements of Λ in its ith row and column are $\hat{\theta}$. By using graph Fourier transform, the original feature matrix x (in which x_i denotes node i's feature vector) is projected into orthonormal space as $\hat{x}$, where the basis is formed by U, the eigenvectors of normalized Laplacian matrix above, and with x can be restored as $x = \hat{x} U$ by inverse graph Fourier transformation. Here, we come to the definition of graph convolution of input x with a filter $g \in R^n$:

$$\mathbf{x}^*{}_G == \mathbf{U}(\mathbf{U}^T \mathbf{x} \odot \mathbf{U}^T \mathbf{g})$$

where $\odot$ denotes the element-wise product. Filters on the graph can be defined as $\mathbf{g}_\theta = \mathrm{diag}(\mathbf{U}^T\mathbf{g})$ and the previous formula is rewritten as:

$$\mathbf{x} *_G \mathbf{g}_\theta = \mathbf{U}\mathbf{g}_\theta\mathbf{U}^T\mathbf{x}$$

It seems a good solution to the convolution on graph structure, while directly learns the eigenvalues of U^T, but it is not appropriate for: (1) Generalization problems, that is permutation of the graph results in change of eigenbasis and learnable filters cannot be applied to graphs with different structures. (2) Eigen-decomposition computationally complex as $O(n^3)$. Kipf et al. then reduced the complexity by approximately learning g_θ. What they did is based on ChebNet promoted by Defferrard et al. [92]. Cheb-Net replaced g_θ with $T_i(\mathbf{x}) = 2\mathbf{x}T_{i-1}(\mathbf{x}) - T_{i-2}(\mathbf{x})$ by Chebyshev polynomials of Λ, where $\widetilde{\Lambda} = 2\Lambda/\lambda_{\max} - \mathbf{I_n}$. Here the Chebyshev polynomials adopted are obtained from recurrent equations: $T_i(\mathbf{x}) = 2\mathbf{x}T_{i-1}(\mathbf{x}) - T_{i-2}(\mathbf{x})$ with $T_0(x) = 1$ and $T_1(x) = x$. It can be induced that $T_i(\widetilde{\mathbf{L}}) = \mathbf{U}T_i(\widetilde{\Lambda})\mathbf{U}^T$, now a definition of graph convolution with the form of:

$$\mathbf{x} *_G \mathbf{g}_\theta = \sum_{i=0}^{K} \theta_i T_i(\widetilde{\mathbf{L}})\mathbf{x}$$

with $\widetilde{\mathbf{L}} = 2\mathbf{L}/\lambda_{\max} - \mathbf{I_n}$, where K denotes the number of layers. By projecting the spectrum into $[-1, 1]$ linearly, the filters are defined spatially. It then can independently extract the local features regardless of the graph structures, which is why we said that there is no clear boundaries between spectral and spatial methods in practice. GCN simplified ChebNet further by bringing in a first-order approximation of its Chebyshev polynomials. With assumption $K = 1$, $\lambda_{\max} = 2$, and $\theta = \theta_0 = -\theta_1$, graph convolution can be expressed as:

$$\mathbf{x} *_G \mathbf{g}_\theta = \theta\left(\mathbf{I_n} + \mathbf{D}^{-1/2}\mathbf{A}\mathbf{D}^{-1/2}\right)\mathbf{x}$$

which further extended to multichannel inputs and outputs as:

$$\mathbf{H} = \mathbf{X} *_G \mathbf{g}_\Theta = f(\overline{\mathbf{A}}\mathbf{X}\Theta)$$

where $\overline{\mathbf{A}} = \mathbf{I_n} + \mathbf{D}^{-1/2}\mathbf{A}\mathbf{D}^{-1/2}$ (a normalized trick to replace A).

Attention is considered one of the most elegant mechanisms in deep learning frameworks, which we have already explained in Section 2.3. Unsurprisingly, there are also attempts at adapting this mechanism for GNNs, as the second "flavor" of attention-based GNNs such as: MoNet [95], GAT [96], and GaAN [97]. As aforementioned, spectral-based convolution depends on the structure of the graph itself; therefore, features learned are limited within the isomorphic graphs. Practically, methods are indeed spatially based by which convolution is directly defined on the graph rather than graph spectral. GAT is a typical case where multihead attention mechanisms were used on graph embedding learning (see Fig. 6). Specifically, a graph attention layer has inputs of $\mathbf{h} = \{h_1, h_2, ..., h_N\}$, $h_i \in R^F$ + and outputs of $\mathbf{h} = \{h_1, h_2, ..., h_N\}$, $h_i \in R^F$ +, where N denotes number of nodes and F, F' denote dimensions of feature vectors. A mask trick is introduced to only compute node j's importance to node i without considering graph structure. A masked self-attention operation is applied to inputs as $e_{ij} = a(\mathbf{W}h_i, \mathbf{W}h_j)$, with a a projection from $R^{F'} \times R^{F'} \to R$ and $W \in R^{F' \times F}$ a weight matrix shared by all the h_i. By multiplying a shared weight W, nodes' features are augmented after projected to a higher dimension. Weighted features of nodes

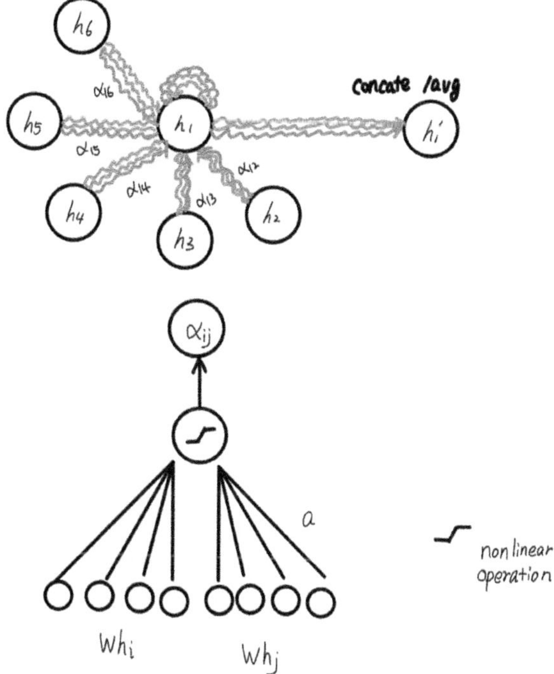

Fig. 6 *Upper*: Multihead attention with $K = 3$ heads (denoted by three different colors) are applied independently by node 1 on its five neighbors. The new embeddings of node 1 h'_1 is calculated by concatenating or averaging aggregated features from each head. *Bottom*: Attention coefficient α_{ij} is obtained by a LeakyReLU activation operated to weighted $(\mathbf{W}h_i, \mathbf{W}h_j)$ calculated from a weight vector a).

i and j are concatenated as input to a single-layer FNN with LeakyReLU activation, resulting in a scalar representing their correlations. Afterwards, softmax is conducted on e_{ij} to get the normalized attention coefficient as α_{ij}. Updated feature of node i is then calculated as

$$h_i' = \sigma\left(\sum_{j \in \mathcal{N}_i} \alpha_{ij} W h_j\right)$$

where $\sigma(\cdot)$ is the activation function. Multihead mechanism is used for improving fitting capacity, which is the same as that in Transformers, namely using multiple W^k to calculate self-attention and concatenating the results as

$$h_i' = \|_{k=1}^{K} \sigma\left(\sum_{j \in \mathcal{N}_s} \alpha_{ij}^k \mathbf{W}^k h_j\right)$$

($\|$) indicates concatenate operation, and $W^k \in R^{T' \times F}$). In final layer for prediction, the authors' choice of averaging is a more sensible way to get latent representation of node i as

$$h_i' = \sigma\left(\frac{1}{K} \sum_{k=1}^{K} \sum_{j \in \mathcal{N}_i} \alpha_{ij}^k \mathbf{W}^k h_j\right)$$

Their model achieved promising results on transductive and inductive tasks for several different datasets. Essentially, GCN and GAT structure are based on leveraging the local stationary of representing the central node by aggregating its neighbors' features, yet in the former adopted Laplacian matrix, the latter tends to the attention coefficient. The same idea is also why there is strictly no difference between spectral and spatial methods as we mentioned. The only difference is that GAT is computed node-wise for iteratively calculating attention coefficients from embeddings of neighbors and the center node, which is free from the Laplacian matrix shackles and more powerful on inductive tasks.

Message passing focuses on computing arbitrary vectors (messages) across edges. In convolutional and attention layer cases, we pass the raw neighbor node features by some constant. Here, target and source vertices collaborate together to compute what the message is. Representative works are interaction networks [98], Message Passing Neural Network (MPNN) [99] and GraphNets [100]. MPNN is, in fact, a framework abstracted from previous models, including GCN and Interaction Network. Given an undirected graph G, node features and edge features are fed into the

MPNN framework for message passing phase and readout phase operation afterwards:

$$m_v^{t+1} = \sum_{w \in N(v)} M_t(h_v^t, h_w^t, c_{vw}) h_v^{t+1} = U_t(h_v^t, m_v^{t+1}) \hat{y} = R(\{h_v^T | v \in G\})$$

Specifically, hidden states of each node are updated over message passing using message functions M_t and update functions U_t. Take a single node h_i and single step t for an explanation: a differentiable learnable function Mt takes the input of source node h_j, $h_j \in N_i$, target node h_i, and edge e_{ij} between them, which is summed as a message vector. Then another function U_t is applied to update the hidden state of node h_i. This message passing and update process is conducted over T time steps parallel with the same function applied to each node. In the readout phase, the final hidden states of all the nodes are fed into a readout function R, which is invariant to the order of nodes. Actually, GCN can be regarded as a form of MPNN, where

$$M(h_v^t, h_w^t) = \tilde{L}_{v,w} h_w^t$$

and

$$U(h_v^t, m_v^{t+1}) = \sigma(m_v^{t+1})$$

(v, w denote node v and node w). In a word, GCN, GTA, and MPNN follow the same idea of representing node i by aggregating information passing interaction of itself and corresponding neighbors, therefore can be interchangeable in form.

3.3 Dynamic GNNs

Dynamic networks change over time, which allow models to leverage not only structural but also temporal patterns. According to Skarding et al. [101], it is defined as: "A graph $G = (V, E)$ where $V = (v, t_s, t_e)$, with v a vertex of the graph and t_s, t_e, respectively, the start and end timestamps for the existence of the vertex (with $t_s \leq t_e$). $E = (u, v, t_s, t_e)$, with u, $v \in V$ and t_s, t_e are, respectively, the start and end timestamps for the existence of the edge (with $t_s \leq t_e$)." It can be viewed from different representation granularity as static or dynamic flexibly. For example, links in a continuous representation can be aggregated into snapshots as discrete representations. Distinct snapshots can be furthermore combined into an edge-weighted representation and finally without any weight information as a static network. Therefore, the dynamic and static concepts are relative in terms of network structures. When we consider from a link dynamics perspective, there are two kinds of dynamic networks under research: temporal networks and evolving networks. Temporal networks are highly dynamic, and each timestamp is nontrivial; links are proper to be treated as an event lasting for periods. In contrast, on evolving networks, links appearance and disappearance are regarded as discrete events on such networks persisting long enough for an instant snapshot to capture enough structure information. Similarly, node dynamics is also another way to distinguish dynamic networks; meanwhile, it can be combined with any kind of link dynamics together.

Dynamic networks are regarded as not merely static GNNs stacked according to the time dimension—but showing different structural properties, which requires well-tailored DGNN models to handle. A good dynamic model catches accurate information on how links are established in time sequences. DGNNs are designed by embedding dynamic graphs into latent spaces to realize link prediction. It is sensible to think of DGNNs as time series encoding with a message passing mechanism from neighboring nodes, thus combining GNNs and RNNs adaptively to construct a DGNN model. By slicing the dynamic network into snapshots as static graphs, discrete DGNNs are capable of adopting GNNs to encode each network snapshot and functions for stacked or interacted snapshots. Narayan and O'N Roe [102] proposed a GCRN-M1 model, which is a combination of GCN and LSTM; they reshaped the matrix as a vector for LSTM. Another model Dynamic-GCN [103] stacked GCN with an LSTM for each node. RNN is used for updating the weights of GCN in EvolveGCN [104]. GAT and Transformers leveraging self-attention are also applied, respectively, on graph snapshots and time dimension as DySAT (see Fig. 7) proposed by Sankar and others [105]. They defined the dynamic graph as sequences of static graph snapshots $G = \{G^1, ..., G^T\}$, where T is the number of time steps. Each snapshot is a weighted undirected graph, including a shared node set V, a link set $\mathcal{E}^t$, and a weighted adjacency matrix A^t at time step t. To learn a latent embeddings combining structural and evolving information $\boldsymbol{e}_v^t \in R^d$ for each node ($v \in V$), they are designed into three components: (1) structural attention, (2) temporal attention, and (3) graph context prediction specifically. Each static graph snapshot (1) learns structural embeddings, then (2) learns temporal embeddings on several static snapshots, and finally (3) through loss function, it encourages nodes within fixed random walks having similar representations for one snapshot. Specifically, for block (1), the one-hot vector for node v and its neighbor u are concatenated after a shared weight matrix W, fed to a weighted (a^T) fully connected layer. Outputs are then multiplied with the

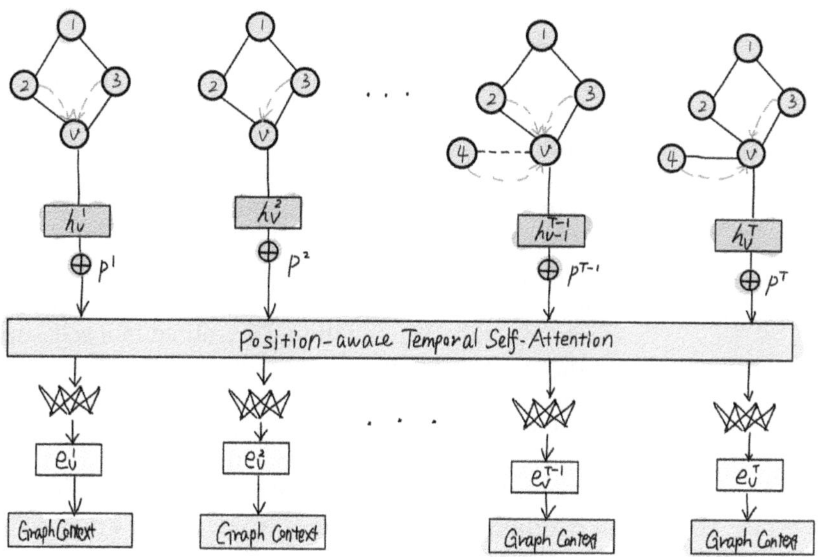

Fig. 7 DySAT model: structural and temporal attention operations are applied sequentially; *dashed black lines* and *dashed green arrows* indicate new links and structural-attention calculated by weighing neighboring nodes.

weight of link (u, v) (A_{uv}), followed by a LeakyReLU nonlinear activation to get output representations e_{uv}. Learned attention coefficients α_{uv} are obtained by softmax over the neighbors of node v. A new representation hv is the result of weighting neighbors embeddings $(W^s x_u)$ by α_{uv}. For block (2), the inputs are node embeddings $(X_v = \{_v^1 + \boldsymbol{p}^1, \boldsymbol{h}_v^2 + \boldsymbol{p}^2, ..., \boldsymbol{h}_v^T + \boldsymbol{p}^T\})$ that are learned for each time step in block (1), adding corresponding position encodings. Then output representation of node v at time t (Z_v with dimensionality F') are calculated by self-attention process with three linear transformation matrices, query key, and value:

$$Z_v = \beta_v(X_v W_v)$$

$$\beta_v^{ij} = \frac{\exp\left(e_v^{ij}\right)}{\sum_{k=1}^{T} \exp\left(e_v^{ik}\right)}$$

$$e_v^{ij} = \left(\frac{\left((X_v W_q)(X_v W_k)^T\right)_{ij}}{\sqrt{F'}} + M_{ij}\right)$$

To capture various facets of network structures, multihead attentions repeating the previous process at structural and temporal level are adopted, with their respective results concatenated for final representations. As we can see, their model takes the most of attention mechanisms to generate a dynamic node representation by jointly learning structural neighbors and temporal dynamics.

Continuous DGNNs commonly adopt RNN structure to update interactive node embeddings. A typical framework for continuous dynamics modeling is Temporal Graph Networks (TGNs) proposed by Rossi et al. [106], which generalizes current models such as Jodie and TGAT (Temporal Graph Attention Networks). In this case, the model is trained in a self-supervised way, predicting future edges using all the information from previous edges. It is essentially an encoder-decoder structure with the encoder part generating temporal node embeddings $z_i(t) = f(i, t)$ for any node i and time t, and the decoding part responsible for a specific task as predicting edge probability based on two node embeddings. Several memories are applied to update the states of nodes chronologically, which is a compressed representation of all the historical interactions of a node as $s_1(t_1)$. Given an interaction between node i (destination) and j (source), a new message will be used to update the memory:

$$\mathbf{m}_i(t) = \text{msg}_\text{s}\left(\mathbf{s}_i(t^-), \mathbf{s}_j(t^-), t, \mathbf{e}_{ij}(t)\right)$$

$$\mathbf{m}_j(t) = \text{msg}_\text{d}\left(\mathbf{s}_j(t^-), \mathbf{s}_i(t^-), t, \mathbf{e}_{ij}(t)\right)$$

Then an aggregator operation for the same node in a batch is applied for each node; take i for example: $\overline{\mathbf{m}}_i(t) = \text{agg}(\mathbf{m}_i(t_1), ..., \mathbf{m}_i(t_b))$. For memory updating, usually an RNN (*mem* operator) is adopted to deal with the previous memory and message: $\mathbf{s}_i(t) = \text{mem}(\overline{\mathbf{m}}_i(t), \mathbf{s}_i(t^-))$. Graph embedding module is for computing the temporal embedding of a node and solves the problem of its memory becoming out of date for not being involved in interaction for a long time. It is formatted as:

$$\mathbf{z}_i(t) = \text{emb}(it) = \sum_{i \in N^k(n+1)} h\left(\mathbf{s}_i(t), \mathbf{s}_j(t), \mathbf{e}_{ij}, \mathbf{v}_i(t), \mathbf{v}_j(t)\right)$$

Each time, it updates memory using interactions from the previous batch, and then calculating node embeddings with the updated memory states and storing the message back to the raw message block for the next batch's memory update. Despite recent works, including the aforementioned, having paved the way for DGNNs, there are still several challenges ahead. For large quantities of nodes with interweaving temporal and topological features, models capable of capturing intricate patterns are still scarce. Future works are expected to deal with diversity, scalability, and continuity. In other words, a good framework could outperform on tasks rising from heterogeneous, large, and dynamic networks. It is possible that Hidden Markov Models (HMMs) or neural symbolic methods implanted inside the framework of DGNNs can acquire more expressive power in relationship reasoning along the time axis.

4. Applications of GNNs on neural data

Since the GNN framework itself is an emerging topic in deep learning, works handling MEG and EEG datasets using GNNs are also in their preliminary stages. We are going to overview some fMRI and EEGs-related studies, most of which adopted GCN structures. Guo et al. [107] employed spectral graph convolutions on prior estimated graphs collected by MEG recording to predict whether the subject views face or object. Similar graph convolution method [108] is also applied to rs-fMRI data and achieved promising results to learn a brain connectivity graph and evaluated it on ABIDE and UK Biobank datasets for autism spectrum disorder and sex classification. Zhao et al. [109] defined an MCI-graph based on the closeness of the collection devices and subject's gender. Here, half of the functional connectivity network matrix collected by fMRI is transformed to a feature vector and attached to the subject node and fed into GCNs for further prediction of MCI disorder, which have obtained a best average accuracy of 85.6%. By applying GNN to fMRI data, Li et al. [108] constructed weighted graphs capturing both local and global interactions. Each node is embedded according to the basic vectors of its community and aggregated with its neighbors' embedding. And then those above threshold values after being projected on pooling vectors are kept for high-score nodes' composed graphs; further MLP operation is applied based on those concatenated representation vectors.

Zhang et al. [97] proposed a model graph-based hierarchical attention model (G-HAM) to resolve EEG-based intention recognition in the subject-independent settings. They used graphs to learn EEG node representations per trial based on positional relationship between nodes, and then attention mechanisms to slices and nodes hierarchically. They built V-graph and D-graph, which is defined on 2D and 3D space, respectively, for each node by multiplying the EEG signals/trial with normalized graph adjacency matrix. By conducting their experiment on a large-EEG dataset with 105 subjects, their model outperformed the baseline models

(EEGNet, AE-XGBoost, etc.). Another study [82] focused on novelty methods of representing EEG signals as a graph based on within-frequency and cross-frequency functional estimates, then using a GCN structure to predict personal identification. EEG signals are band-pass filtered, after which phase lock value is calculated from a specific node and corresponding band. Within- and cross-frequency functional connectivity graphs are calculated and fused into an extended EEG graph representation, which augmented the graph embeddings for later prediction by 3%–4%, yet differences were not observed whether the graph was built on 3D or 2D spaces. Similar GCN structures (GCN-net) were adopted by Lun et al. [110] to detect four-class MI intentions, which also showed robustness to data size when evaluated on different amounts of subjects. Specifically, when increasing subjects from 50 to 100, the accuracy is slightly decreased from 89.75% to 88.14%, proving that graph-based methods can grasp the invariant structural information across subjects. Hybrid models are also combined with GNNs for various tasks. For example, BiLSTM and GCN are applied [111] to extract features for recognizing motor imagery. Followed by a BiLSTM with attention to extract raw EEG signals, the output features are combined with adjacency matrices fed into six GCN layers with respective filters and max-pooling for final prediction. Their experiment has shown 98.81% max GAA compared with previous methods (RNNs, ESI + CNNs). In their study, graphs were constructed by using Absolute Pearson matrix and Graph Laplacian matrix. The previous studies show that GNN, particularly GCN infrastructures, are applied to graphs built based on topological distances or functional correlations, in the form of adjacency matrices calculated by Absolute Pearson Correlation or other methods. However, models are distinguished by whether the graphs are built in a domain adaptive way to represent neural signals properly.

Here, we elaborate on a study [112] in details of how they reasonably constructed their graphs. They promoted a joint graph structure and representation learning network (JGRN) for robust seizure recognition. It uses graph structures to jointly optimize the weights that learns global and local connections together from the perspective of frequencies and channels. Specifically, graph structures are learned with the following process: Nodes with components of frequency info (144 components with 1D PSD features) are extracted, and edges with weights measured by the correlation coefficient between corresponding PSD are defined together to formulate a graph for each record. Sets of graphs for short-term records slices are averaged to get a densely connected graph and then pruned into a sparse graph $\mathcal{G}_s$, which is task-relevant. A noninformative prior graph $\mathcal{G}_s$ is sampled from a Gaussian distribution, and nodes are clustered according to the relationship between each pair of channels (six channels, represented by C) into subgraphs. To learn global structure, a CNN is used to learn the shared representation, and then fully connected layers are adopted to densify $\mathcal{F}^{conv}$, and attention functions are applied to calculate the relative influence $\mathcal{F}_i^a$ of those subgraphs. After reshaping the adjacency matrices $\{A_g^i\}_{i=1,...,C^2}$, a global structure $\mathcal{G}_g$ with adjacency matrix A_g is acquired. Similarly for local structures, CNN f_{deconv} with a logistic Sigmoid function are conducted to get local structure $\mathcal{G}_l$ with A_l. Finally by element-wise product of A_g and A_l, a densely connected graph $\mathcal{G}_d$ is acquired and pruned into a sparse graph $\mathcal{G}_s$. It is advantageous for its robustness over various configurations of dataset and setting that allows space for data augmentation methods, and not asking for a prior graph that may cause problems because of the imbalanced sample distribution.

Considering the relatively small scale acquired neural datasets, schemes were brought up for data augmentation. One way is graph empirical mode decomposition (g-EMD) proposed by Kalaganis et al. [113]. They conducted the Kronecker product operation on graph adjacency matrix W and identity matrix I_E, adding spatial and temporal transform of several layers by matrix $S + S^T (S_{i,j} = \delta_{ij+E})$ into a multiplex representation. Meanwhile, inspired by EMD, which decomposes a given signal into a finite set of Intrinsic Mode Functions (IMFs), a graph signal x is defined with i as a local maximum/minimum whose value is higher/lower than all its neighbors. Then it is interpolated for a new graph signal s, which minimizes the total graph variation; similar iterative processes are conducted to get a decomposition of a sample graph signal into its graph IMFs. Finally, IMFs' components are recollected to combine artificial samples from different epochs with the same class labels. Another way is to generate new graph samples by Neural Structural Learning (NSL, Tensorflow). Raza et al. [114] improved EEGNet with NSL framework. It is a method adaptive to various base neural networks leveraging structured signals together with feature inputs. They augmented training samples (epoched EEG with labels represented as a graph) with corresponding neighbors. Neighbors are implicitly created by adversarial learning, and the neighbor loss is defined as the distance between output prediction of the generated adversarial neighbor and the ground truth label. Combined approach is evidenced better than the sole EEGNet model on MI classification dataset.

5. Discussion

We began this chapter by introducing popular signal recording techniques, including EEG, MEG, and fMRI. To analyze the data collected from these recording modalities and harness their predictive power, traditional signal processing and machine learning methods have been applied for years. Recently, deep learning methods have been used extensively to improve the data's predictive power, and it has shown to have outperformed the traditional ones with high encoding and decoding accuracies. Therefore, we reviewed this promising branch of machine learning families by introducing the deep learning framework from its basic structures to an attractive direction of GNNs. First, we elaborated on CNNs, RNNs, and attention mechanisms as the foundation of other derived models, with their ideas mathematically expounded and their applications to brain datasets exemplified. CNNs and RNNs are usually adapted as hybrid methods, sometimes with attention mechanisms, to capture both spatial and temporal information efficiently. Then we showed the promises of a new direction through GNNs, where we focused on how the concept of convolution operation on CNNs is transferred to the case of graph networks. Specifically, we clarified three flavors of layers in GNNs: (1) spectral layers, (2) attentional layers, and (3) message passing layers. In fact, they are both based on the same idea of embedding nodes based on message passing across neighboring nodes, which is also intuitively the way convolution in graphs is conducted. Furthermore, we expanded the content as DGNNs, which we assume are vital to deal with real-time data on graphs. However, DGNNs are still considered spuriously continuous for most of the models. We also introduced research using GNNs for neural signal processing in recent years. Attempts have been made primarily on EEG and fMRI datasets, but few studies also tried to apply these methods to other types of recordings. We have shown evidence that hybrid and graph-based neural networks are promising directions in this field, and it outperforms the basic neural network models.

As stated earlier, deep learning methods outperform other methods for its strong representation capability and model flexibility. Different structures are developed for different data types. CNNs are effective at embedding spatial pixels, RNNs are suitable for time-series sequences, and GNNs achieve better results on non-Euclidean space, which provide appropriate templates for data structured naturally. Due to the fast progress in the current state of the art in high-performance hardware, attention of the research and engineering community has reinvigorated into the field of deep learning, which in turn guarantees consistent efficiency and performance for the future.

Traditional methods such as decision trees and symbolic methods are more interpretable but show less accuracy compared with its deep learning counterparts. It seems there exists a trade-off between accuracy and interpretability. Deep learning, despite its performance, is highly dependent on the configuration of hyperparameters, model optimization parameters, and network structural parameters. According to Das and Rad [115]:

> A deep learning model f is considered a black-box if the model parameters and the network architectures are hidden from the end-user.

Models developed within a deep learning framework are highly likely to fall into this black-box paradigm, which results in lack of reliability and validity. They also suffered from adversarial network attacks because of their sensitivity to large quantities of parameters. Any small changes to input features (even if not perceived by the human eye) could drop the performance of the deep learning model or the model could train itself to completely different parameters that were not intended by the operators. So, developing trustworthy and unbiased algorithms is very important for understanding and exploiting neural signals properly. For example, user experience is a key consideration when designing BCI systems, and models are required to be consistent across similar data inputs across environment and subjects. Human-understandable algorithms make it possible for users to make decisions based on feedback from the interfaces. Moreover, prediction of major brain diseases from collected neural activity datasets also need to be consistent with expert knowledge because a decision made by unreliable algorithms may bring unexpected public health risks. Therefore, it is important to include explainability and interpretability of results along with the predictive outputs as an evaluation standard of various deep learning methods. However, only a few studies [82, 108, 112, 113] have emphasized and given reasoning of their models. Often, explainability is deemed as a secondary requirement, and it is often traded with the purpose of reaching high accuracy.

Another limitation comes from the data scarcity, especially labeled data. Deep learning is data thirsty, which demands large numbers of samples for generalization. Whether the model will give us valuable results or not relies closely on the input data. However, it is expensive and time-consuming to collect signals with current recording equipment. A typical example is fMRI, which costs £35 on average if running consistently for half an hour. The fact is that we can only access limited data resources despite being submerged by big data. Deep learning, considering the model width and depth, needs to be carefully adapted to the relatively small datasets of various neural signals. However, the effectiveness of deep learning methods comes from their "deep" layers of hierarchical features representation. The lack of large benchmarks and standards of data acquisition procedures have inhabited the power of deep learning methods. On the contrary, this also raises challenges for (1) using self-supervised methods to pretrain on benchmark datasets and then transfer the embeddings learned for specific tasks to a newer task; (2) emphasizing domain-adapted deep learning models that involve prior knowledge and reasoning into the neural network structures, meanwhile still keeping its continuous information transmitting mechanisms; and (3) representing the online generated data stream effectively (including neural signals), which commonly happens in practical settings, such as in BCI.

With the surge of various frameworks and studies compensating for the theoretically explainability of deep learning and cross-disciplinary attention from neuroscience-related communities, we are expecting several breakthroughs in the following aspects:

- Tailoring deep learning infrastructures to be more domain-adapted and small-scale neural signal data effectively.
- Exploring deep learning methods for other types of neural signal recordings at various levels, such as MEG, electrocorticography, spikes, and more.
- Combining data from various recordings and representing them into some common latent space for data augmentation.
- Incorporating hybrid methods (such as domain adaptation, transfer learning, semisupervised learning, and generative method) and domain knowledge from neuroscience with GNN to develop explainable models.
- Creating data processing pipelines for neural signal processing under deep learning framework that could be leveraged on small and practical-purpose data.

References

[1] D. Pei, R. Vinjamuri, Introductory chapter: methods and applications of neural signal processing, in: Advances in Neural Signal Processing, IntechOpen, 2020, https://doi.org/10.5772/intechopen.93335.

[2] R.T. Schirrmeister, J.T. Springenberg, L.D.J. Fiederer, M. Glasstetter, K. Eggensperger, M. Tangermann, F. Hutter, W. Burgard, T. Ball, Deep learning with convolutional neural networks for EEG decoding and visualization, Hum. Brain Mapp. 38 (2017) 5391–5420, https://doi.org/10.1002/hbm.23730.

[3] Y. Roy, H. Banville, I. Albuquerque, A. Gramfort, T.H. Falk, J. Faubert, Deep learning-based electroencephalography analysis: a systematic review, J. Neural Eng. 16 (2019) 051001, https://doi.org/10.1088/1741-2552/ab260c.

[4] A. Craik, Y. He, J.L. Contreras-Vidal, Deep learning for electroencephalogram (EEG) classification tasks: a review, J. Neural Eng. 16 (2019) 031001, https://doi.org/10.1088/1741-2552/ab0ab5.

[5] J.A. Livezey, J.I. Glaser, Deep learning approaches for neural decoding: from CNNs to LSTMs and spikes to fMRI, ArXiv (2020). https://arxiv.org/abs/2005.09687.

[6] D. Zhang, K. Chen, D. Jian, L. Yao, Motor imagery classification via temporal attention cues of graph embedded EEG signals, IEEE J. Biomed. Health Inform. 24 (2020) 2570–2579, https://doi.org/10.1109/JBHI.2020.2967128.

[7] L. Zhang, M. Wang, M. Liu, D. Zhang, A survey on deep learning for neuroimaging-based brain disorder analysis, Front. Neurosci. 14 (2020), https://doi.org/10.3389/fnins.2020.00779.

[8] L.I. Smith, A tutorial on Principal Components Analysis (Computer Science Technical Report No. OUCS-2002-12), 2002. Available from: http://hdl.handle.net/10523/7534.

[9] J.V. Stone, Independent component analysis, in: N. Balakrishnan, T. Colton, B. Everitt, W. Piegorsch, F. Ruggeri, J.L. Teugels (Eds.), Wiley StatsRef: Statistics Reference Online, Wiley, 2015, https://doi.org/10.1002/9781118445112.stat06502.pub2.

[10] R.H. Myers, D.C. Montgomery, A tutorial on generalized linear models, J. Qual. Technol. 29 (3) (2018) 274–291.

[11] I. Steinwart, A. Christmann, Support Vector Machines, Information Science and Statistics, Springer-Verlag, New York, 2008, https://doi.org/10.1007/978-0-387-77242-4.

[12] A. Tharwat, T. Gaber, A. Ibrahim, A.E. Hassanien, Linear discriminant analysis: a detailed tutorial, AI Commun. 30 (2017) 169–190, https://doi.org/10.3233/AIC-170729.

[13] K. Priddy, P.E. Keller, Artificial Neural Networks – An Introduction, Tutorial Text Series, SPIE, 2005.

[14] Y. LeCun, Y. Bengio, G. Hinton, Deep learning, Nature 521 (2015) 436–444, https://doi.org/10.1038/nature14539.

[15] Y. Bengio, O. Delalleau, N. Roux, The curse of highly variable functions for local kernel machines, Adv. Neural Inf. Process. Syst. 18 (2005) 1–8.

[16] W.S. McCulloch, W. Pitts, A logical calculus of the ideas immanent in nervous activity, Bull. Math. Biophys. 5 (1943) 115–133, https://doi.org/10.1007/BF02478259.

[17] F. Rosenblatt, The Perceptron, a Perceiving and Recognizing Automaton Project Para, Cornell Aeronautical Laboratory, 1957.

[18] Y. Lecun, A theoretical framework for back-propagation, in: Proceedings of the 1988 Connectionist Models Summer School, CMU, Pittsburgh, PA, 1988, pp. 21–28.

[19] Y. Lecun, L. Bottou, Y. Bengio, P. Haffner, Gradient-based learning applied to document recognition, Proc. IEEE 86 (1998) 2278–2324, https://doi.org/10.1109/5.726791.

[20] Y. Bengio, R. Ducharme, P. Vincent, C. Janvin, A neural probabilistic language model, J. Mach. Learn. Res. 3 (2003) 1137–1155.

[21] A. Krizhevsky, I. Sutskever, G.E. Hinton, ImageNet classification with deep convolutional neural networks, in: Proceedings of the 25th International Conference on Neural Information Processing Systems – Volume 1 (NIPS'12), Curran Associates Inc., Red Hook, NY, USA, 2012, pp. 1097–1105.

[22] I.J. Goodfellow, J. Pouget-Abadie, M. Mirza, B. Xu, D. Warde-Farley, S. Ozair, A.C. Courville, Y. Bengio, Generative Adversarial Nets, NIPS, 2014.

[23] Y. LeCun, Deep Learning Hardware: Past, Present, and Future, in: Presented at the 2019 IEEE International Solid-State Circuits Conference—(ISSCC), 2019, pp. 12–19, https://doi.org/10.1109/ISSCC.2019.8662396.

[24] D.H. Hubel, T.N. Wiesel, Receptive fields, binocular interaction and functional architecture in the cat's visual cortex, J. Physiol. 160 (1) (1962) 106–154, https://doi.org/10.1113/jphysiol.1962.sp006837.

[25] Y. LeCun, et al., Backpropagation applied to handwritten zip code recognition, Neural Comput. 1 (4) (1989) 541–551, https://doi.org/10.1162/neco.1989.1.4.541.

[26] K. He, X. Zhang, S. Ren, J. Sun, Deep residual learning for image recognition, in: 2016 IEEE Conference on Computer Vision and Pattern Recognition (CVPR), IEEE, 2016, pp. 770–778.

[27] A. Krizhevsky, I. Sutskever, G.E. Hinton, ImageNet classification with deep convolutional neural networks, Commun. ACM 60 (2017) 84–90, https://doi.org/10.1145/3065386.

[28] M. Schuster, K.K. Paliwal, Bidirectional recurrent neural networks, IEEE Trans. Signal Process. 45 (1997) 2673–2681, https://doi.org/10.1109/78.650093.

[29] J.J. Hopfield, Neural networks and physical systems with emergent collective computational abilities, Proc. Natl. Acad. Sci. USA 79 (1982) 2554–2558, https://doi.org/10.1073/pnas.79.8.2554.

[30] M.I. Jordan, Serial order: a parallel distributed processing approach, California University, San Diego, La Jolla (USA). Institute for Cognitive Science, 1986. Technical report, June 1985–March 1986 (No. AD-A-173989/5/XAB; ICS-8604).

[31] J.L. Elman, Finding structure in time, Cogn. Sci. 14 (1990) 179–211, https://doi.org/10.1207/s15516709cog1402_1.

[32] S. Hochreiter, J. Schmidhuber, Long short-term memory, Neural Comput. 9 (1997) 1735–1780, https://doi.org/10.1162/neco.1997.9.8.1735.

[33] P.J. Werbos, Backpropagation through time: what it does and how to do it, Proc. IEEE 78 (1990) 1550–1560, https://doi.org/10.1109/5.58337.

[34] K. Cho, B.V. Merrienboer, Ç. Gülçehre, D. Bahdanau, F. Bougares, H. Schwenk, Y. Bengio, Learning phrase representations using RNN encoder–decoder for statistical machine translation, in: Proceedings of the 2014 Conference on Empirical Methods in Natural Language Processing (EMNLP), Doha, Qatar, Association for Computational Linguistics, 2014, pp. 1724–1734.

[35] S. Sarraf, G. Tofighi, Deep learning-based pipeline to recognize Alzheimer's disease using fMRI data, in: Presented at the 2016 Future Technologies Conference (FTC), 2016, pp. 816–820, https://doi.org/10.1109/FTC.2016.7821697.

[36] F. Ramzan, M.U. Khan, A. Rehmat, S. Iqbal, T. Saba, A. Rehman, Z. Mehmood, A deep learning approach for automated diagnosis and multi-class classification of Alzheimer's disease stages using resting-state fMRI and residual neural networks, J. Med. Syst. 44 (2019), https://doi.org/10.1007/s10916-019-1475-2.

[37] A.M.S. Aradhya, A. Ashfahani, Deep network optimization for rs-fMRI Classification, in: Presented at the 2019 International Conference on Data Mining Workshops (ICDMW), 2019, pp. 77–82, https://doi.org/10.1109/ICDMW.2019.00022.

[38] L. Zou, J. Zheng, C. Miao, M.J. Mckeown, Z.J. Wang, 3D CNN based automatic diagnosis of attention deficit hyperactivity disorder using functional and structural MRI, IEEE Access 5 (2017) 23626–23636, https://doi.org/10.1109/ACCESS.2017.2762703.

[39] H. Choi, Functional connectivity patterns of autism spectrum disorder identified by deep feature learning, ArXiv (2017). https://arxiv.org/abs/1707.07932.

[40] F.J. Martinez-Murcia, A. Ortiz, J.M. Górriz, J. Ramírez, F. Segovia, D. Salas-Gonzalez, D. Castillo-Barnes, I.A. Illán, A 3D convolutional neural network approach for the diagnosis of Parkinson's disease, in: J.M. Ferrández Vicente, J.R. Álvarez Sánchez, F. de la Paz López, J. Toledo Moreo, H. Adeli (Eds.), Natural and Artificial Computation for Biomedicine and Neuroscience, Lecture Notes in Computer Science, Springer International Publishing, Cham, 2017, pp. 324–333, https://doi.org/10.1007/978-3-319-59740-9_32.

[41] M.N.I. Qureshi, J. Oh, B. Lee, 3D-CNN based discrimination of schizophrenia using resting-state fMRI, Artif. Intell. Med. 98 (2019) 10–17, https://doi.org/10.1016/j.artmed.2019.06.003.

[42] X. Li, N.C. Dvornek, X. Papademetris, J. Zhuang, L.H. Staib, P. Ventola, J.S. Duncan, 2-Channel convolutional 3D deep neural network (2CC3D) for fMRI analysis: ASD classification and feature learning, in: Presented at the 2018 IEEE 15th International Symposium on Biomedical Imaging (ISBI 2018), 2018, pp. 1252–1255, https://doi.org/10.1109/ISBI.2018.8363798.

[43] M. Khosla, K. Jamison, A. Kuceyeski, M.R. Sabuncu, 3D convolutional neural networks for classification of functional connectomes, in: D. Stoyanov, Z. Taylor, G. Carneiro, T. Syeda-Mahmood, A. Martel, L. Maier-Hein, A. Madabhushi (Eds.), Deep Learning in Medical Image Analysis and Multimodal Learning for Clinical Decision Support, 2018, pp. 137–145, https://doi.org/10.1007/978-3-030-00889-5_16.

[44] M. Khosla, K. Jamison, A. Kuceyeski, M.R. Sabuncu, Ensemble learning with 3D convolutional neural networks for functional connectome-based prediction, NeuroImage 199 (2019) 651–662, https://doi.org/10.1016/j.neuroimage.2019.06.012.

[45] H. Vu, H.-C. Kim, M. Jung, J.-H. Lee, fMRI volume classification using a 3D convolutional neural network robust to shifted and scaled neuronal activations, NeuroImage 223 (2020) 117328, https://doi.org/10.1016/j.neuroimage.2020.117328.

[46] T.-E. Kam, H. Zhang, Z. Jiao, D. Shen, Deep learning of static and dynamic brain functional networks for early MCI detection, IEEE Trans. Med. Imaging 39 (2020) 478–487, https://doi.org/10.1109/TMI.2019.2928790.

[47] X. Zhang, L. Yao, X. Wang, J.J.M. Monaghan, D. Mcalpine, Y. Zhang, A survey on deep learning-based non-invasive brain signals: recent advances and new frontiers, J. Neural Eng. (2020), https://doi.org/10.1088/1741-2552/abc902.

[48] S. Sakhavi, C. Guan, S. Yan, Parallel convolutional-linear neural network for motor imagery classification, in: Presented at the 2015 23rd European Signal Processing Conference (EUSIPCO), 2015, pp. 2736–2740, https://doi.org/10.1109/EUSIPCO.2015.7362882.

[49] Y.R. Tabar, U. Halici, A novel deep learning approach for classification of EEG motor imagery signals, J. Neural Eng. 14 (2016) 016003, https://doi.org/10.1088/1741-2560/14/1/016003.

[50] T. Dharamsi, P. Das, T. Pedapati, G. Bramble, V. Muthusamy, H. Samulowitz, K.R. Varshney, Y. Rajamanickam, J. Thomas, J. Dauwels, Neurology-as-a-service for the developing world, ArXiv (2017). https://arxiv.org/abs/1711.06195.

[51] S. Sakhavi, C. Guan, Convolutional neural network-based transfer learning and knowledge distillation using multi-subject data in motor imagery BCI, in: Presented at the 2017 8th International IEEE/EMBS Conference on Neural Engineering (NER), 2017, pp. 588–591, https://doi.org/10.1109/NER.2017.8008420.

[52] Z. Tang, C. Li, S. Sun, Single-trial EEG classification of motor imagery using deep convolutional neural networks, Optik 130 (2017) 11–18, https://doi.org/10.1016/j.ijleo.2016.10.117.

[53] R. Zafar, S.C. Dass, A.S. Malik, Electroencephalogram-based decoding cognitive states using convolutional neural network and likelihood ratio based score fusion, PLoS ONE 12 (2017) e0178410, https://doi.org/10.1371/journal.pone.0178410.

[54] G. Gao, L. Shang, K. Xiong, J. Fang, C. Zhang, X. Gu, EEG classification based on sparse representation and deep learning, NeuroQuantology (2018), https://doi.org/10.14704/NQ.2018.16.6.1666.

[55] I. Loshchilov, F. Hutter, SGDR: stochastic gradient descent with warm restarts, ArXiv (2017). https://arxiv.org/abs/1608.03983.

[56] U.R. Acharya, S.L. Oh, Y. Hagiwara, J.H. Tan, H. Adeli, Deep convolutional neural network for the automated detection and diagnosis of seizure using EEG signals, Comput. Biol. Med. 100 (2018) 270–278, https://doi.org/10.1016/j.compbiomed.2017.09.017.

[57] J. Zhou, W. Xu, End-to-end learning of semantic role labeling using recurrent neural networks, in: Proceedings of the 53rd Annual Meeting of the Association for Computational Linguistics and the 7th International Joint Conference on Natural Language Processing (volume 1: Long Papers). Presented at the ACL-IJCNLP 2015, Association for Computational Linguistics, Beijing, China, 2015, pp. 1127–1137, https://doi.org/10.3115/v1/P15-1109.

[58] A. Page, C. Shea, T. Mohsenin, Wearable seizure detection using convolutional neural networks with transfer learning, in: Presented at the 2016 IEEE International Symposium on Circuits and Systems (ISCAS), 2016, pp. 1086–1089, https://doi.org/10.1109/ISCAS.2016.7527433.

[59] Y. Hao, H.M. Khoo, N. von Ellenrieder, N. Zazubovits, J. Gotman, DeepIED: an epileptic discharge detector for EEG-fMRI based on deep learning, NeuroImage Clin. 17 (2018) 962–975, https://doi.org/10.1016/j.nicl.2017.12.005.

[60] I. Ullah, M. Hussain, E.-H. Qazi, H. Aboalsamh, An automated system for epilepsy detection using EEG brain signals based on deep learning approach, Expert Syst. Appl. 107 (2018) 61–71, https://doi.org/10.1016/j.eswa.2018.04.021.

[61] N.D. Truong, A.D. Nguyen, L. Kuhlmann, M.R. Bonyadi, J. Yang, S. Ippolito, O. Kavehei, Convolutional neural networks for seizure prediction using intracranial and scalp electroencephalogram, Neural Netw. 105 (2018) 104–111, https://doi.org/10.1016/j.neunet.2018.04.018.

[62] Q. Zhang, Y. Liu, Improving brain computer interface performance by data augmentation with conditional. Deep Convolutional Generative Adversarial Networks, ArXiv (2018). https://arxiv.org/abs/1806.07108.

[63] C. Zhang, S. Bengio, M. Hardt, B. Recht, O. Vinyals, Understanding deep learning (still) requires rethinking generalization, Commun. ACM 64 (3) (2017) 107–115, https://doi.org/10.1145/3446776.

[64] L. Chu, R. Qiu, H. Liu, Z. Ling, T. Zhang, J. Wang, Individual recognition in schizophrenia using deep learning methods with random forest and voting classifiers: insights from resting state EEG streams, ArXiv (2018). https://arxiv.org/abs/1707.03467.

[65] G. Ruffini, D. Ibañez, M. Castellano, L. Dubreuil-Vall, A. Soria-Frisch, R. Postuma, J.-F. Gagnon, J. Montplaisir, Deep learning with EEG spectrograms in rapid eye movement behavior disorder, Front. Neurol. 10 (2019), https://doi.org/10.3389/fneur.2019.00806.

[66] O. Tsinalis, P.M. Matthews, Y. Guo, S. Zafeiriou, Automatic sleep stage scoring with single-channel EEG using convolutional neural networks, ArXiv (2016). https://arxiv.org/abs/1610.01683.

[67] A. Patanaik, J.L. Ong, J.J. Gooley, S. Ancoli-Israel, M.W.L. Chee, An end-to-end framework for real-time automatic sleep stage classification, Sleep 41 (2018), https://doi.org/10.1093/sleep/zsy041.

[68] H. Phan, F. Andreotti, N. Cooray, O.Y. Chén, M. De Vos, Joint classification and prediction CNN framework for automatic sleep stage classification, IEEE Trans. Biomed. Eng. 66 (2019) 1285–1296, https://doi.org/10.1109/TBME.2018.2872652.

[69] S. Chambon, M.N. Galtier, P.J. Arnal, G. Wainrib, A. Gramfort, A deep learning architecture for temporal sleep stage classification using multivariate and multimodal time series, IEEE Trans. Neural Syst. Rehabil. Eng. 26 (2018) 758–769, https://doi.org/10.1109/TNSRE.2018.2813138.

[70] A. Vilamala, K.H. Madsen, L.K. Hansen, Deep convolutional neural networks for interpretable analysis of EEG sleep stage scoring, in: 2017 IEEE 27th International Workshop on Machine Learning for Signal Processing (MLSP), IEEE, 2017, pp. 1–6.

[71] A. Sors, S. Bonnet, S. Mirek, L. Vercueil, J.-F. Payen, A convolutional neural network for sleep stage scoring from raw single-channel EEG, Biomed. Signal Process. Control 42 (2018) 107–114, https://doi.org/10.1016/j.bspc.2017.12.001.

[72] S. Roy, A. Chowdhury, K. McCreadie, G. Prasad, Deep learning based inter-subject continuous decoding of motor imagery for practical brain-computer interfaces, Front. Neurosci. 14 (2020) 918, https://doi.org/10.3389/fnins.2020.00918.

[73] S. Alhagry, A. Aly, R. El-Khoribi, Emotion recognition based on EEG using LSTM recurrent neural network, Int. J. Adv. Comput. Sci. Appl. 8 (2017), https://doi.org/10.14569/IJACSA.2017.081046.

[74] K.M. Tsiouris, V.C. Pezoulas, M. Zervakis, S. Konitsiotis, D.D. Koutsouris, D.I. Fotiadis, A long short-term memory deep learning network for the prediction of epileptic seizures using EEG signals, Comput. Biol. Med. 99 (2018) 24–37, https://doi.org/10.1016/j.compbiomed.2018.05.019.

[75] N.C. Dvornek, P. Ventola, K.A. Pelphrey, J.S. Duncan, Identifying autism from resting-state fMRI using long short-term memory networks, in: Machine Learning in Medical Imaging, MLMI Workshop, vol. 10541, 2017, pp. 362–370, https://doi.org/10.1007/978-3-319-67389-9_42.

[76] J.G. Makin, D.A. Moses, E.F. Chang, Machine translation of cortical activity to text with an encoder-decoder framework, Nat. Neurosci. 23 (2020) 575–582, https://doi.org/10.1038/s41593-020-0608-8.

[77] M.R. Rezaei, A.K. Gillespie, J.A. Guidera, B. Nazari, S. Sadri, L.M. Frank, U.T. Eden, A. Yousefi, A comparison study of point-process filter and deep learning performance in estimating rat position using an ensemble of place cells, in: Presented at the 2018 40th Annual International Conference of the IEEE Engineering in Medicine and Biology Society (EMBC), 2018, pp. 4732–4735, https://doi.org/10.1109/EMBC.2018.8513154.

[78] S. Yoo, S. Woo, Z. Amad, Classification of three categories from prefrontal cortex using LSTM networks: fNIRS study, in: Presented at the 2018 18th International Conference on Control, Automation and Systems (ICCAS), 2018, pp. 1141–1146.

[79] A. Hasasneh, N. Kampel, P. Sripad, N.J. Shah, J. Dammers, Deep learning approach for automatic classification of ocular and cardiac artifacts in MEG data, J. Eng. 2018 (2018) e1350692, https://doi.org/10.1155/2018/1350692.

[80] D. Dash, P. Ferrari, J. Wang, Decoding imagined and spoken phrases from non-invasive neural (MEG) signals, Front. Neurosci. 14 (2020), https://doi.org/10.3389/fnins.2020.00290.

[81] W. Li, X. Lin, X. Chen, Detecting Alzheimer's disease Based on 4D fMRI: an exploration under deep learning framework, Neurocomputing 388 (2020) 280–287, https://doi.org/10.1016/j.neucom.2020.01.053.

[82] M. Wang, H. El-Fiqi, J. Hu, H.A. Abbass, Convolutional neural networks using dynamic functional connectivity for EEG-based person identification in diverse human states, IEEE Trans. Inf. Forensics Secur. 14 (2019) 3259–3272, https://doi.org/10.1109/TIFS.2019.2916403.

[83] C. Spampinato, S. Palazzo, I. Kavasidis, D. Giordano, N. Souly, M. Shah, Deep learning human mind for automated visual classification, in: 2017 IEEE Conference on Computer Vision and Pattern Recognition (CVPR), IEEE, 2017, pp. 4503–4511, https://doi.org/10.1109/CVPR.2017.479.

[84] M.C. Tjepkema-Cloostermans, R.C.V de Carvalho, M.J.A.M. van Putten, Deep learning for detection of focal epileptiform discharges from scalp EEG recordings, Clin. Neurophysiol. 129 (2018) 2191–2196, https://doi.org/10.1016/j.clinph.2018.06.024.

[85] H.-I. Suk, C.-Y. Wee, S.-W. Lee, D. Shen, State-space model with deep learning for functional dynamics estimation in resting-state fMRI, NeuroImage 129 (2016) 292–307, https://doi.org/10.1016/j.neuroimage.2016.01.005.

[86] X. Zhang, L. Yao, D. Zhang, X. Wang, Q.Z. Sheng, T. Gu, Multi-person brain activity recognition via comprehensive EEG signal analysis, in: Proceedings of the 14th EAI International Conference on Mobile and Ubiquitous Systems: Computing, Networking and Services, MobiQuitous 2017, Association for Computing Machinery, New York, NY, 2017, pp. 28–37, https://doi.org/10.1145/3144457.3144477.

[87] A.B. Said, A. Mohamed, T. Elfouly, K. Harras, Z.J. Wang, Multimodal deep learning approach for joint EEG-EMG data compression and classification, in: Presented at the 2017 IEEE Wireless Communications and Networking Conference (WCNC), 2017, pp. 1–6, https://doi.org/10.1109/WCNC.2017.7925709.

[88] D. Bahdanau, K.H. Cho, Y. Bengio, Neural machine translation by jointly learning to align and translate, Paper presented at 3rd International Conference on Learning Representations, ICLR 2015, San Diego, United States, 2015.

[89] A. Vaswani, N. Shazeer, N. Parmar, J. Uszkoreit, L. Jones, A.N. Gomez, Ł. Kaiser, I. Polosukhin, Attention is all you need, in: Proceedings of the 31st International Conference on Neural Information Processing Systems (NIPS'17), Curran Associates Inc., Red Hook, NY, USA, 2017, pp. 6000–6010.

[90] M.M. Bronstein, J. Bruna, T. Cohen, P. Velivckovi'c, Geometric deep learning: grids, groups, graphs, geodesics, and gauges, ArXiv (2021). https://arxiv.org/abs/2104.13478.

[91] J. Bruna, W. Zaremba, A.D. Szlam, Y. LeCun, Spectral networks and locally connected networks on graphs, CoRR (2014). http://arxiv.org/abs/1312.6203.

[92] M. Defferrard, X. Bresson, P. Vandergheynst, Convolutional neural networks on graphs with fast localized spectral filtering, Proceedings of the 30th International Conference on Neural Information Processing Systems (NIPS'16), Curran Associates Inc., Red Hook, NY, USA, 2016, pp. 3844–3852.

[93] T.N. Kipf, M. Welling, Semi-supervised classification with graph convolutional networks, ArXiv (2017). https://arxiv.org/abs/1609.02907.

[94] F. Wu, T. Zhang, A.H. Souza, C. Fifty, T. Yu, K.Q. Weinberger, Simplifying graph convolutional networks, ArXiv (2019). http://arxiv.org/abs/1902.07153.

[95] F. Monti, D. Boscaini, J. Masci, E. Rodolà, J. Svoboda, M.M. Bronstein, Geometric deep learning on graphs and manifolds using mixture model CNNs, in: 2017 IEEE Conference on Computer Vision and Pattern Recognition (CVPR), IEEE, 2017, pp. 5425–5434.

[96] P. Veličković, G. Cucurull, A. Casanova, A. Romero, P. Liò, Y. Bengio, Graph attention networks, ArXiv (2018). https://arxiv.org/abs/1710.10903.

[97] D. Zhang, L. Yao, K. Chen, S. Wang, P.D. Haghighi, C. Sullivan, A graph-based hierarchical attention model for movement intention detection from EEG signals, IEEE Trans. Neural Syst. Rehabil. Eng. 27 (2019) 2247–2253, https://doi.org/10.1109/TNSRE.2019.2943362.

[98] P. Battaglia, R. Pascanu, M. Lai, D.J. Rezende, K. Kavukcuoglu, Interaction networks for learning about objects, relations and physics, Proceedings of

the 30th International Conference on Neural Information Processing Systems (NIPS'16), Curran Associates Inc., Red Hook, NY, USA, 2016, pp. 4509–4517.

[99] J. Gilmer, S.S. Schoenholz, P.F. Riley, O. Vinyals, G.E. Dahl, Neural message passing for Quantum chemistry, in: Proceedings of the 34th International Conference on Machine Learning – Volume 70 (ICML'17), JMLR.org, 2017, pp. 1263–1272.

[100] P.W. Battaglia, J.B. Hamrick, V. Bapst, A. Sanchez-Gonzalez, V. Zambaldi, M. Malinowski, A. Tacchetti, D. Raposo, A. Santoro, R. Faulkner, C. Gulcehre, F. Song, A. Ballard, J. Gilmer, G. Dahl, A. Vaswani, K. Allen, C. Nash, V. Langston, C. Dyer, N. Heess, D. Wierstra, P. Kohli, M. Botvinick, O. Vinyals, Y. Li, R. Pascanu, Relational inductive biases, deep learning, and graph networks, ArXiv (2018). https://arxiv.org/abs/1806.01261.

[101] J. Skarding, B. Gabrys, K. Musial, Foundations and modelling of dynamic networks using dynamic graph neural networks: a survey, IEEE Access 9 (2021) 79143–79168, https://doi.org/10.1109/ACCESS.2021.3082932.

[102] A. Narayan, P.H.O.N. Roe, Learning graph dynamics using deep neural networks, in: IFAC-Pap., 9th Vienna International Conference on Mathematical Modelling, vol. 51, 2018, pp. 433–438, https://doi.org/10.1016/j.ifacol.2018.03.074.

[103] F. Manessi, A. Rozza, M. Manzo, Dynamic graph convolutional networks, Pattern Recognit. 97 (2020) 107000, https://doi.org/10.1016/j.patcog.2019.107000.

[104] A. Pareja, G. Domeniconi, J. Chen, T. Ma, T. Suzumura, H. Kanezashi, T. Kaler, T.B. Schardl, C.E. Leiserson, EvolveGCN: evolving graph convolutional networks for dynamic graphs, Proc. AAAI Conf. Artif. Intell. 34 (4) (2020) 5363–5370, https://doi.org/10.1609/aaai.v34i04.5984.

[105] A. Sankar, Y. Wu, L. Gou, W. Zhang, H. Yang, DySAT: Deep neural representation learning on dynamic graphs via self-attention networks, Proceedings of the 13th International Conference on Web Search and Data Mining, Association for Computing Machinery, New York, NY, USA, 2020, pp. 519–527, https://doi.org/10.1145/3336191.3371845.

[106] E. Rossi, B.P. Chamberlain, F. Frasca, D. Eynard, F. Monti, M.M. Bronstein, Temporal graph networks for deep learning on dynamic graphs, ArXiv (2020). https://arxiv.org/abs/2006.10637.

[107] Y. Guo, H. Nejati, N.-M. Cheung, Deep neural networks on graph signals for brain imaging analysis, in: 2017 IEEE International Conference on Image Processing (ICIP), IEEE, 2017, pp. 3295–3299, https://doi.org/10.1109/ICIP.2017.8296892.

[108] X. Li, Y. Zhou, S. Gao, N. Dvornek, M. Zhang, J. Zhuang, S. Gu, D. Scheinost, L. Staib, P. Ventola, J. Duncan, BrainGNN: interpretable brain graph neural network for fMRI analysis, bioRxiv 2020.05.16.100057 (2020), https://doi.org/10.1101/2020.05.16.100057.

[109] X. Zhao, F. Zhou, L. Ou-Yang, T. Wang, B. Lei, Graph convolutional network analysis for mild cognitive impairment prediction, in: Presented at the 2019 IEEE 16th International Symposium on Biomedical Imaging (ISBI 2019), 2019, pp. 1598–1601, https://doi.org/10.1109/ISBI.2019.8759256.

[110] X. Lun, S. Jia, Y. Hou, Y. Shi, Y. Li, H. Yang, S. Zhang, J. Lv, GCNs-Net: a graph convolutional neural network approach for decoding time-resolved EEG motor imagery signals, ArXiv (2020). https://arxiv.org/abs/2006.08924.

[111] Y. Hou, S. Jia, S. Zhang, X. Lun, Y. Shi, Y. Li, H. Yang, R. Zeng, J. Lv, Deep feature mining via attention-based BiLSTM-GCN for human motor imagery recognition, ArXiv (2020). https://arxiv.org/abs/2005.00777.

[112] Q. Lian, Y. Qi, G. Pan, Y. Wang, Learning graph in graph convolutional neural networks for robust seizure prediction, J. Neural Eng. 17 (2020) 035004, https://doi.org/10.1088/1741-2552/ab909d.

[113] F.P. Kalaganis, N.A. Laskaris, E. Chatzilari, S. Nikolopoulos, I. Kompatsiaris, A data augmentation scheme for geometric deep learning in personalized brain-computer interfaces, IEEE Access 8 (2020) 162218–162229, https://doi.org/10.1109/ACCESS.2020.3021580.

[114] H. Raza, A. Chowdhury, S. Bhattacharyya, S. Samothrakis, Single-trial EEG classification with EEGNet and neural structured learning for improving BCI performance, in: Presented at the 2020 International Joint Conference on Neural Networks (IJCNN), 2020, pp. 1–8, https://doi.org/10.1109/IJCNN48605.2020.9207100.

[115] A. Das, P. Rad, Opportunities and challenges in explainable artificial intelligence (XAI): a survey, ArXiv (2020). https://arxiv.org/abs/2006.11371.

10

Improved extraction of the extreme thermal regions of breast IR images

Mahnaz Etehadtavakol[a,b], Zahra Emrani[c], and E.Y.K. Ng[d]

[a]Department of Medical Physics, School of Medicine, Isfahan University of Medical Sciences, Isfahan, Iran. [b]Poursina Hakim Digestive Diseases Research Center, Isfahan University of Medical Sciences, Isfahan, Iran. [c]Medical Image and Signal Processing Research Center, Isfahan University of Medical Sciences, Isfahan, Iran. [d]School of Mechanical and Aerospace Engineering, College of Engineering, Nanyang Technological University, Singapore, Singapore

1. Introduction

These days, with state-of-the-art infrared cameras that can indicate the thermal profile of the human body quite accurately, thermal imaging has been reevaluated and compared to other medical procedures as a complementary method to identify breast abnormalities. The thermal imaging system is driven by displaying specified skin temperature. It is a radiation-free and safe approach to analyze physiological performance related to the controlled skin temperature. This approach detects infrared radiation correlated to the temperature profile of described body areas. Thomas Tierney, in 1972, declared that, "The medical specialists expressed that thermography, at this time, is in advance of the exploratory state as a diagnostic method in the coming fields: (1) Female breast pathology, (2) Extracranial vessel disorder, (3) Peripheral vascular disorder, (4) Musculoskeletal damage" [1,2]. This advanced method has been employed for early identification of anomalies in female breasts. It recognizes thermal abnormalities like hot areas associated with skin's increased superficial temperatures. Increased blood flow and elevated metabolism in tissues with cancer treatment is highly correlated. Vascular proliferation corresponding to tumor-related angiogenesis results in increasing vascular flow. Cancerous cells develop a chemical that certainly increases the expansion of blood vessels nourishing the

Advanced Methods in Biomedical Signal Processing and Analysis. https://doi.org/10.1016/B978-0-323-85955-4.00002-8
Copyright © 2023 Elsevier Inc. All rights reserved.

area where the tumor is located. Despite this, the sympathetic nervous system essentially controls normal blood vessels, but, under these conditions, the blood vessels are dilated and disabled. Blood vessel dilation as well as increasing blood flow in the area due to angiogenesis surely introduces more heat, which is detectable by an infrared camera. Many researches have indicated that thermal imaging has the potential to detect heat indications years before traditional methods can detect abnormalities in womens' breasts [3–14].

It contributes functional details on thermal and vascular status of the tissue. These functional developments occur sooner than the onset of structural developments progress in a malignant situation. It is worth mentioning that physiological developments in cells occur prior to pathological developments [15]. Thermal imaging or thermography is radiation free, and breast tissues are not compressed. It is an absolutely safe system for early detection of breast cancer. Image segmentation techniques have a crucial performance to map extreme thermal areas in clinical infrared images. In breast thermal images, shape, size, and boundaries of the segmented extreme thermal areas are helpful to detect abnormalities and perhaps tumor types. As of yet, several methods are used to segment different areas, exclusively the extreme thermal areas from breast thermal images [16–18]. For medical professionals, observing the extreme thermal areas, possibly areas of suspect, of a thermal image in real time could be valuable.

Lazy snapping procedure can be useful in that aspect, which is very fast, user friendly, and easy. Coarse and fine-scale processing are separated by applying this interactive image technique. It achieves object condition and comprehensive transformation easily [19]. Moreover, lazy snapping provides quick evaluation, dividing the separated contour to the precise object's edges intelligently despite of the presence of unclear or low-contrast borders. A direct user interface (UI) approach is applied to guide adjustable control for the users.

This chapter is presented as follows: Section 2 explains the method of procedure, Section 3 illustrates the test results, and the findings are finalized in Section 4.

2. Methodology

Image cutout is an approach to remove an object in a picture from its background. For many years, image cutout has been considered. With the onset of digital imaging, an individual pixel level has become available to accurately determine the foreground and background. The role of image cutout is in defining the foreground part and the background part. When the user is required to specify each area of the foreground separately with pixel accuracy, it is a dull and frustrating task. Two main approaches that enhance standard pixel-level selection methods for general image cutout are (1) boundary-based and (2) region-based. Both tools obtain aspects of the image that the computer can recognize, like color constancy. Then the computer uses them to conduct the foreground qualification process. In boundary-based methods, the user is allowed to mark the boundary with a disclosing curve to cut out the foreground. The method enhances the curve in a piecewise style when the user determines the object edges. Although it is more effortless than just choosing pixels manually with the usual selection means, these methods still require enormous user's attention, and the user must cautiously control the curve. In region-based approaches, the user is allowed to miss clues as to which sections of the image are background or foreground beyond the bordering regions or accurately marking the pixels. Commonly, clicking or dragging on background or foreground pixels are clues that can be done quickly and easily. Then, depending on the user's input clues, a basic optimization procedure could obtain the actual object edges. Region-based approaches also let the user perform at any scale they desire. However, the region-based approaches have a problem in which, sometimes, the procedures do not obtain the preferred background or foreground. For example, obscured regions, low-contrast borders, and other unclear sections can be highly tiring to be identified.

Lazy snapping is a new coarse-to-fine (UI) design for image cutout. It involves two actions: first, a fast object marking action and, second, a straightforward boundary choosing action. In the first action, object marking defines the desired object by a few marking lines. It performs at a coarse scale. The second action or boundary choosing allows the user to choose the object's edges by easily clicking and dragging polygon vertices. It performs at a finer scale. Consequently, it has the benefits of region-based as well as boundary-based methods in two actions. The first action is direct and fast for object context indication, even though the second action is simple and effective for controlling a detailed boundary [20]. Permitting the user to define the foreground against the background of an object is an important task. Lines and curves can be employed by the user to demonstrate the enlargement of the desired object rather than following the boundary of the object. The user marks down several lines on the image by dragging the mouse cursor by holding a button to determine the extreme thermal area. The color likeness inside the questionable area as well as the gradient along the boundary are maximized to optimize the borders of the area, and consequently, an interactive graph cut procedure is supported by this approach.

2.1 Graph theory

A graph is denoted by a set of elements in which some linked connections are found between some pairs. A graph is represented mathematically as $G=(V,E)$ where E describes a group of edges and V describes a group of vertices. A set of nodes, V, and a set of directed edges, E, that ties nodes are involved in a directed weighted graph. Pixels, voxels, or some features are usually associated to nodes. We intend to solve a labeling problem in this research [20]. Assume a unique label x_i ($i \in V$) for each node that is denoted, such that if $x_i \in$ foreground then $x_i = 1$, whereas if $x_i \in$ background, then $x_i = 0$.

The solution $X = \{x_i\}$ is computed by applying optimization theory. $E(X)$ or Gibbs energy as described in Eq. (1) is minimized in the optimization section.

$$E(X) = \sum_{i \in V} E_l(x_i) + \lambda \sum_{(i,j) \in \varepsilon} E_p(x_i, x_j) \tag{1}$$

where $E_l(x_i)$ and $E_p(x_i, x_j)$ are denoted as the likelihood energy and the prior energy, respectively. The cost when the label of node i is x_i is explained by the likelihood energy, while the cost when the labels of adjacent nodes i and j are x_i and x_j, respectively, is explained by the prior energy. Moreover, the likelihood energy or E_l encodes the color likeness of a node and indicates either the node associates to the background or the foreground [21].

Following steps are required to obtain E_l: (1) by K means classifier, the seed colors of the foreground and the background are separated, (2) mean of the foreground colors and the background colors sets are obtained and called $\{K^F_m\}$ and $\{K^B_n\}$, respectively, and (3) minimum distances, d, are obtained as follows [22]:

$$d_i^F = \min_m \|G(i) - \{K^F_m\}\| \text{ and } d_i^B$$
$$= \min_n \|G(i) - \{K^B_n\}\|, \text{respectively}$$

where $G(i)$ is the color, and m and n are the number elements in the foreground and in the background, respectively. Hence $E_l(x_i)$ can be computed as Eq. (2):

$$\begin{cases} E_l(x_i = 1) = 0 & E_l(x_i = 0) = \infty & \forall i \in F \\ E_l(x_i = 1) = \infty & E_l(x_i = 0) = 0 & \forall i \in B \\ E_l(x_i = 1) = \dfrac{d_i^F}{d_i^F + d_i^B} & E_l(x_i = 0) = \dfrac{d_i^B}{d_i^F + d_i^B} & \forall i \in U \end{cases} \tag{2}$$

where U is the unpredictable section and presented as $U = V - \{F \cup B\}$. Prior energy or E_p is described by the energy due to the gradient along the edges of the object. E_p is controlled by the color gradient between two nodes i and j, hence, we have $E_p(x_i, x_j)$ as:

$$E_p(x_i, x_j) = |x_i - x_j| \cdot \frac{1}{G_{ij} + 1} \tag{3}$$

where $G_{ij} = \|G(i) - G(j)\|^2$ is the L_2-Norm, observing that $|x_i - x_j|$ contributes the gradient detail exclusively along the segmentation border. Apart from that, E_p is an indication when distinctive labels are denoted for adjacent nodes. Greater E_p implies two node colors are very much alike, hence, the edge is unlikely on the object border. Boykov and Kolmogorov introduced the maxflow procedure [21] that was employed for minimization of $E(X)$ in Eq. (1).

A lazy snapping approach flow chart is demonstrated in Fig. 1. As shown, at first, marked seeds in each part of the foreground and background areas were chosen. Then, the likelihood energy, $E_l(x_i)$, and the prior energy, $E_p(x_i, x_j)$, were computed, and therefore, the Gibbs energy was calculated. Last, maximization of the Gibbs energy was done by employing maxflow procedure.

3. Experimental results and discussion

Results regarding the procedure implementation on nine breast thermograms having different breast abnormalities were presented to show medical professionals who are attentive how to discover the capability of the lazy snapping process for segmenting irregular parts in real time. Inflammations, cancerous tissues, and cysts appeared as extreme thermal regions in breast thermograms. Three malignant tumors, four benign tumors, and two mammary cysts cases were depicted as follows.

3.1 Case 1: Breast cancer

A thermal image of a cancerous breast is shown in Fig. 2A. The tumor area, which is the extreme thermal area, was segmented by lazy snapping technique and is shown in Fig. 2B.

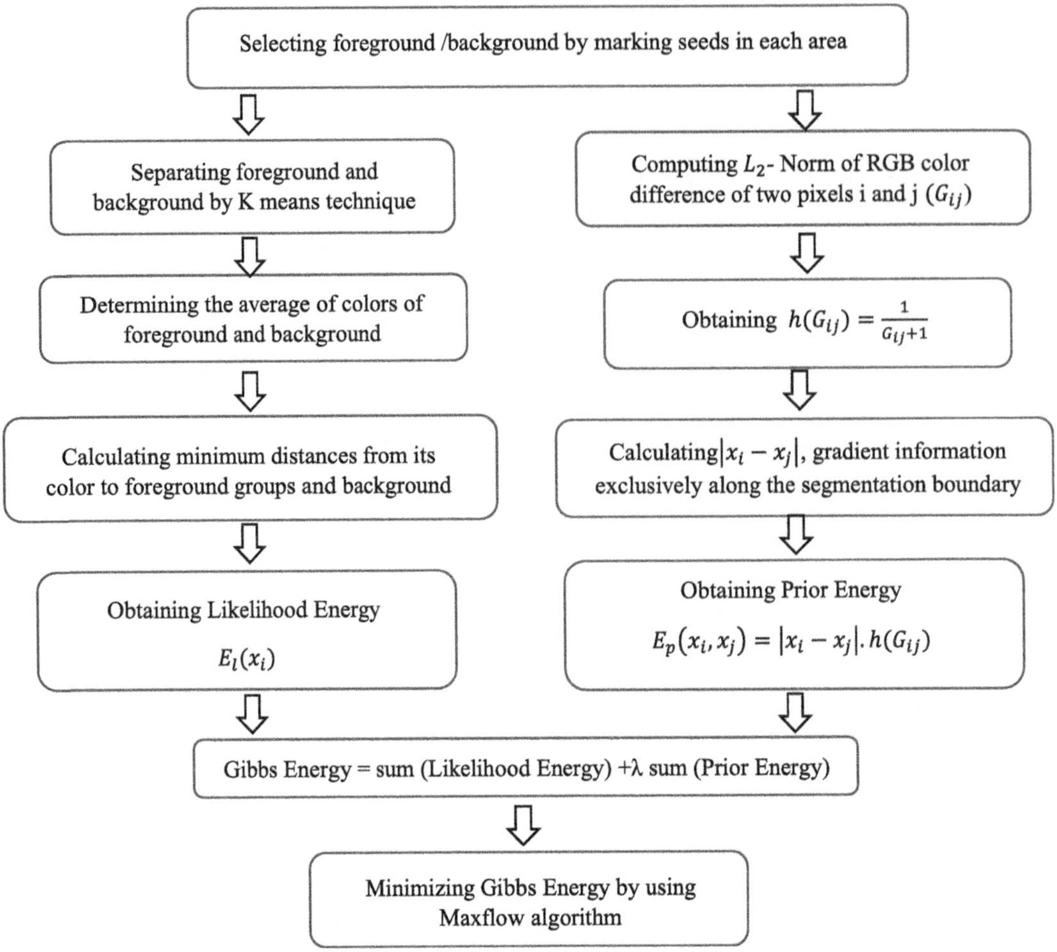

Selecting foreground /background by marking seeds in each area
Separating foreground and background by K means technique
Determining the average of colors of foreground and background
Calculating minimum distances from its color to foreground groups and background
Obtaining Likelihood Energy
$E_l(x_i)$
Computing L_2- Norm of RGB color difference of two pixels i and j (G_{ij})
Obtaining $h(G_{ij}) = \frac{1}{G_{ij}+1}$
Calculating $|x_i - x_j|$, gradient information exclusively along the segmentation boundary
Obtaining Prior Energy
$E_p(x_i, x_j) = |x_i - x_j| . h(G_{ij})$
Gibbs Energy = sum (Likelihood Energy) +λ sum (Prior Energy)
Minimizing Gibbs Energy by using Maxflow algorithm

Fig. 1 Lazy snapping flow chart.

FLIR
36
29
Trefl=23 Tatm=24 Dst=0.4 FOV 23
06/02/06 10:58:21 -10 - +55 e=1.00
°C
(a)
(b)

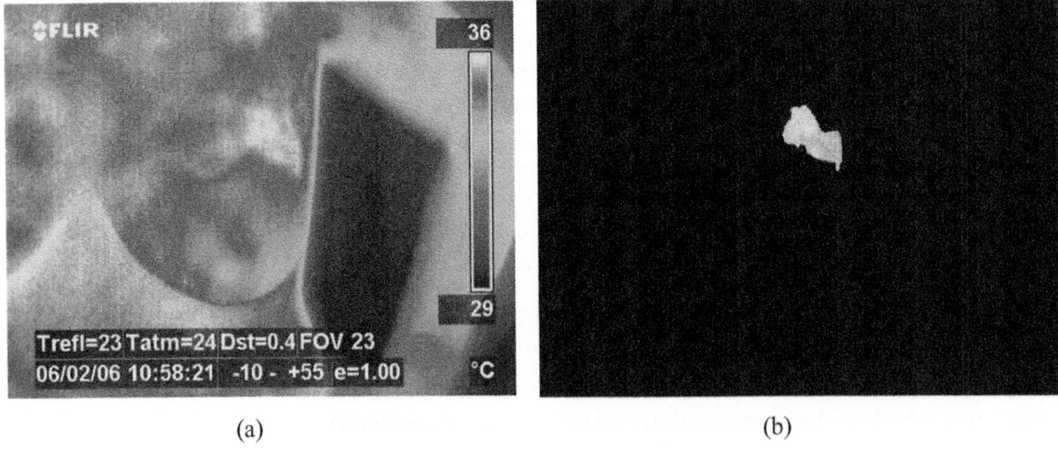

Fig. 2 A cancerous breast (case 1) [Prof. Santos and Prof. Rita dataset]. (A) Thermal image and (B) segmented suspicious region (7 s).

3.2 Case 2: Breast cancer

Thermal image of a female with breast cancer was illustrated. Fortunately, by using thermography, the malignancy was correctly identified. Her thermal image and the tumor or the extreme thermal area segmented by lazy snapping are shown in Fig. 3A and B, respectively.

3.3 Case 3: Mammary cysts

Thermal image of a middle-aged female having mammary cysts in her left breast is shown. Breast cysts can be considered as fluid-filled sacs inside the breast, which are generally not malignant. It usually appears like a grape or water-filled balloon; however, occasionally it is firm. The time taken to segment the extreme thermal region for this case was less than 5 s.

Her thermal image and segmented cysts by lazy snapping are presented in Fig. 4A and B, respectively.

3.4 Case 4: Mammary cysts

Thermal image of a female in middle age is shown. She had mammary cysts in her left breast. Her thermal image is presented in Fig. 5A. The extreme thermal area or suspicious regions segmented by lazy snapping procedure are presented in Fig. 5B. It took us less than 5 s to extract the area.

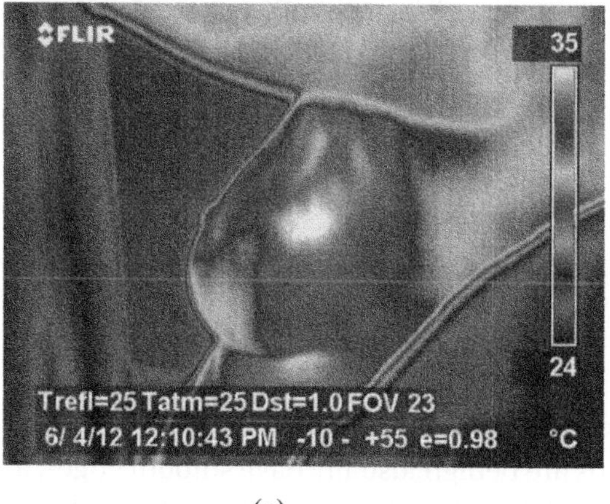

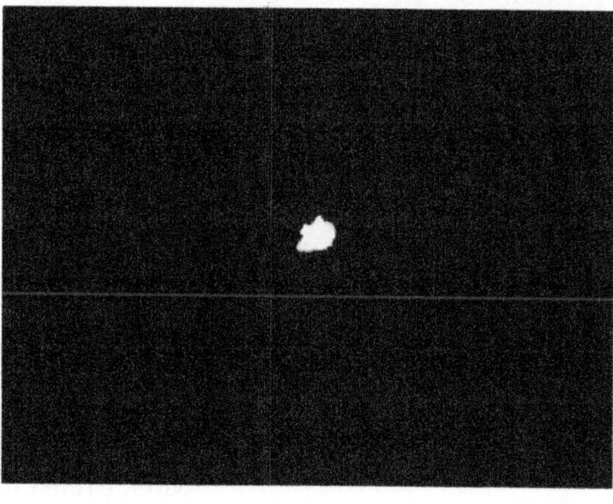

(a) (b)

Fig. 3 A cancerous subject (case 2) [Prof. Santos and Prof. Rita dataset]. (A) Thermal image and (B) extracted tumor area (5 s).

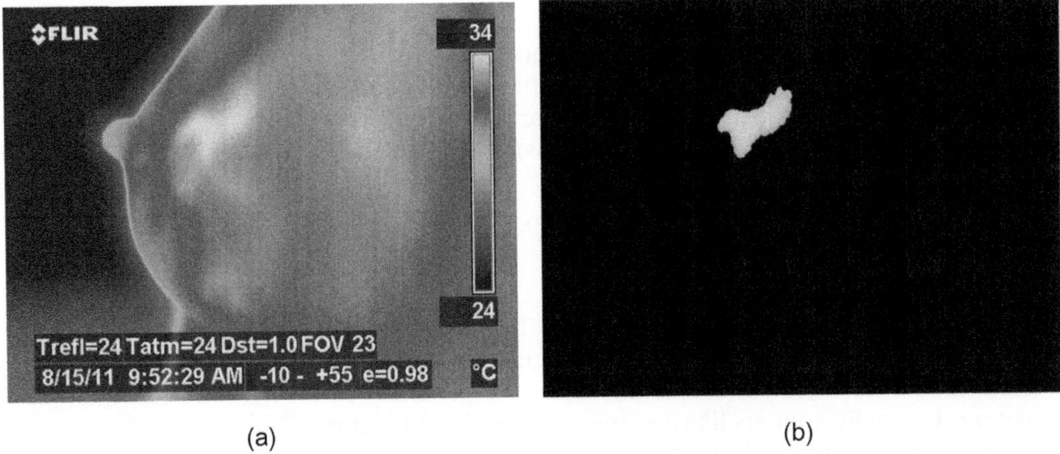

(a)   (b)

Fig. 4 A subject with mammary cysts (case 3) [Prof. Santos and Prof. Rita dataset]. (A) Thermal image and (B) segmented suspicious region (<5 s).

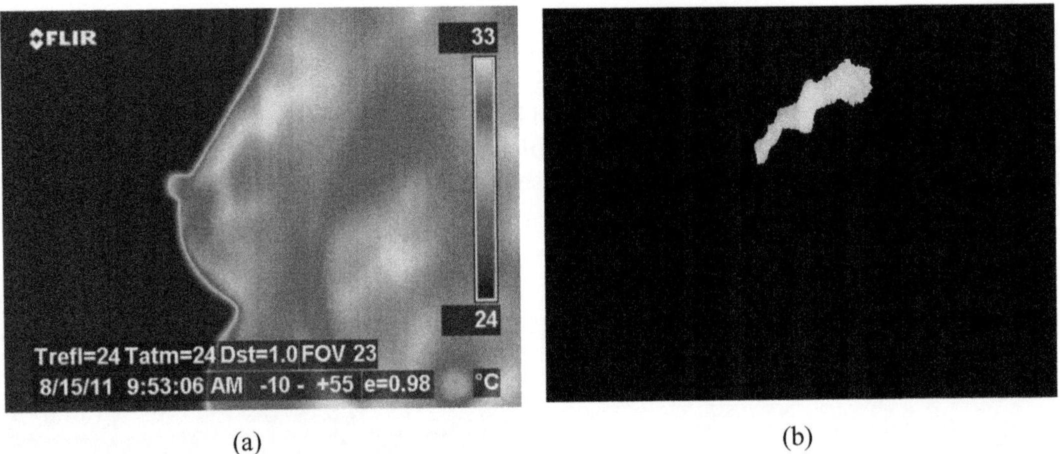

(a)   (b)

Fig. 5 A subject with mammary cysts (case 4) [Prof. Santos and Prof. Rita dataset]. (A) Thermal image and (B) segmented suspicious region (<5 s).

3.5 Case 5: Benign tumor

Most breast lumps are benign, usually have smooth edges, and can be moved slightly when one pushes against them. They are often found in both breasts. Thermal image of a woman in middle age is shown. She had a benign tumor in her right breast. It took us less than 5 s to segment hot spots in her thermogram.

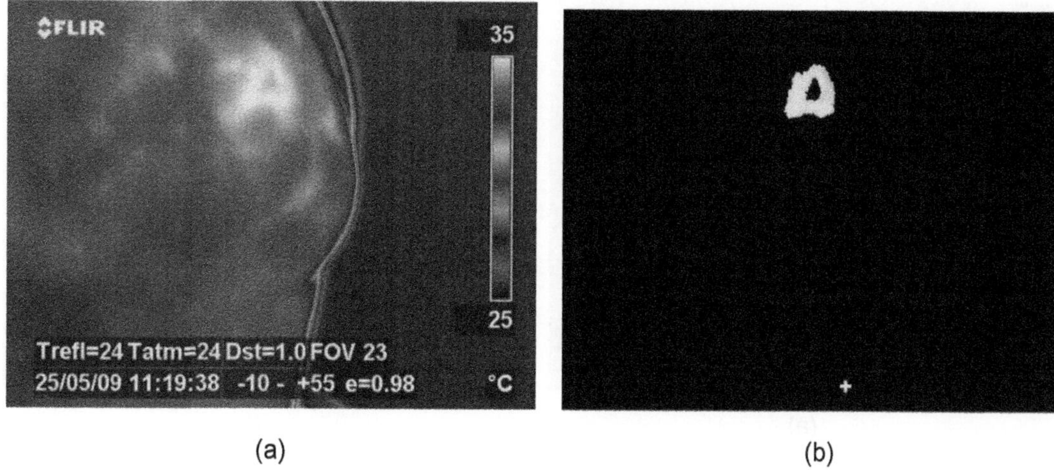

(a)   (b)

Fig. 6 A subject with benign tumor (case 5) [Prof. Santos and Prof. Rita dataset]. (A) Thermal image and (B) segmented suspicious region (<5 s).

Her thermal image and the segmented hot spots by lazy snapping procedure are included in Fig. 6A and B, respectively.

3.6 Case 6: Benign tumors (multiple)

Thermal image of a female is shown. She had several benign tumors in her right breast. It took us only 5 s to extract the hot spots in her thermogram.

Her thermal image and the extracted suspicious regions by lazy snapping procedure are included in Fig. 7A and B, respectively.

3.7 Case 7: Benign tumors

Thermal image of a female in middle age is presented. She had several benign tumors in her left breast. Extracting the extreme thermal sites in her thermogram took us less than 5 s.

Her thermal image is demonstrated in Fig. 8A. The extracted inflamed parts are depicted in Fig. 8B.

3.8 Case 8: Benign tumors

Thermal image of a female in middle age is shown. Her problem was a benign tumor in her right breast. The time taken to segment the hot areas in her thermogram was less than 5 s.

Her thermal image is illustrated in Fig. 9A. Also, the suspicious area segmented by lazy snapping procedure is included in Fig. 9B.

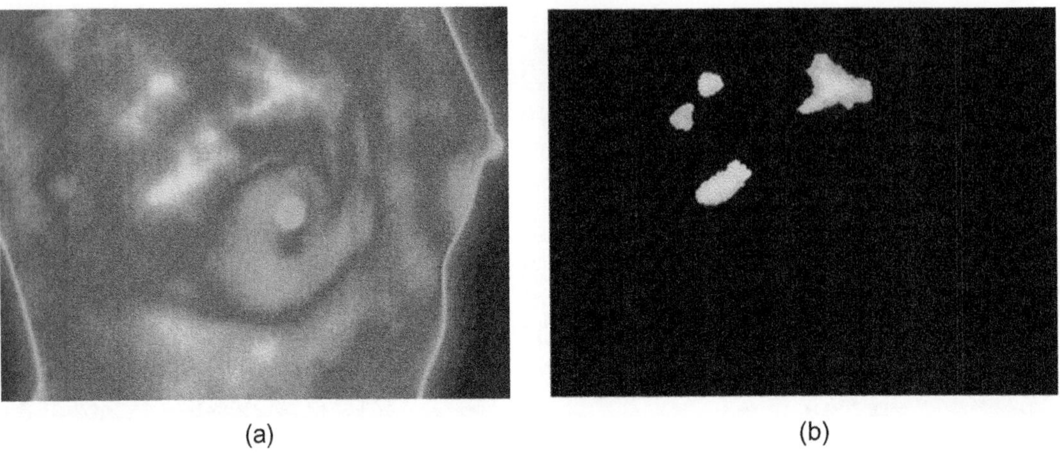

(a)   (b)

Fig. 7 A subject with multiple benign tumors (case 6) [Prof. Santos and Prof. Rita dataset]. (A) Thermal image and (B) segmented suspicious region (5 s).

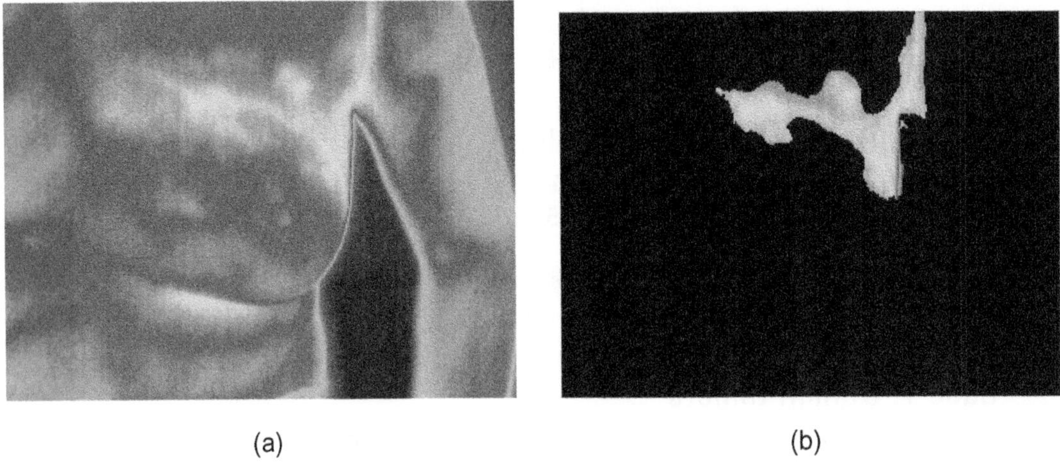

(a)   (b)

Fig. 8 A benign tumor subject (case 7) [Prof. Santos and Prof. Rita dataset]. (A) Thermal image and (B) segmented suspicious region (<5 s).

3.9 Case 9: Advanced cancer

A thermal image of a subject with advanced cancer is illustrated in Fig. 10A. Her cancer was in her right breast. By lazy snapping, the suspicious region was extracted for 10 s. The segmented tumor is included in Fig. 10B. As observed, the segmented regions were not accurate enough. Small areas with narrow and sharp

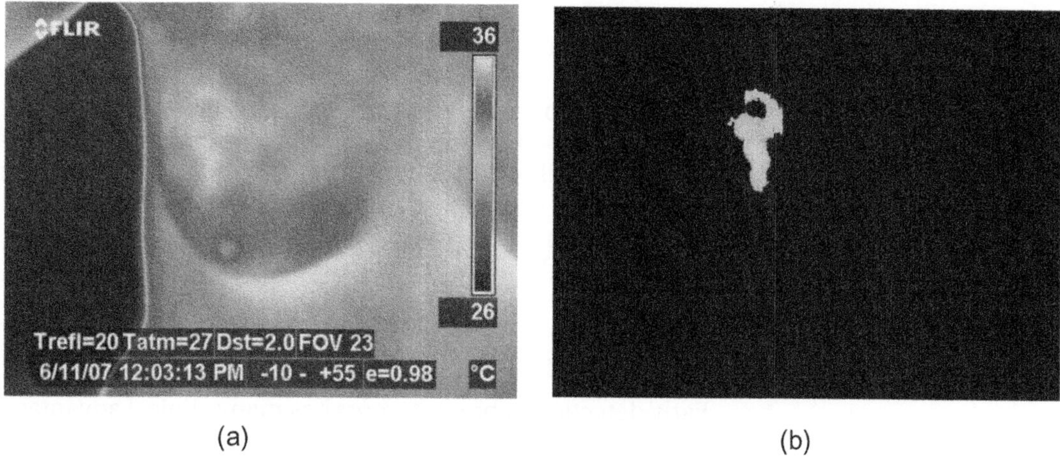

(a)   (b)

Fig. 9 A subject with benign tumor (case 8) [Prof. Santos and Prof. Rita dataset]. (A) Thermal image and (B) segmented suspicious region (<5 s).

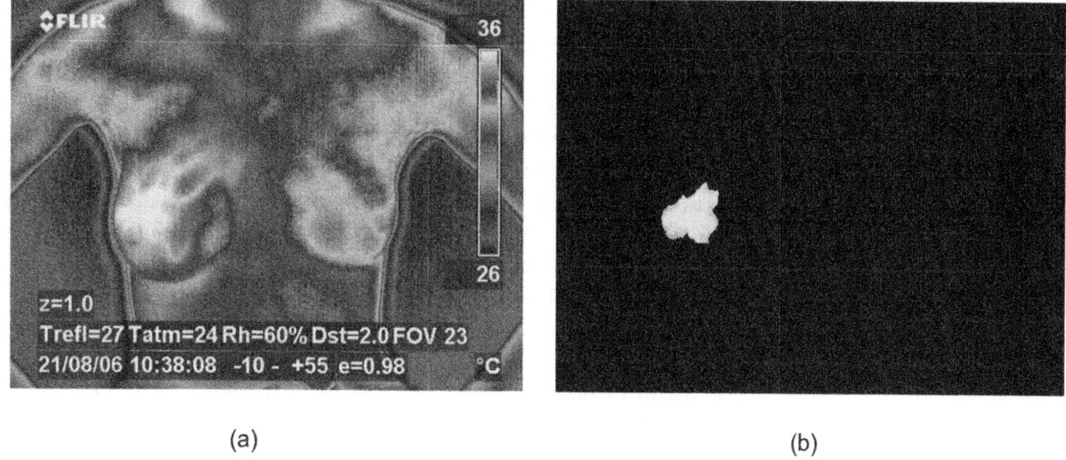

(a)   (b)

Fig. 10 An advanced cancerous subject (case 9) [Prof. Santos and Prof. Rita dataset]. (A) Thermal image and (B) segmented tumor (10 s).

edges sometimes cannot be segmented accurately. This case presented a limitation for employing lazy snapping to segment doubtful regions in breast thermal images.

As seen, the inflamed tumor areas were successfully segmented in the cancer cases, mammary cysts, and benign tumors cases, respectively. A related point to consider is that implementing the procedure was sufficiently fast to be conceded as a quick evaluation. The time taken varied from less than 5 to 10 s for each of these nine cases. Segmentation procedures such as fuzzy c means, level set, K means, and mean shift procedures were used by the authors to segment breast thermograms in their previous studies [17,18,23–26]. Nonetheless, lazy snapping procedure was more user-friendly and could contribute to a quicker evaluation. Moreover, a case with low accuracy was illustrated in this study to show a limitation of this procedure for cases containing small suspicious areas with narrow and sharp edges.

4. Conclusion

Early detection of breast tumors has many clinical advantages, such as treating primary tumors without surgery and considering more treatment options. Psychologically, it is more approachable to the patients since their chance of survival will be increased. Thermography is a technique with the potential to detect breast abnormalities earlier than other methods. Extreme thermal sites in breast thermal images have susceptibility to be suspicious. Accordingly, segmenting these areas in breast thermal images is beneficial. Lazy snapping procedure was employed in this study to segment doubtful, inflamed regions in thermal images for early breast cancer detection. Nine cases were included to demonstrate our findings. The time taken to see the results of these nine cases varied from less than 5 to 10 s. The procedure was quite user-friendly and quick as well. Furthermore, different segmentation procedures such as fuzzy c means, level set, K means, and mean shift procedures were used by the authors to extract suspicious regions in breast thermal images. It is worthwhile to mention that, when comparing them, lazy snapping was quicker and can promptly support results for medical professionals in real time. The authors believe that lazy snapping procedure is capable of being employed to segment extreme thermal regions in breast thermal images quickly with easily detailed transformation.

Acknowledgments

We would like to thank Prof. Wellington Pinheiro dos Santos and Prof. Rita for letting us share their breast dataset.

References

[1] W.C. Amalu, Infrared Imaging Review, 2017. http://www.breastthermography.com/infrared_imaging_review.htm. (Accessed 2017).

[2] M. Etehadtavakol, E.Y.K. Ng, An overview of medical infrared imaging in breast abnormalities detection, in: E.Y.K. Ng, M. Etehadtavakol (Eds.), Application of Infrared to Biomedical Sciences, Springer Nature Science, 2017, pp. 45–57, https://doi.org/10.1007/978-981-10-3147-2.

[3] E.Y.K. Ng, A review of thermography as promising non-invasive detection modality for breast tumour, Int. J. Therm. Sci. 48 (5) (2009) 849–855.

[4] E.Y.K. Ng, L.N. Ung, F.C. Ng, L.S.G. Sim, Statistical analysis of healthy and malignant breast thermography, J. Med. Eng. Technol. 25 (6) (2001) 253–263.

[5] J.F. Head, F. Wang, C.A. Lipari, R.L. Elliott, The important role of infrared imaging in breast cancer, IEEE Eng. Med. Biol. Mag. 19 (3) (2000) 52–57.

[6] M. Gautherie, C.M. Gros, Breast thermography and cancer risk prediction, J. Cancer 45 (1) (1980) 51–56.

[7] A.M. Stark, The value of risk factors in screening for breast cancer, Eur. J. Surg. Oncol. 11 (2) (1985) 147–150.

[8] J.F. Head, R.L. Elliott, Infrared imaging: making progress in fulfilling its medical promise, IEEE Eng. Med. Biol. Mag. 21 (6) (2002) 80–85.

[9] M.A. Santana, J.M.S. Pereira, F.L. Silva, N.M. Lima, F.N. Sousa, G.M.S. Arruda, R.C.F. Lima, W.W.A. Silva, W.P. Santos, Breast cancer diagnosis based on mammary thermography and extreme learning machines, Res. Biomed. Eng. 34 (1) (2018) 45–53.

[10] J.H. Vasconcelos, W.P. Santos, R.F. Lima, Analysis of methods of classification of breast thermography images to determine their viability in the detection of cancer, IEEE Lat. Am. Trans. 16 (6) (2018) 1631–1637.

[11] N.A. Espíndola, L.A. Bezerra, L.C. Santos, R.C.F. Lima, Estimating breast thermophysical parameters by the use of mapping surface temperatures measured by infrared images, IEEE Lat. Am. Trans. 16 (10) (2018) 2617–2624.

[12] M.C. Araujo, R.M.C.R. Souza, R.C.F. Lima, T.M.S. Filho, An interval prototype classifier based on a parameterized distance applied to breast thermographic images, Med. Biol. Eng. Comput. 55 (6) (2017) 873–884.

[13] M.C. Araujo, R.C.F. Lima, R.M.C.R. Souza, Interval symbolic feature extraction for thermography breast cancer detection, Expert Syst. Appl. 41 (15) (2014) 6728–6737.

[14] M. Etehadtavakol, E.Y.K. Ng, Breast thermography as a potential non-contact method in early detection of cancer: a review, J. Mech. Med. Biol. 13 (2) (2013) 1330001.

[15] Sat, N.D. Kaur, The Complete Natural Medicine Guide to Breast Cancer, Robert Rose, 2003.

[16] M. Etehadtavakol, E.Y.K. Ng, Color segmentation of breast thermograms, in: E.Y.K. Ng, M. Etehadtavakol (Eds.), Application of Infrared to Biomedical Sciences, Springer Nature Science, 2017, pp. 69–77.

[17] M. Etehadtavakol, S. Sadri, E.Y.K. Ng, Application of K-and fuzzy c-means for color segmentation of thermal infrared breast images, J. Med. Syst. 34 (1) (2010) 35–42.

[18] N. Golestani, M. Etehadtavakol, E.Y.K. Ng, Level set method for segmentation of infrared breast thermograms, EXCLI J. 13 (2014) 241–251.

[19] Y. Li, J. Sun, C.K. Tang, H.Y. Shum, Lazy snapping, in: Proceeding SIGGRAPH '04, Association for Computing Machinery's Special Interest Group on Computer Graphics and Interactive Techniques, 2004, pp. 303–308.

[20] S. Geman, D. Geman, Stochastic relaxation, Gibbs distributions, and the Bayesian restoration of images, IEEE Trans. Pattern Anal. Mach. Intell. PAMI-6 (6) (1984) 721–741.

[21] Y. Boykov, V. Kolmogorov, An experimental comparison of min-cut/max-flow algorithms for energy minimization in vision, IEEE Trans. PAMI 26 (9) (2004) 1124–1137.

[22] R.O. Duda, P.E. Hart, D.G. Stork, Pattern Classification, second ed., Wiley Press, 2001, https://doi.org/10.1007/BF01237942.

[23] S. Kermani, N. Samadzadehaghdam, M. Etehadtavakol, Automatic color segmentation of breast infrared images using a Gaussian mixture model, Optik 126 (21) (2015) 3288–3294.

[24] N. Samadzadehaghdam, M. Moradiamin, M. Etehadtavakol, E.Y.K. Ng, Designing and comparing different color map algorithms for pseudo-coloring breast thermograms, J. Med. Imag. Health Informatics 3 (4) (2013) 487–493.

[25] E.Y.K. Ng, M. Etehadtavakol, Application of Infrared to Biomedical Sciences, Springer Nature Science, 2017, https://doi.org/10.1007/978-981-10-3147-2.

[26] M. Etehadtavakol, Z. Emrani, E.Y.K. Ng, Rapid extraction of the hottest or coldest regions of medical thermographic images, Med. Biol. Eng. Comput. 57 (2) (2019) 379–388.

11

New metrics to assess the subtle changes of the heart's electromagnetic field

I. Chaikovsky[a], M. Primin[a], I. Nedayvoda[a], A. Kazmirchuk[b], Yu. Frolov[a], and M. Boreyko[a]

[a]Glushkov Institute for Cybernetics of National Academy of Science of Ukraine, Kyiv, Ukraine. [b]National Military Medical Clinical Center "GVKG", Kyiv, Ukraine

1. Introduction

Effective diagnosis of heart disease remains one of New metrics to assess the subtle changes?>the main tasks of clinical medicine due to the high prevalence and socioeconomic importance of diseases such as cardiovascular diseases, which in recent decades has become a pandemic [1]. In most European countries, cardiovascular diseases account for around 300 deaths per 100,000 people. Clearly, there is a need to improve methods for heart diseases detection. Which applies to noninvasive methods that are most accessible and safe.

Analysis of the electrical activity of the heart is still the most common, affordable, and cheapest method of objective examination of the heart. However, the sensitivity and specificity of routine electrocardiographic examination are not high enough. It is known, for example, that a resting ECG, assessed by its routine criteria, remains normal in approximately 50% of patients with chronic coronary heart disease, including during episodes of chest discomfort [2]. Improving diagnostics is possible only based on innovative technologies.

Over many years, the Glushkov Institute of Cybernetics of NAS of Ukraine developed a number of modern information technologies based on new software and hardware complexes for the analysis of both electric and magnetic components of the

Advanced Methods in Biomedical Signal Processing and Analysis. https://doi.org/10.1016/B978-0-323-85955-4.00005-3
Copyright © 2023 Elsevier Inc. All rights reserved.

electromagnetic field of the heart. The basis of the development of these modern means of functional diagnostics, and especially their implementation in the practice of treatment and prevention facilities, is a new scientific direction of the Institute, i.e., clinical cybernetics.

Clinical cybernetics is a branch of science whose subject is the development and application of automated information systems and technologies that support the adoption of all possible types of medical decisions, namely diagnostic, prognostic, and tactical—related to the tactics of patients in the broadest sense of the word—which all take place in clinical medicine. Thus, the central feature of clinical cybernetics is clinical information technology (IT), which is a combination of up-to-date methods and equipment bound in a chain that provides collection, storage, preprocessing, interpretation, conclusion, and dissemination of information [3].

At the output of technology, an information product is formed that meets the needs of a particular subject area, using a "dictionary" of this subject area. In IT related to clinical cybernetics, such automatically occurring products are diagnostic reports, forecast reports, and personalized preventive measures reports, including different kinds of treatment.

Many clinical IT include the development of technical means for recording and analyzing biological information in the form of program and apparatus complexes (PAC), for example, the IT analyzes of the electric generator of the heart developed in Glushkov Institute of Cybernetics of National Academy of Science of Ukraine. The development of diagnostic tools is primarily a constant increase in the "distributive" capacity of diagnostic methods, i.e., the ability to detect increasingly subtle changes in the function being studied by one method or another.

Such opportunities appear due to the progress of technical means of measuring a particular function, and even more due to the development of IT; in other words, the creation of new metrics, i.e., numerical indicators that can assess previously unavailable aspects of various organs and systems of the human body. As a result, first, ways are opened to increase the diagnostic accuracy of a method within the traditional application scenarios for this method, and second, the usual methods are beginning to be used in new areas.

The purpose of this chapter is to give some examples of innovative information technologies introduced into our practice. They are used for registration and evaluation of slight electromagnetic field changes of a heart, thus providing early diagnosis of severe heart malfunctions.

2. Information technology of magnetocardiography: Basis, technical means, diagnostic metrics

2.1 Definition and short essay on the history of magnetocardiography

Magnetocardiography (MCG) is a method of noninvasive, electrophysiological examination of the human heart. This method consists of noncontact registration—over the patient's thorax—of the values of the parameters of the magnetic field generated by the electrical activity of the myocardium during the cardiac cycle, and reconstruction and analysis of the spatiotemporal characteristics of electrical sources in the volume of the myocardium found after solving the inverse problem.

The history of MCG begins in 1963, when Baule and McFee measured the parameters of the magnetic field of the human heart using induction sensors containing more than 2 million turns of copper wire at the University of New York (Faculty of Medicine, Syracuse, USA). The first studies of MCG on similar equipment were carried out in the USSR in 1966. A breakthrough in the field of MCG came in 1970 when Cohen of the Massachusetts Institute of Technology for the first time registered human MCG using a Superconductive Quantum Interference Device (SQUID) magnetometer. Currently, MCG laboratories operate in the USA, Germany, China, Korea, Italy, Finland, Great Britain, Russia, Ukraine, Japan, Taiwan, India, etc.

Compared with the potential methods of heart examination, the conducting volume of the human body is "transparent" to the magnetic field of the heart and practically does not affect the magnitude of the signal recorded by the magnetometric system. Thus, when measuring the MCG, we receive information directly about the currents in the heart, and when registering an ECG, we receive information about the currents flowing in the human body and indirectly in the heart.

By measuring the parameters of the magnetic field of the heart in the air over the patient thorax, we can correctly reconstruct the spatial distribution of its sources in the heart according to these data. One can then "see" the very first changes in the spatial structure of ion currents, which are precursors of subsequent pathology.

Developing supersensitive equipment is only part of the problem of contactless diagnostics. Another essential component of high technology, which determines the possibility and success of the application of such systems, is the developing of IT for the interpretation of magnetometric measurements data. This requires theoretical studies and the development of new mathematical models and methods to restore the space–time image of the distribution of the field sources in the human heart.

Thus, magnetocardiographic technology is provided by technical and software tools, combined and developed in a diagnostic complex. Magnetocardiographic systems, which were developed in Germany, Finland, Japan, Korea, etc., can work only in special magnetically shielded rooms, the cost of which is comparable to or higher than the cost of the diagnostic systems themselves.

A series of diagnostic magnetocardiographic software-hardware complexes, "MAGSCAN," which do not require special equipment and magnetic shielding of the compartment, has been created in V.M. Glushkov Institute of Cybernetics. Developing these complexes opens up the possibility of their widespread use in ordinary city clinics. These devices are examples of new medical technology and belong to the products combining a number of high technologies, such as superconducting microelectronics, quantum magnetometry, composite materials technology, mathematical methods of data processing and analysis, IT, statistical methods of process recognition, and clinical cardiology.

Manufactured diagnostic systems have successfully passed state technical and clinical tests in Ukraine and China.

2.2 Technical means: Magnetometric complex

Magnetocardiographic complex "MAGSCAN" provides nine channels for magnetocardiosignal (MCS) recording and three reference channels, which are used in the system of electronic noise suppression. Each channel for MCG registration comprises the second-order axial gradiometer ($\partial^2 B_z / \partial z^2$), consisting of a wire-wound magnetic flux transformer mounted on a graphite base 20 mm in diameter and connected to a DC-SQUID placed in a capsule. The reference channels are in the form of a vector SQUID magnetometer, which consists of three separate DC-SQUIDs arranged on the respective sides of the cube. Nine recording MCG channels based on DC-SQUIDs are placed in a fiberglass cryostat with helium at the nodes of a square grid (Fig. 1; 3×3) with a 40-mm step between the centers of the receiving coils of the gradiometers.

In the process of the MCG examination, the patient's chest is moved relative to the fixed cryostat with a measuring module sequentially in four spatial positions. The movement is performed in such a way that, after the location of centers of the flux

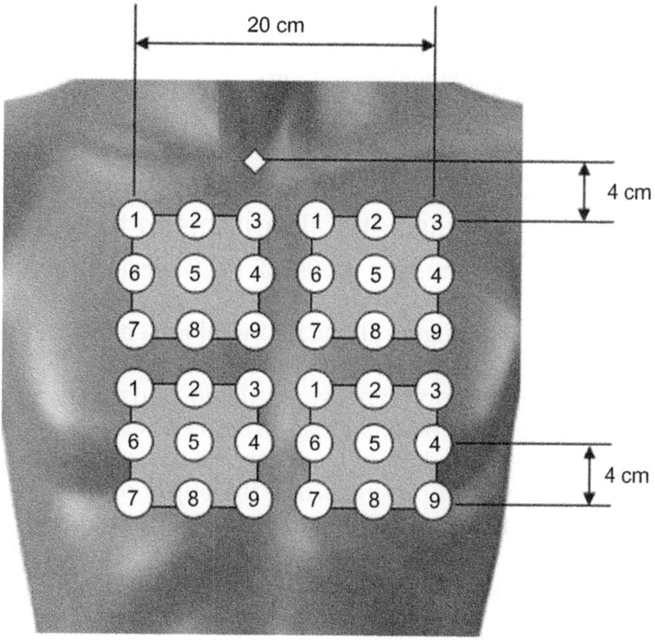

Fig. 1 Arrangement of MCG recording channels and positions of the measuring module in relation to the patient's chest.

transformer of MCG, recording channels form a system of 36 points in the plane (6×6 along mutually perpendicular directions with a step of 4 cm; Fig. 1). Fig. 1 shows a diagram of the points of MCS registration in relation to the patient's chest and its "binding" to the anatomical landmarks (at *jugular foci*).

MCS registration by nine channels takes about 1 min in each of the four positions for the accumulation of 30–60 cardiocycles to achieve the maximum signal-to-noise ratio by averaging. Note that an increase in the number of channels to several dozen means an increase in the cost of both the system itself and the consumption of expensive consumable material, i.e., liquid helium. Therefore, the potential market for such multichannel systems is limited. In addition, an increase in the number of channels does not mean a proportional decrease in the patient's examination time, since a certain time is needed to prepare them and the system for examination, and this takes at least 5 min. Therefore, to optimize the price/quality balance of the diagnostic procedure, a measuring module was designed with nine signal and three reference channels, which reduces the number of registration points to four and reduces the examination time for each patient to 5–7 min; 15 L of liquid helium is enough for 7 days of continuous work. The final step in this phase of the investigation involves recording MCG registration data to the database and executing signal preprocessing in an automatic mode.

2.3 The consecutive steps, electrophysiological basis, and algorithms of the MCG-signal analysis

In the first steps of MCG development, the MCG analysis methods reproduced the ECG analysis methods; it was used without changing all the names of ECG peaks, segments, and intervals. The morphological features of MCG at different points of the measurements plane were studied, and a few amplitude-temporal criteria for the diagnosis of some disease symptoms were found and described. It is necessary to understand that the peculiarity of MCG processing is that the object of study is one averaged cardio complex at given points of the measurements plane (in our case, the number of points is 36: 6×6 grid with 4 cm between the points placed along the mutually perpendicular axis). During the ECG analysis, the subject of study is the temporal sequence of complexes of determined number of ECG leads (it is also possible to perform them in one averaged complex, but the information about the spatial distribution of the signal will absent). Therefore the direct transfer of ECG analysis methods into an MCG analysis prevents its use, in this case, the main advantage of MCG, which the high sensitivity of this method to the changes of spatial–temporal distribution of currents density vector or to the changes of distributions of measured values of the heart's magnetic field in the borders of the measurements area. As a result, it is necessary to take the next step in the development of MCG analysis and interpretation methods: the development of new computer analysis methods directed to the study of spatial (in the borders of measurements area) and temporal (in the sequence of discontinuous temporal points $t_1 \ldots t_n$ of the cardiocycle) characteristics of an MCG signal.

Computer processing of MCG starts from digital data processing with digital filtration and averaging of cardiocycles as mean stages; averaging (accumulation) of MCG cardiocycles supposes their synchronization with respect to some temporal moment of support at any recurring QRS complex. Moreover, binding to the support point inside already averaged cardiocycles is necessary for the synchronization of MCG measurements at different space points made at different time intervals (in our case, four positions of a nine-channel measuring module). Since ECG and MCG are caused by the activity of the same electrophysiological sources, the support time moments and cardiocycle borders are chosen from the second standard ECG lead. All the processes are made automatic, but in case of need, manual correction of all the filtration and averaging parameters is possible. As a result of initial processing, the file with temporal sampling of averaged cardiocycles is created for every type of QRS complex and for every 36 points of space where MCG recording was performed (Fig. 2).

After averaging, the cardiocycle includes the complete P-QRS-T complex with the segments of base (zero) line before and after the complex. The averaged cardiocycles are synchronized with all the measurements points, and MCG curves are recorded to files with 1000 Hz frequency. In other words, the interval between the samplings is 1 ms for any sampling moment (time point on the MCG curve in 1 ms), thus it is possible to construct a map of spatial distribution of measured field characteristics. The construction and analysis of the dynamic sequence of the spatiotemporal distribution of the values of the parameters of the magnetic field of the patient's heart within the measurement grid (magnetic map) for the selected times of the averaged cardiac cycle is one of the main visual stages of the MCG analysis. Fig. 3 shows an example of the sequence of the magnetic maps during an ST-T interval for a healthy patient and for a patient with ischemia heart disease

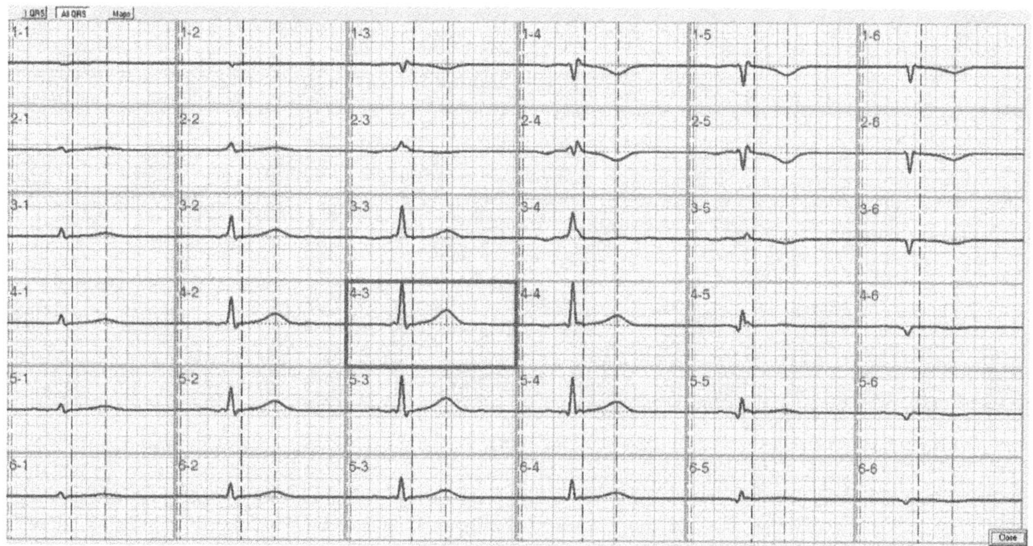

Fig. 2 Averaged MCG cardiocycles in 36 points of rectangular measurements grid: an example of the representation on the computer screen.

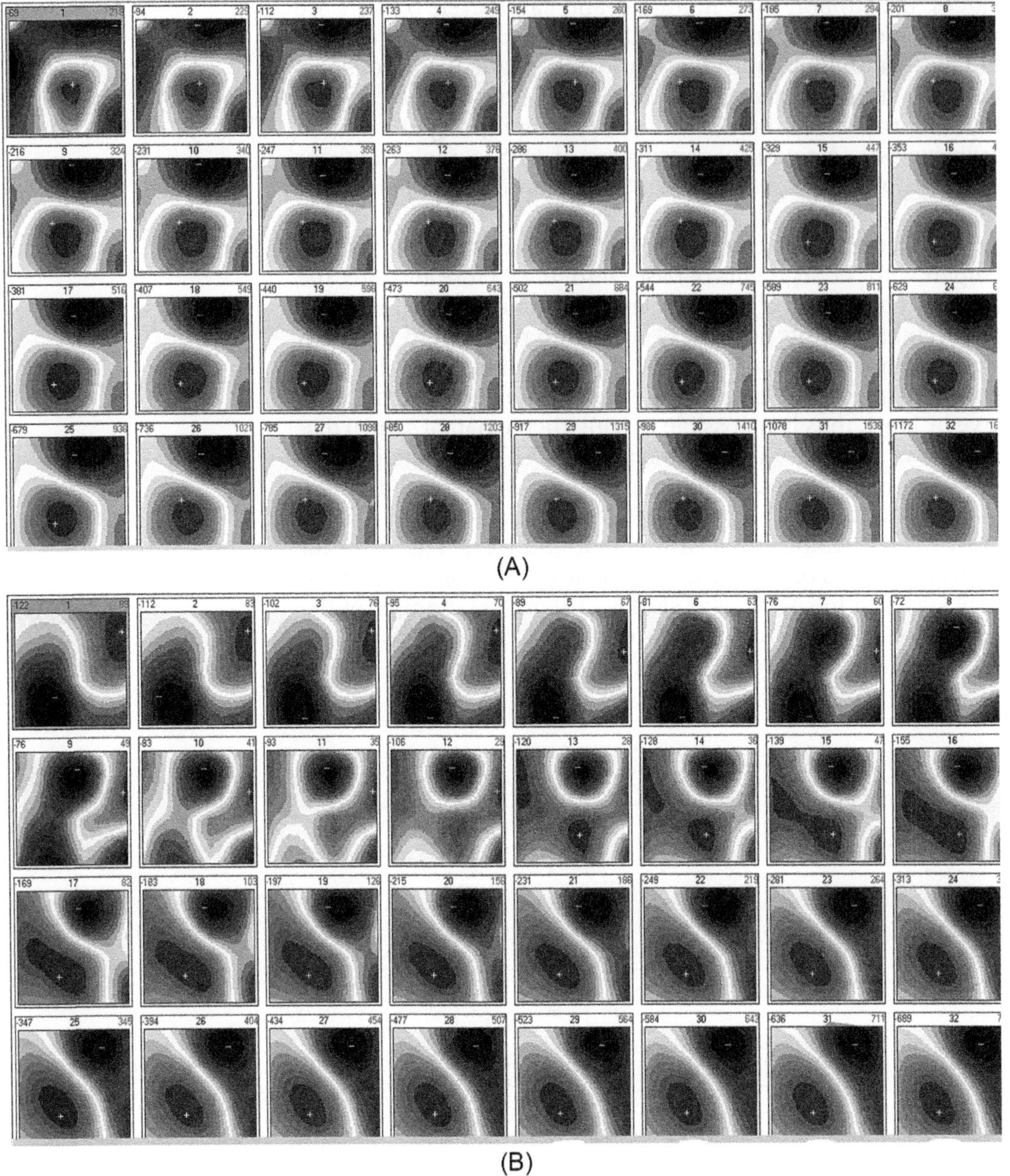

(A)

(B)

Fig. 3 Heart magnetic field distribution (ST-T interval) in the norm (A) and in the case of left coronary artery occlusion (B). Note that, in this presentation, the adaptive step between the isolines is used. This step is adjusted depending on the values of maximum and minimum of every separate map, and these values are indicated by *red* (gray in the print version) and *blue colors* (dark gray in the print version) over every map. (For interpretation of the references to color in this figure legend, the reader is referred to the web version of this article.)

(IHD). Each map from Fig. 3 represents the measured magnetic field distribution not only in the given 36 points of measurement plane but also in the points of the finer grid. The signal values in these lattice points (not corresponding to the initial 36 points) are calculated using interpolation methods.

During the study of the ventricular repolarization process, the known electrophysiological model is used as the hypothesis. This model supposes that the beginning of the ST-T interval clashes with the start of a slow repolarization phase (action potential plateau). If all parts of the myocardium simultaneously enter this phase, then in the very beginning of the ST segment, we will get the maps of "normal" structure (two extremums: positive and negative); the maps are symmetrical with respect to the diagonal, and the maximal positive values exceed the negative in absolute meaning (in the limits of 1.3–2.3) over all the ST-T interval. However, even in the norm, some heterogeneity (dispersion) of repolarization may be observed on the first part of the ST. It becomes apparent in the fact that the first few magnetic field distribution maps (and currents maps as well) have a modified structure compared with all other maps from the ST-T interval. At the increase of heterogeneity level because of the change of action potential shape (for example, because of ischemia or others pathological processes), the number of myocardium areas with unfinished depolarization can increase. It leads to an increase of map's quantity with abnormal field distribution. If after some time all the myocardium areas are in the same action potential phase, then the recovery of the field distribution map's structure happens. It is possible to estimate the heterogeneity durability and nature of the magnetic maps during the visual analysis of the MCG of investigated patient and/or using the special magnetocardiograph software. For the study and analysis of the homogeneity of the heart ventricular repolarization processes using the magnetocardiograph MAGSCAN, the program block Spcwin.exe was developed and used. After the start of this program, the MCG analysis in the ST-T interval is performed according to a special algorithm.

The reconstruction and analysis of magnetic field sources distributed in the heart volume is performed on the next stage of the MCG study. After the start of the program block to solve the magnetostatics inverse problem for the dipole model of MCG, signal source performs the solution and analysis of the magnetostatics inverse problem for the "punctated" (focal) pathologies for given time moments from chosen cardiocycle interval. By its mathematical nature, the transformation methods of MCG information (for this stage of the study) correspond to the solution of the so-named magnetostatics inverse problem for the dipole model of the magnetic signal source. The authors of IT "MAGSCAN" have proposed using a biomagnetic signal source, the so-named magnetic dipole, to find the problem solution in the form of simple algebraic equations (ratios). The developed method is realized in the form of program blocks of magnetocardiograph and is successfully used in cardio-hospitals to find the location of an arrhythmia source in the heart. To connect the results of magnetic field source localization with the anatomical reference points in the heart, metal rings of 10-mm diameter were used. These coils were fixed on the patient's thorax over the problem place. The coordinates of this place have been calculated during processing of the measurements data of the MCG signal. The metal coils are distinguishable in the X-ray during surgery (Fig. 4).

The accuracy of calculation of coordinate of focal magnetic field source is better than 3 mm. In the next stage, the magnetostatics' inverse problem solution for several independent magnetic field sources distributed in the heart was found and realized by the software [4]. In other words, the program "MAGSCAN-09" makes it possible to find and noninvasively localize the position of several simultaneously existing pathology zones.

When analyzing data from a magnetocardiographic study, it is often required to solve the inverse problem. In this case, it is assumed that the location of the observation points (in the air,

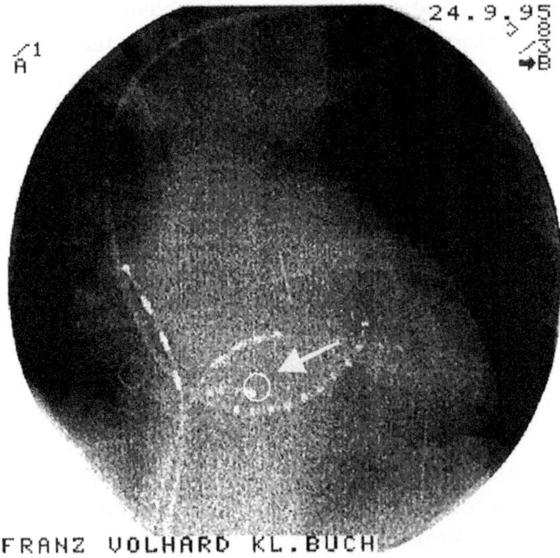

Fig. 4 The view of an X-ray scanner screen during high-frequency ablation of additional conduction underway in WPW syndrome. The arrow shows the position of a 10-mm diameter metal coil against a background of the heart. The coordinates of this coil are defined during MCG signal analysis, and the point inside the coil is the catheter position during ablation.

above the patient's chest) is known. At each observation point, the values of the output signal of the SQUID gradiometer are known (measured). Based on these data, it is required to restore the spatial configuration of the source of the MCS, for example, to determine the distribution of the current density vectors (CDVs).

2.4 Inverse problem statement

Let us assume that the model in the form of one [5,6] or N [4] magnetic dipoles can be correctly applied to describe the magnetic field. Then the solution of the inverse problem of magnetostatics can be obtained in the form of analytical methods. These algorithms have no restrictions on the area of application.

Choosing a field source model is an exacting task. To solve it, it is necessary to analyze the conditions for registering a magnetic signal. Suppose that the source of the field is the CDVs $\mathbf{j}(\mathbf{r}')$, which are located at points $\mathbf{r}'$ of a homogeneous infinite space V. Then the magnetic induction vector $B(r)$ at a point in the surrounding space $\mathbf{r}$ (in air) is determined by the Biot-Savard law:

$$\mathbf{B(r)} = \frac{\mu_0}{4\pi} \int_V \frac{[\mathbf{j}(\mathbf{r}') \times (\mathbf{r} - \mathbf{r}')]}{|\mathbf{r} - \mathbf{r}'|^3} dV. \tag{1}$$

It is known that the use of the results of magnetometric measurements to reconstruct (determine) CDVs, arbitrarily distributed in a three-dimensional volume, is indistinct. Let us further assume that the CDVs have a two-dimensional structure. Then, under the appropriate conditions, you can get a unique solution to the problem. The areas of application of the described approach are calculations of the distribution of electric currents in slices of active biological tissue and the study of various physical systems (microcircuits, welding places of aircraft parts) using nondestructive methods [7].

So, let's assume that the CDVs $\mathbf{j}(\mathbf{r}')$ are in a thin layer in the XOY plane. The observation points are in the $z = r_z$ plane, parallel to the XOY plane, as shown in Fig. 5.

Suppose that the quasistatic current distribution satisfies the condition div $\mathbf{j} = 0$. Then using Eq. (1), we obtain for the magnetic induction vector at each measurement point:

$$B_z(\mathbf{r}) = \frac{\mu_0}{4\pi} \int_V \frac{\left[j_x(\mathbf{r}) \times (y - y') \right]}{|\mathbf{r} - \mathbf{r}'|^3} dV$$

$$-\frac{\mu_0}{4\pi} \int_V \frac{\left[j_y(\mathbf{r}') \times (x - x') \right]}{|\mathbf{r} - \mathbf{r}'|^3} dV \tag{2}$$

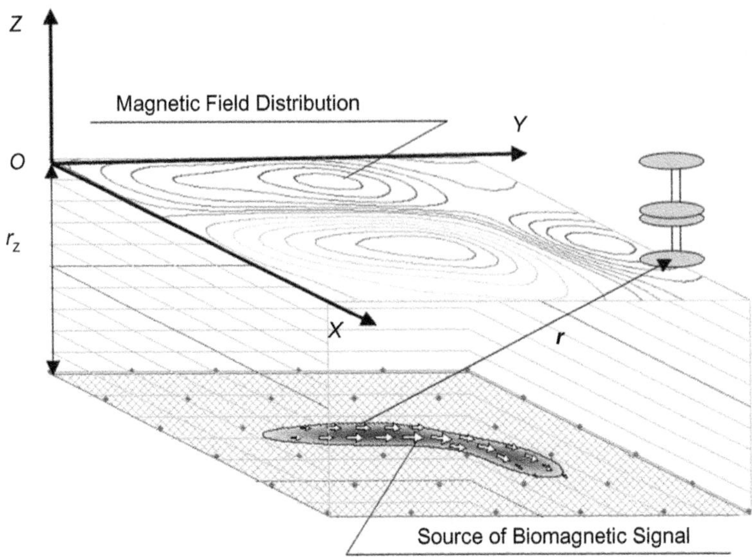

Fig. 5 The relative position of the pickup coil of the magnetic flux transformer of the SQUID gradiometer, the plane where the characteristics of the magnetic signal are registered, and the source of the magnetic signal in the form of a planar system of currents.

Then the inverse problem can be formulated as follows: Assuming that the source of the magnetic field is distributed in the plane $z=r_z$ and creates a magnetic field at the points of the plane $z=0$ (observation plane), the magnetic induction vector described by Eq. (2) is required to find the spatial configuration of the plane system currents, which at the points of the observation plane creates a magnetic field corresponding to the measurement results.

2.5 Algorithm for solving the inverse problem of magnetostatics for a 2D field source

For a 2D distribution of currents, we obtain from Eq. (1) the following expression for the field component, for example, B_x at the observation point:

$$B_x(x, yz) = \frac{\mu_0 r_z}{4\pi} \int\limits_{-\infty}^{+\infty} \int\limits_{-\infty}^{+\infty} \frac{j_y(x'y')}{\left[(x - x')^2 + (y - y')^2 + r_z^2\right]^{3/2}} dx' dy' \quad (3)$$

We further define the double Fourier transform as follows [8]:
The direct transform:

$$f(k_x, k_y z) = \int\limits_{-\infty}^{+\infty} \int\limits_{-\infty}^{+\infty} f(x, yz) \exp\left(-i k_x x - i k_y y\right) dx dy; \qquad (4)$$

The inverse transform:

$$f(x, yz) = \frac{1}{4\pi^2} \int\limits_{-\infty}^{+\infty} \int\limits_{-\infty}^{+\infty} f(k_x, k_y z) \exp\left(i k_x x + i k_y y\right) dk_x dk_y \qquad (5)$$

In Eqs. (4) and (5), $f(x, y, z)$ and $f(k_x, k_y, z)$ are a function of coordinates and its Fourier image and k_x and k_y are components of the wave vector $\mathbf{k}$.

The values of the Fourier images $b_x(k_x, k_y, r_z) = F|B_x|$ of the components of the magnetic induction vector and $j_y(k_x, k_y) = F|j_y|$ the CDV are obtained from Eq. (3) using the convolution theorem [8]:

$$b_x(k_x, k_y r_z) = g(k_x, k_y r_z) j_y(k_x k_y),$$

where $g(k_x, k_y, r_z)$ is the Fourier image of the Green's function $g(x - x', y - y', r_z) = g(\mathbf{r})$:

$$g(\mathbf{r}) = \frac{\mu_0 r_z}{4\pi} \frac{1}{\left[(x - x')^2 + (y - y')^2 + r_z^2\right]^{3/2}}. \qquad (6)$$

For the Fourier transform of the Green's function, we obtain from Eq. (6) using the direct Fourier transform in Eq. (4):

$$g(\mathbf{r}) \Rightarrow g(k_x, k_y, r_z) = (\mu\mu_0/2) \exp\left(-k r_z\right),$$

where $k = (k_x^2 + k_y^2)^{1/2}$ is the magnitude of the propagation vector.
Similarly, expressions can be obtained for other components of the field vector in the wave plane:

$$F[B_y] = b_y(k_x, k_y, r_z) = -(\mu_0/2) \exp\left(-k \cdot r_z\right) F\left[j_y\right]$$

$$F[B_z] = b_z(k_x, k_y, r_z) = i(\mu_0/2) \exp\left(-k \cdot r_z\right) \left(\frac{k_y}{k} F[j_x] - \frac{k_x}{k} F[j_y]\right)$$

$$\qquad (7)$$

In MCG, the output signal of a gradiometer (axial or planar) is most often proportional to the values of z, which is the component of the magnetic field induction vector. The values depend on the linear combination of the j_x and j_y CDV components. The continuity condition div $\boldsymbol{j}=0$ in the wave plane is obtained using the direct integral Fourier transform:

$$- i \cdot k_x \cdot F\left[j_x\right] - i \cdot k_y \cdot F\left[j_y\right] = 0.$$

Thus, the "measured" $F[B_z]$ values and components of the CDV in the wave plane are related by the following algebraic expressions:

$$F\left[j_x\right] = g_x \cdot F[B_z], \tag{8}$$

$$F\left[j_y\right] = g_y \cdot F[B_z], \tag{9}$$

$$g_x = -i \cdot 4\pi/\mu_0 \exp\left(k \cdot r_z\right) \cdot k_y/2k,$$

$$g_y = i \cdot 4\pi/\mu_0 \exp\left(k \cdot r_z\right) \cdot k_x/2k.$$

The values of the components of the CDV in each coordinate system XYZ can be determined from the known values of the coordinate r_z and Fourier—the image of the zth component of the magnetic induction vector—using the inverse Fourier transform.

Suppose that in Eqs. (8) and (9), the values of the coordinate r_z are known—the distance between the measurement plane, the plane in which the CDV is determined, and the Fourier values—the image of the zth component of the magnetic induction vector. Then the values of the components of the CDV in each coordinate system XYZ can be determined using the inverse Fourier transform. In this case, the procedure for restoring the spatial structure of the CDV in the plane will be unambiguous. The values of the r_z coordinate can be determined by direct measurement in nondestructive testing methods or found from tomography data (coordinates of the pathological focus in the study of the brain, magnetoencephalography, MEG).

In the study of MCG, we have developed and used a "step-by-step" algorithm, which is implemented in the form of software and instrumental tools of a magnetocardiograph [9–11]. At the first step, a spatial analysis of the distribution of the characteristics of the MCS in the measurement plane is carried out, the "most distant" from the source points are selected, an analytical solution of the inverse problem is performed at the selected points, and the location and integral parameters of the "effective" field source are determined from the obtained results [6]. In the second step, a plane parallel to the measurement plane and located at the depth of the "effective" source (coordinate rz), is selected. In this plane (in the heart, "cutting" the heart), the spatial configuration of the field source is determined in the form of a system of CDVs using the double integral Fourier transform.

Thus, the analysis of the processes of polarization and depolarization of the ventricular system of the human heart is realized by analyzing its "image." The spatial configuration of the system of currents distributed in the plane is used as the initial information. The plane of the source of the magnetic signal is a secant for the heart and is parallel to the plane where the characteristics of the magnetic signal are recorded.

2.6 Consideration of the spatial configuration of the magnetic flux transformer: Axial and planar gradiometers

The scheme for magnetometric information transformation is determined by the model of the field source (in our case, a two-dimensional current layer), the mathematical method for solving the inverse problem, and the measurement algorithm. This is because the SQUID sensor does not directly register a magnetic field. For indirect measurements, the SQUID is connected to a magnetic flux transformer in the form of a loop, for example, from a superconducting wire (Fig. 1). In most of the known problems, the magnetic field is created both by a "useful" source (in MCG, these are the values of the parameters of the magnetic field of the heart) and by "external" sources. Consequently, superconducting screens cannot be used to shield magnetic fields from "external" sources. Proceeding from this, the main method of dealing with noises is the implementation of the receiving coil of the flux transformer in the form of a gradiometer of the first or higher orders [7]. In other words, the SQUID magnetic flux transformer is made in the form of a set of identical turns, which are spaced apart and included in the differential electrical circuit. If the distance to the field source is much greater than the distance between the coils (distant sources, including magnetic noise), then the magnetic field is relatively uniform, and the fluxes in the receiving turns have equal values and are oppositely directed. If the distance to the field source is comparable to the values of the distance between the coils, then the magnetic field has a high spatial inhomogeneity and gives different fluxes in the receiving turns. As a result, a nonzero total flux is formed at the input of the SQUID sensor, which is recorded by the magnetometric system.

Let us assume, as before, that the plane $z=0$ is "secant" for the volume of the magnetic field source (in the human heart). The direction of the OZ axis coincides with the normal to the measurement plane $z=z_0$. Then most of the existing designs of magnetic flux transformers of SQUID-gradiometric system (single-channel or multichannel) can be divided into two groups.

1) SQUID gradiometers, in which all receiving coils are in the plane $z=z_0$ and are switched on according to one of the following schemes:

$$d_{lx} = B_z(x - l, yz_0) - B_z(x + l, yz_0);$$
$$d_{ly} = B_z(x, y - lz_0) - B_z(x, y + lz_0),$$

where l is the distance (base) between the turns of the flux transformer along the X and Y axes, respectively. In this case, the output signals of the SQUID gradiometer d_{lx} and d_{ly} are proportional to the corresponding difference in the components of the magnetic field created by the source at the observation point. Such magnetic flux transformers can be made in planar technology, including those based on high-temperature superconductors (HTSC).

2) The normal to the surface of all receiving coils is directed along the OZ axis, the coaxial coils are in the planes $z=z_0$, $z=z_0+l$, $z=z_0+2L$, and are connected in such a way that the output signal of the first order gradiometer is proportional to the value:

$$d_{1z} = B_z(x, yz_0) - B_z(x, yz_0 + l) \tag{10}$$

And the output signal of the second-order gradiometer is proportional to the value:

$$d_{2z} = B_z(x, y, z_0) - 2B_z(x, y, z_0 + l) + B_z(x, y, z_0 + 2l). \tag{11}$$

Data processing within the framework of the proposed algorithm has no peculiarities even if the normal to the surface of all receiving coils is directed along the OX axis, and the output signal of the gradiometer is proportional to:

$$d_{lzx} = B_x(x, yz_0) - B_x(x, yz_0 + l),$$

or

$$d_{lxx} = B_x(x - l, yz_0) - B_x(x + l, yz_0).$$

As noted, the first step in the analysis of a magnetocardiogram involves the localization of an "effective" magnetic source [4]. If a magnetic dipole model is used for a biomagnetic signal source, then an analytical solution of the inverse problem can be performed for the selected observation points. This method is based on the properties of the tensors of the first (D_1) and second (D_2) spatial derivatives of vector $\mathbf{B}$. In a homogeneous, nonmagnetic, nonconducting medium, these tensors are symmetric and have no trace (at the measurement points div $\mathbf{B}=0$ and curl $\mathbf{B}=0$). Their eigenvalues are real and different, and the eigenvectors are independent and orthogonal. Tensors are diagonal in a coordinate system based on eigenvectors. The parameters of the field source are found first in the "new" coordinate system (using algebraic relations) and then in the given coordinate system (by means of a reverse transition). Investigations [5,6] show that, for the analytical solution of the problem of localizing the source of the magnetic field in this formulation (magnetic dipole), a six-channel magnetometric system is sufficient, for example, a magnetometric system of five first-order gradiometers (three off-diagonal $\partial B_x/\partial y$, $\partial B_x/\partial z$, $\partial B_y/\partial z$, and two diagonal $\partial B_x/\partial x$, $\partial B_y/\partial y$) and a B_x magnetometer (to determine distance to source), or a magnetometric system of five second-order gradiometers (three off-diagonal $\partial^2 B_z/\partial x\partial z$, $\partial^2 B_z/\partial y\partial z$, $\partial^2 B_z/\partial x\partial y$ and two diagonal $\partial^2 B_z/\partial y^2$, $\partial^2 B_z/\partial z^2$) and the first-order gradiometer $\partial B_z/\partial z$ (to determine the distance to the source).

Since magnetocardiographs based on the second-order SQUID gradiometers with axial magnetic flux transformers are used to measure the values of the parameters of the magnetic field of the heart, in open space, the measurement data at the given points of the plane are homogeneous and do not correspond to the initial data for the analytical solution of the inverse problem (vector of magnetic induction and its spatial derivatives of the first and second order). Therefore, these quantities must be determined from the measurement data, considering the spatial configuration of the magnetic flux transducer and the features of the measurement algorithm. In other words, in the process of preliminary processing of the measurement data, it is necessary to solve the following problem: According to the results of measurements of the biomagnetic signal $Bs = \{d_{1z}, d_{1x}, d_{1y}, d_{1zx}, d_{1xx}, d_{2z}\}$ at the nodes (measurement points) of a flat regular lattice, "restore" the values of the zth component of the magnetic induction vector, taking into account the design of the SQUID magnetic flux transformer-gradiometer, determine the values of the components B_x, B_y of vector $\mathbf{B}$, its first (D_1; $D_1 = \partial B_i/\partial r_j$; i, $j = x$, y, z)

and (or) second (D_{2x}, D_{2y}, D_{2z}; $\partial^2 B_z/\partial r_i \partial r_j$) spatial derivatives at each observation point.

We will assume that an arbitrary system of currents is in the volume V of space. The magnetic field of this source has no break points at an arbitrary point in space outside the volume V. The lines of force are always closed. Hence it follows that, in the observation plane $z=z_0$ with unlimited dimensions, the integral of the parameter Bs of the biomagnetic signal (of any of the above) is equal to zero. Therefore, there is a Fourier transform F [Bs], and its values at given points of the wave plane (k_x, k_y, 0) can be found using the double integral Fourier transform. The values of the Fourier images of the quantities d_{1x}, d_{1y}, d_{1xx} and the corresponding component of the vector $\boldsymbol{B}$ are related by the algebraic relations:

$$\begin{aligned}
&F[B_z] = 2i\mathrm{F}\,[d_{1x}]/\sin\,(k_x \cdot l) = 2i\mathrm{F}\big[d_{1y}\big]/\sin\,(k_y \cdot l);\\
&F[B_x] = 2i\mathrm{F}\,[d_{1xx}]/\sin\,(k_x \cdot l), \quad k_x, k_y \neq 0.
\end{aligned} \tag{12}$$

Similarly, using Eq. (4) and the accepted conditions, we obtain for the Fourier transform of the vector $\boldsymbol{B}$:

$$\begin{aligned}
F[B_z] &= \mathrm{F}[d_{1z}]/[1 - \exp\,(-k \cdot l)\\
&= \mathrm{F}[d_{2z}]/[1 - 2\exp\,(-k \cdot l) + \exp\,(-2k \cdot l);\\
F[B_x] &= \mathrm{F}[d_{1zx}]/[1 - \exp\,(-k \cdot l).
\end{aligned} \tag{13}$$

Using the inverse transformation of Eq. (5), at each observation point, we obtain the values of the vector $\boldsymbol{B}$, taking into account the spatial configuration of the magnetic flux transformer.

The obtained information is sufficient to solve the second part of the problem, which is to determine the values of the magnetic induction vector and its spatial derivatives of the first D_1 and second D_{2x}, D_{2y}, D_{2z} orders. The observation points are in a homogeneous, nonmagnetic, nonconductive environment. The indicated tensors are symmetric and have no trace (curl $\boldsymbol{B}=0$, div $\boldsymbol{B}=0$). It follows that the Fourier transforms of the components of the magnetic induction vector are linearly dependent and are determined through the values of the Fourier transform of the zth (or xth in the case of Eqs. (12) and (13)) component from simple algebraic relations:

$$F[dB_z/dx] = ik_x F[B_z],$$

$$F[dB_z/dy] = ik_y F[B_z],$$

$$F[dB_z/dz] = -ikF[B_z],$$

$$ik_xF[B_x] + ik_yF[B_y] - ikF[B_z] = 0,$$

$$ik_xF[B_z] - k_xF[B_x] = 0,$$

$$-ik_yF[B_z] - ikF[B_y] = 0,$$

$$ik_yF[B_x] - ik_xF[B_y] = 0.$$

From this, in the wave plane, we obtain

$$F[\partial B_x/\partial x] = k_x{}^2F[B_z]/k, \quad F[\partial B_y/\partial y] = k_y{}^2F[B_z]/k,$$

$$F[\partial B_x/\partial y] = k_xk_yF[B_z]/k, \quad F[\partial B_x/\partial z] = ik_xF[B_z],$$

$$F[\partial B_y/\partial z] = ik_yF[B_z], \quad F[\partial^2 B_z/\partial x^2] = -k^2{}_xF[B_z],$$

$$F[\partial^2 B_z/\partial y^2] = -k^2{}_yF[B_z], \quad F[\partial^2 B_z/\partial x\partial y] = -k_yk_xF[B_z],$$

$$F[\partial^2 B_z/\partial x\partial z] = -ikk_xF[B_z], \quad F[\partial^2 B_z/\partial y\partial z] = -ikk_yF[B_z].$$

The implementation of the inverse transformation of Eq. (5) gives the values of the magnetic induction vector and all its independent spatial derivatives of the first and second order at the given points of the measurement plane. The values of the Fourier transforms of the indicated parameters of the magnetic field are also known at given points of the wave plane. Thus, we have obtained a complete data set for spatial analysis of the biomagnetic signal.

2.7 Application of the algorithm for the analysis of the magnetocardiosignal

A schematic diagram of the conversion and spatial analysis of the MCS is shown in Fig. 6.

Fig. 6 shows a diagram of the algorithm for processing the results of measurements of a magnetocardiogram using an axial SQUID gradiometer of the second order. In this case, the algorithm uses both analytical (exact) expressions when solving the problem of localizing a dipole source and when solving the problem of reconstructing a flat layer of currents. An exception is the stages of the implementation of the direct (4) and inverse (5) Fourier transforms (transitions from the laboratory

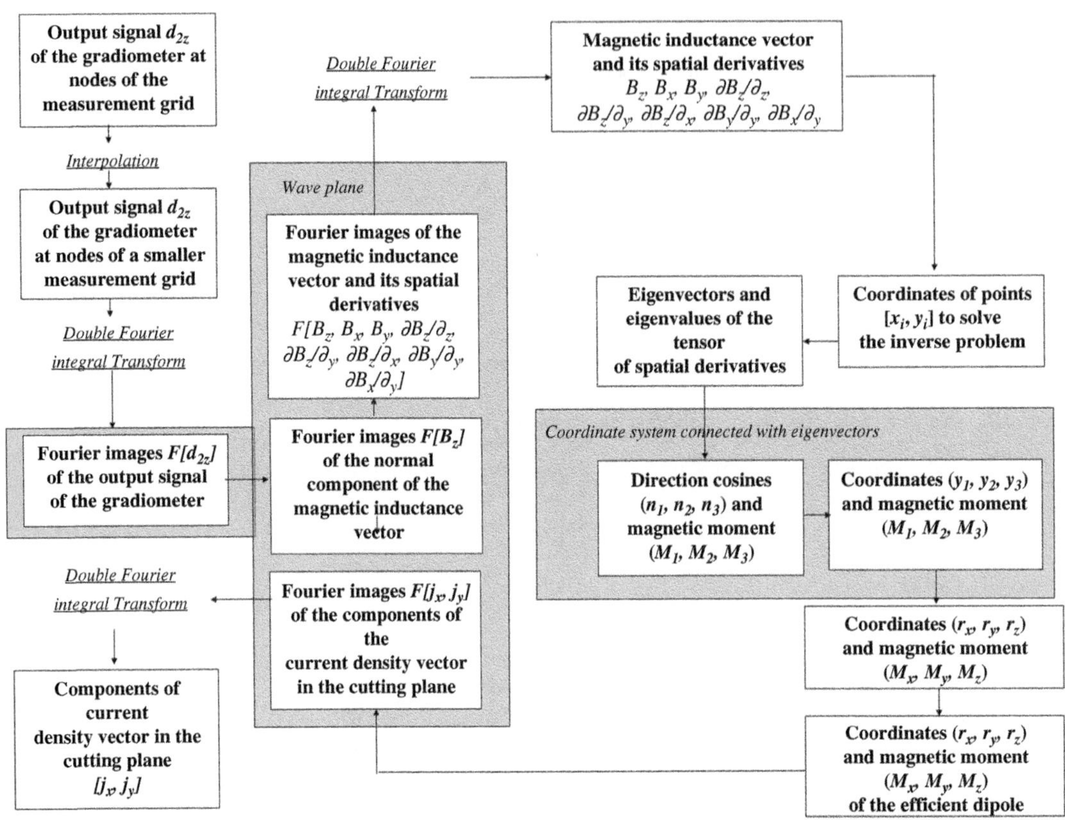

Fig. 6 Block diagram of the "step-by-step" analysis of the magnetocardiosignal algorithm; solution of the inverse problem in the dipole model and in the model of the system of current density vectors distributed in the plane.

coordinate system XYZ to the wave plane and the inverse transformation).

At the first stage, direct transformation (4) is realized for distribution of the output signal of the SQUID gradiometer (proportional to d_2). In this case, a systematic error arises, which is largely associated with the limited dimensions of the observation area in the $z = z_0$ plane. To reduce it, it is necessary to make corrections to the algorithm, taking into account the possible distribution of the magnetic field at points of the plane that are located outside the observation area.

Consider points in the measurement plane that are located at a distance greater than three times the size of the measurement grid. Investigations [12] showed that, at these points, the output signal of the SQUID gradiometer approaches zero (decreases almost to zero). The values of the cardiomagnetic signal at the boundaries of the measurement area are known (measured). If we assume that the cardiomagnetic signal decreases linearly with distance, then the corresponding integrals can be calculated analytically (exactly). The obtained values are then used to correct the results of calculating the Fourier transforms of the parameters of the magnetic signal. Alternatively, a different approach can be used. At the first stage of data transformation, the problem of localizing the dipole source of the field is solved. Suppose that the magnetic field at an arbitrary point of the measurement plane $z = z_0$ outside the measurement area is created by the indicated dipole. Then, in the dipole approximation, it is possible to calculate the value of the output signal of the SQUID gradiometer at the specified point (according to the known configuration of the magnetic flux transformer). The implementation of the direct transformation (4), considering the obtained values, gives practically exact values of the Fourier images of the magnetic field.

The analytical algorithm for calculating the Fourier values of the image of the measured signal Bs is as follows:

1. We will assume that the observation area consists of N_{ij} squares with side L (i, j is the number of "areas" along the OX and OY axes, respectively).
2. Suppose that the magnetic field Bs_{ij} does not change within an arbitrary "area" with numbers i, j ($Bs_{ij} = const$). Then, from the direct transformation relations (4), we obtain analytical (exact) expressions for the Fourier transform of the measured data:

$$F\left[Bs_{ij}\right] = 4 \cdot Bs_{ij} \cdot \exp\left[-i \cdot k_x x_i - i \cdot k_y y_i\right]$$

$$\frac{\sin\left(k_x \cdot L/2\right) \cdot \sin\left(k_y \cdot L/2\right)}{k_x k_y},$$

when $k_x, k_y \neq 0$;

$$F\left[Bs_{ij}\right] = 2 \cdot B_{ij} \cdot \exp\left[-i \cdot k_x x_i\right] \cdot L \cdot$$

$$\frac{\sin\left(k_x \cdot L/2\right)}{k_x},$$

when $k_y = 0$, $k_x \neq 0$;

$$F\left[Bs_{ij}\right] = Bs_{ij} \cdot L^2,$$

when $k_x, k_y = 0$.

3. Based on the results obtained, we find the values of the Fourier transform of the z-th component of the magnetic induction vector using relations of Eqs. (10) and (11) according to the known (given) design of the flux transformers

The magnetic field is recorded using a SQUID gradiometer, where the pickup coils have a radius R ($R=0.8 \div 1.5\,cm$). This means that it is necessary to refine the values of the parameters $g_x(k)$, $g_y(k)$ (taking into account the radius of the turns) when implementing the calculation algorithm of Eqs. (8) and (9) of the Fourier transforms of the components of the CDV.

Consider a circular coil with radius R, for which the normal vector to its area is directed along the OZ axis. Let us define the function of turns $G(x,y)$; its value is equal to the number of turns of the coil in the vicinity of an arbitrary point of the plane with coordinates $(x, y, 0)$. If we neglect the diameter of the wire itself, then for a coil of N identical turns, we get:

$$\begin{aligned} G(\rho) &= N, \quad \rho < R, \\ G(\rho) &= 0, \quad \rho > R, \end{aligned} \tag{14}$$

where ρ is the radial coordinate in the XOY plane.

From here, we obtain the following expression for the magnetic flux $[Fcy]_p(x,y)$ through the receiving coil:

$$\Phi_p(xy) = \int\limits_{-\infty}^{+\infty} \int\limits_{-\infty}^{+\infty} G(x - x'y - y')B(x'y')dx'dy'$$

In the wave plane, the convolution of two functions can be written as the product of their Fourier transforms:

$$[\mathrm{Fcy}]_p(k_x k_y) = G(k_x k_y)B(k_x k_y), \tag{15}$$

where $[Fcy]_p(k_x,k_y)$ and $B(k_x,k_y)=F[B_z]$ are Fourier images of the magnetic flux and vertical component of the magnetic inductance vector and $G(k_x,k_y)$ is the Fourier image of the function of turns.

From Eq. (15), it follows that, in the wave plane, the magnetic flux through the pickup coil can be represented as a convolution of the coil area and the magnetic induction vector. Using Eq. (4), we obtain the expression for the filtration of the Fourier transform of the magnetic field in an explicit form, taking into account radius R of the coil:

$$g_x = -i\, 4\pi/\mu_0 \exp{(kr_z)}k_y RN/J_1(kR),$$

$$g_x = i\, 4\pi/\mu_0 \exp{(kr_z)}k_x RN/J_1(kR),$$

where $i = \sqrt{-1}$ and $J_1(kR)$ is the Bessel function.

Let us show that the properties of the filtering function are related to the spatial resolution of the magnetic flux transformer coil. The value $G(0)$ in Eq. (15) is equal to the area of the loop πR^2 (or $\pi R^2 N$, if the number of loops is N); the Bessel function $J_1(kR)$ is approximately equal to $kR/2$ for small values of the argument [8,13]. The Bessel function $J_1(kR)$ has an oscillating character and infinitely many zeros; the first zero is located at $k_1 = 3.83/R$, the second at $k_2 = 7.02/R$ [8]. Since the Fourier transforms of currents are inversely proportional to the Bessel function, they can go to infinity at the indicated points. Let us assume that k_{max} is the highest spatial frequency, above which the Fourier spectrum of the magnetic signal is practically zero (at the level of calculation accuracy). Then, to avoid singularity points, the requirement must be met: the radius R of the receiving coil must be much less than $3.83/k_{max}$. When designing magnetocardiographic systems, the radius R is usually chosen so that the output signal of the gradiometer is proportional to the magnetic field (the magnetic field is almost constant over the area of the receiving coil). In addition, at an arbitrary moment of the cardiocycle, the values of the cutoff frequency k_{max} do not exceed unity, if the grating spacing in the wave plane is determined as $2\pi/L$, where $L = 20$ cm is the size of the observation area and, therefore, certainly less than $3.83/R$.

It is important to note that there is "magnetic noise" in the actual results of magnetic measurements, which excludes division by zero. However, some information may be lost (some frequency components cannot be determined) if the level of the useful signal becomes less than $G(k_x, k_y)$. Then it is possible to "amplify the noise components" when implementing the inverse transformation (5) to determine the components of the CDV. One of the options for solving this problem can be the use of the Hanning window in the frequency domain [13].

Let us assume that the Fourier transforms of the biomagnetic signal and CDVs are given at an arbitrary point of the wave plane and have no singularities and break points. Then, for the points where $F[B_z] \neq 0$, the following algorithm is implemented:

1) In the wave plane, we select a given number of elementary areas in such a way that, within each area, the Fourier transform of the magnetic signal does not change (it can be considered constant).

2) Analytically (exactly) calculate the value of the inverse transformation integral (5) of the functions g_x, g_y for each elementary area of the wave plane centered at the point with the current coordinates $(k_x, k_y, 0)$.

3) We calculate the sum (over elementary areas) of the products of the Fourier image F $[B_z]$ in the center of the area by the corresponding integral of the functions g_x, g_y, and from the obtained values, we calculate the value of the current density in the measurement plane using standard techniques that allow us to eliminate the mutual influence of neighboring region's spectrum under commutative convolution.

As an example, consider the results of processing a biomagnetic signal from a healthy patient. The cardiomagnetic signal was recorded in an unshielded room using a nine-channel magnetometric system. The measuring channels were the second-order axial SQUID gradiometers [11]. The nodal points Q, R, S, J, and T were selected for display. For each nodal point, magnetic maps are shown in Fig. 7A: the distribution of the magnetic field in the measurement plane. On magnetic maps, the arrow shows the projection of the source of the field of the dipole model localized in the heart. Fig. 7C shows the results of the implementation of the procedure for restoring the source of the cardiomagnetic signal in the form of a system of plane currents. The value of the z-coordinate of a plane parallel to the measurement plane and that is a secant for the heart is given in text form. Fig. 7B shows the averaged cardiocycle at one of the measurement points. In the form of lines (marks), the location of the nodal points for which the procedure for restoring the source of the cardiomagnetic signal was implemented is shown.

The developed algorithm for solving the inverse problem is implemented as a block of programs and is the basis for the information and diagnostic technology of the magnetocardiographic system. After the launch of this program, the solution and analysis of the inverse problem of magnetostatics for pathologies associated with changes in electrophysiological characteristics in a large volume of the myocardium is performed; identification of patients with coronary heart disease (IHD), monitoring of cardiac patients after (or during) different courses of treatment, and localization of the coronary artery basin, which is the cause of IHD, etc.

Fig. 8 shows an example of a few versions of data representation during the work of program block "MAGSCAN" in "step-by-step" mode of MCG data processing.

To analyze the MCS, one can use the maps of the magnetic field distribution and the corresponding maps of the distribution of the

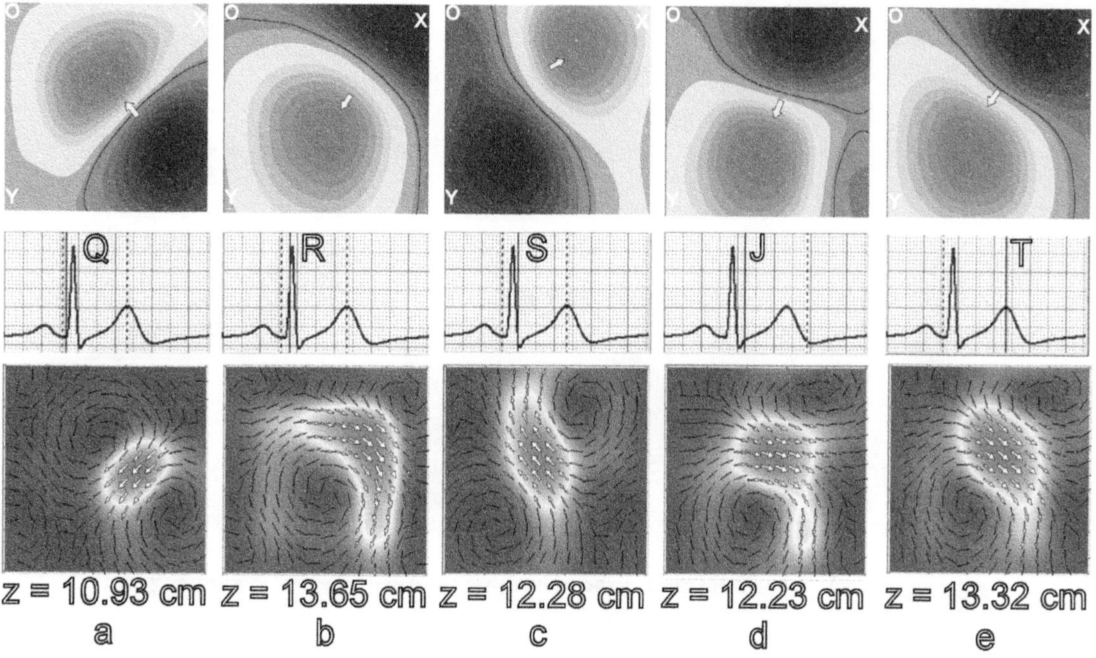

Fig. 7 Example of solving the inverse problem of magnetostatics for a field source in the form a two-dimensional distribution of the current density vector.

CDV obtained after solving the inverse problem. The maps of the distribution of currents give more complete and correct information in relation to the maps of the distribution of the values of the parameters of the magnetic field within the boundaries of the measurement area. On the one hand, the solution of the inverse problem in the form of the found spatial distribution of the CDV in a plane parallel to the measurement plane unambiguously corresponds to the measured magnetic field of the heart for a given moment of the cardiocycle and, thus, excludes the influence of anthropometric characteristics in different people on the analysis results. On the other hand, the map of the distribution of currents obtained after solving the inverse problem makes it possible to interpret local electrical processes in the myocardium in accordance with their real distribution. Note that the study of the distribution maps of the CDV in the MCG has no analogues in electrocadiographic diagnostics, and their analysis is the basis for the development of a diagnostic conclusion.

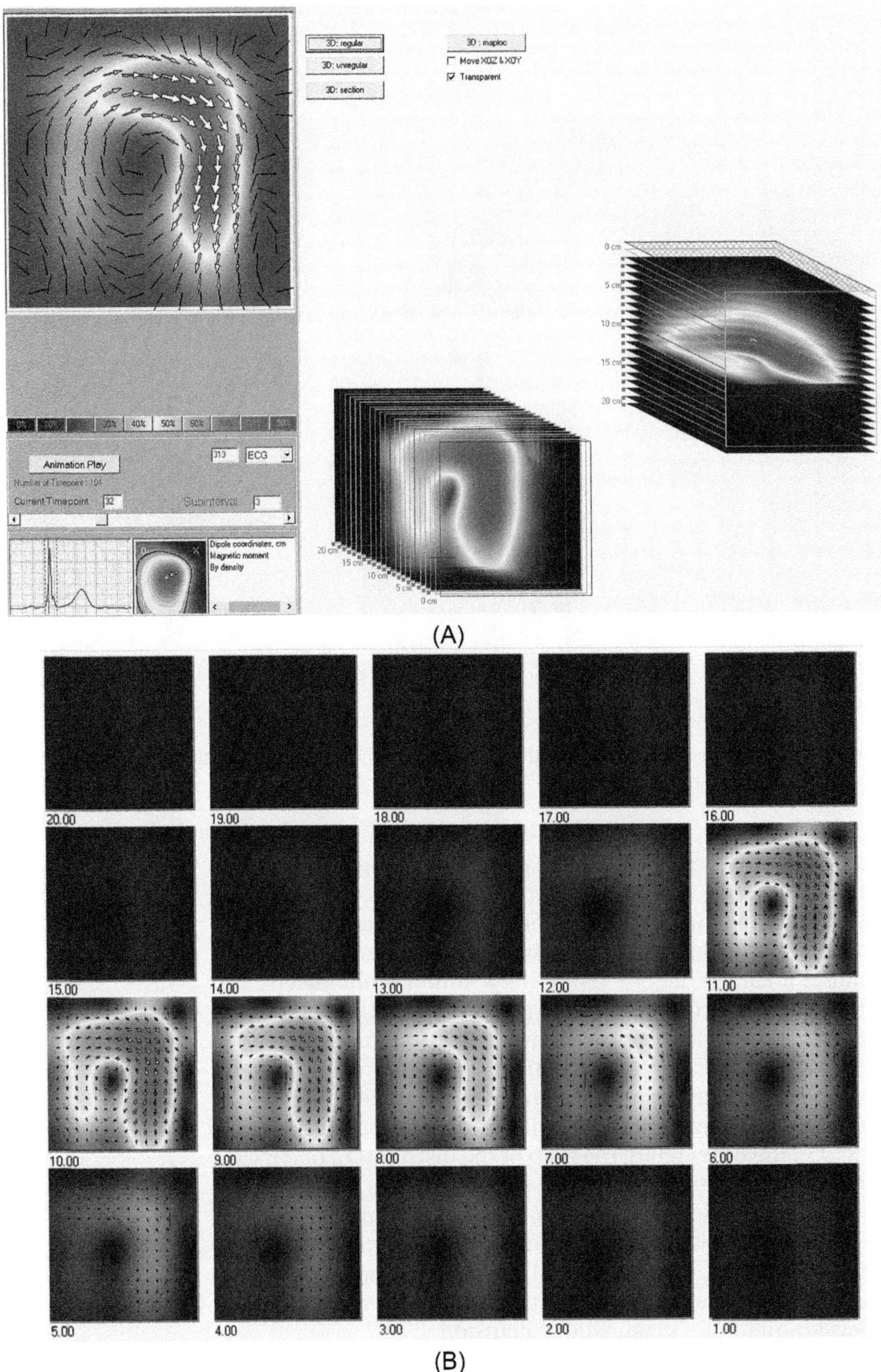

Fig. 8 Examples of data imaging of MCG processing during the inverse problem solution in "step-by-step" mode: (A) and (B) layer-to-layer inverse problem solution for a given cardiocycle time moment and representation of this solution over corresponding layers of tree-dimensional heart volume;

(Continued)

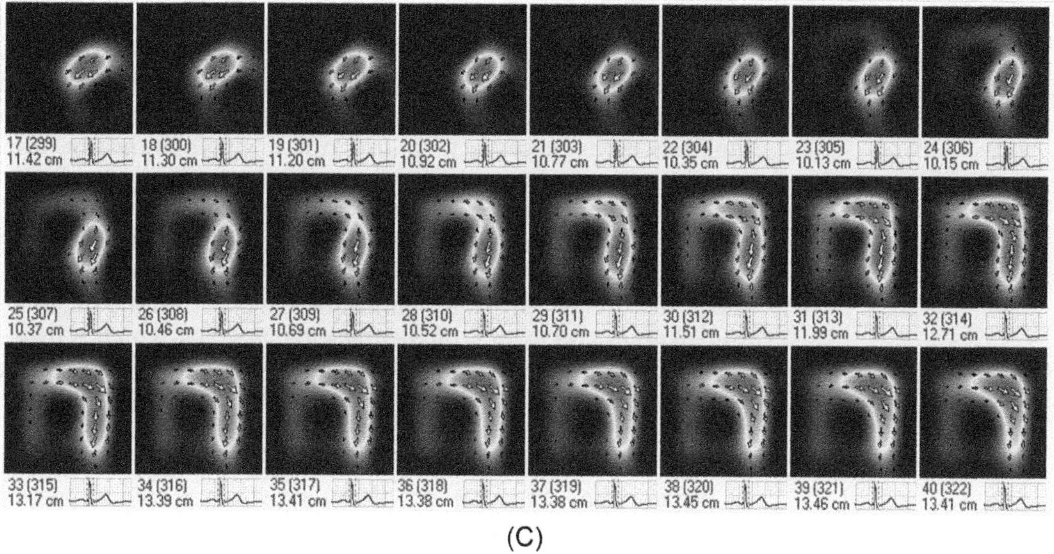

(C)

Fig. 8, cont'd (C) the sequence of distribution maps of current density vectors over analyzed cardiocycle time interval.

3. Metrics and information technologies for the analysis of magnetocardiographic data based on two-dimensional visualization of the solution of the inverse problem of magnetostatics

Note that the fundamental novelty of the proposed analysis of MCG data is the use of a new methodological approach—to assess the dynamics of changes in current density during the cardiocycle using maps sequentially arranged in time (dynamic mapping). This approach has identified several new MCG indicators, which, on one hand, have a clear electrophysiological meaning, and on the other, they exclude the impact on research results of technical and design features of the MCG system used due to the analysis of relative values.

At the next stage, the analysis of the dynamics of the selected parameters of CDVs in the selected time intervals of the cardiocycle (QRS, ST-T, T_{a-e}) with an arbitrary or specified time step (4–10 ms).

CDV instant maps and sets of such maps during cardiocycle intervals are the main diagnostic image and object of analysis in MCG. Each individual map and, even more so, set of maps during a certain phase of the cardiocycle contains multifaceted information. Therefore, to take full advantage of the method for analysis, it is necessary to use not a single indicator but a combination.

One of the methods of analysis of the spatial structure of the current distribution map is based on the concept of "proper" direction [14]. For each CDV, the normal direction is known. Normal direction is the sector within the pie chart from 0 degrees to 180 degrees and from -180 degrees to 0 degrees, which is used in the ECG. In this direction, CDV is considered normal (appropriate). In this case, the "appropriate" direction has a clear link to the interval of the cardiocycle to which this map belongs. Thus, during ventricular repolarization (from point J to the end of the T wave) the direction in the sector of 10–80 degrees is "appropriate." It is known that, during ventricular depolarization, the excitation sequentially covers the interventricular septum, anterior-apical area, lateral wall, and posterior-inferior region of the left ventricle. Each of these phases of depolarization has its own "appropriate" direction of CDVs (Fig. 9). The quantitative parameter of this type of analysis is a 100% normalized anomaly index (abnormality index—AI). This indicator is the ratio of the sum of the lengths of the vectors directed in the correct, "appropriate" direction for each moment of time to the sum of the lengths of the vectors that are different from the "appropriate" direction. From the electrophysiological point of view, this indicator reflects the ratio of ion fluxes flowing in the "appropriate" direction and in a direction different from the "appropriate."

The next stage of the analysis is the assessment of the processes of de- and repolarization of the ventricles in general. The average AI values $AIQRS_{total}$ (during the QRS complex) and $AIST_{Ttotal}$ (during the ST-T interval) are calculated.

Another group of indicators is designed to assess the homogeneity of the repolarization process, which is the similarity of the spatial structure of the maps and the smoothness of the curve of the total current. These indicators correspond to the curve of arithmetic sums of values of all CDVs for each instantaneous map during the studied interval.

To quantify the homogeneity of the spatial structure of maps over time, the correlation (similarity) C_{cor} coefficient between

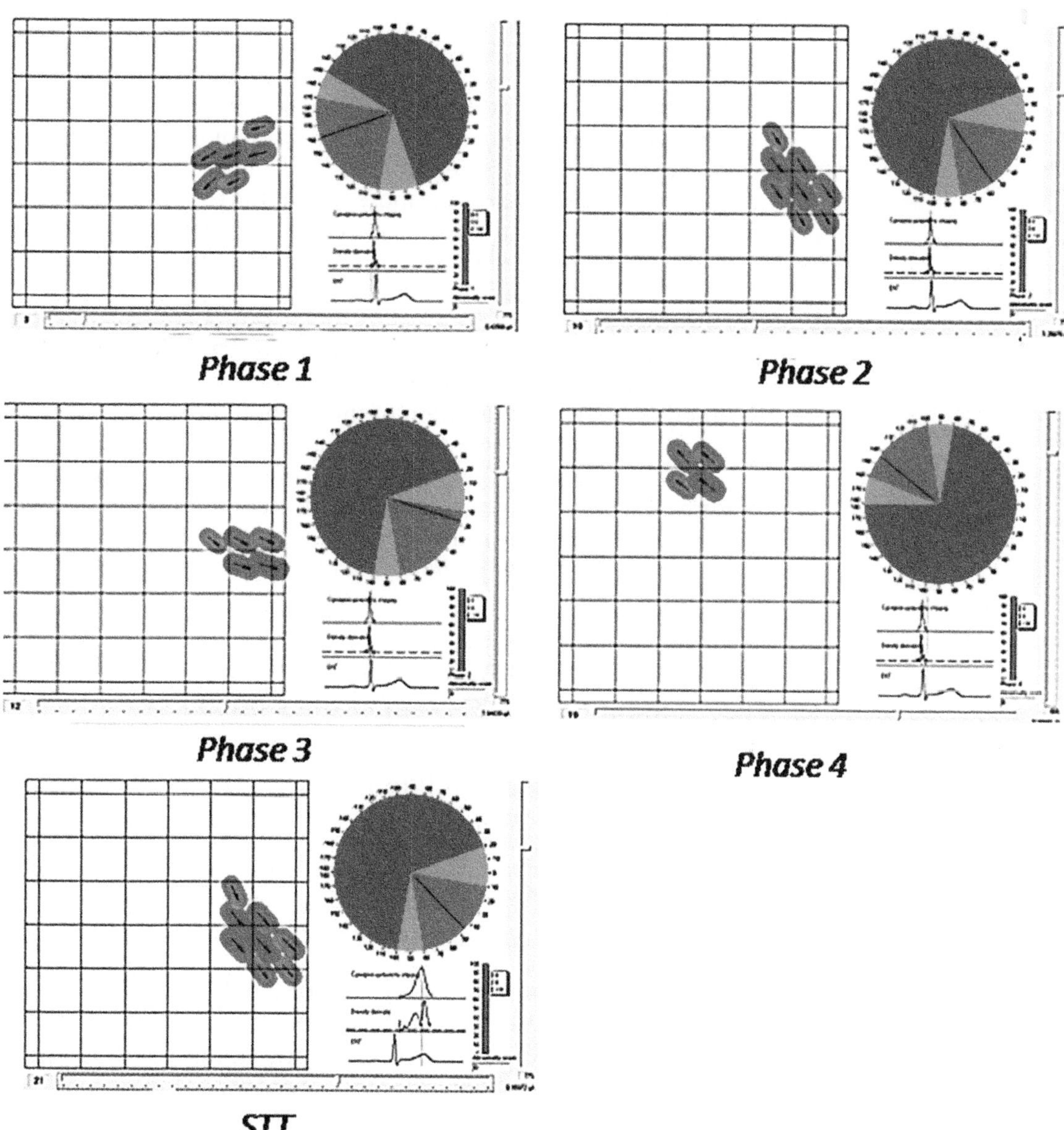

Fig. 9 Distribution maps of CDV of a healthy volunteer (*left*) and pie charts (*right*) of depolarization: interventricular septum (phase 1), anterior wall and apex of the left ventricle (phase 2), lateral wall of the left ventricle (phase 3), basal myocardium (phase 4), as well as ventricular repolarization (ST-T).

all maps during the ST-T interval is calculated. To estimate the smoothness of the curve of changes in the total current, the shape of this curve is analyzed. The duration A_{Dur} (in % to the total duration of the ST-T interval) of the section of this curve from its beginning to the inflection point (to the moment of the beginning of its monotonic growth) is determined. The higher the C_{cor} value and the lower the A_{dur} value, the more similar the CDV maps are within the ST-T interval and the higher the homogeneity of the repolarization process. Decreases in C_{cor} values and increases in A_{dur} almost always occur due to the initial part of the ST segment. The duration of one initial segment corresponds to the time during which some areas of the myocardium are in a later phase of the transmembrane action potential compared to neighboring areas. In other words, the duration of this section reflects the degree of regional heterogeneity of repolarization.

The calculation of the previous set of temporal and spatial features is based on a key electrophysiological concept: the increase of electrical unhomogeneity (heterogeneity) of the myocardium in the occurrence of pathological processes, such as ischemia.

3.1 Clinical approbation of metrics of analysis of magnetocardiographic data based on two-dimensional visualization of the solution of the inverse problem of magnetostatics. Multicenter research

The purpose of using any diagnostic parameter is to formulate a clinically significant diagnostic conclusion:

a) the decision on the presence or absence of a pathological process and

b) in the case of a process, to determine the severity.

The set of indexes has a higher diagnostic accuracy than a single index. Thus, there is a problem of forming from a set of parameters of a single complex indicator. This indicator synthesizes various aspects of the information contained in each indicator. Such an indicator can be created based on the method of linear discriminant analysis (LDA). As a result, a discriminant function is automatically built. If the value of the function is greater than the threshold, the results of the MCG test are positive; if less, it's negative.

Another empirical-statistical approach used to form a comprehensive index is calculated on the basis of scores. When using this approach, the values of all quantitative indicators are a priori divided into ranges. When the value of an individual indicator falls into the appropriate range, it is given a certain number of points. Then the number of points of all indicators is summed. If the sum of points exceeds a certain threshold, the MCG test is considered positive; if contrary, it's negative. If the test is positive, the number of points determines the severity of the pathology on the principle; the higher the score, the more pronounced the pathology. Such scores are widely used in electrocardiography (Sylvester score, Freuleher score, CIIS, and others), as well as to assess the results of the test with dosed exercise (Duke's index). We have created an integrated point criterion of the additive type for the diagnosis of myocardial ischemia using MCG. The value of this criterion was recently investigated by us in two multicenter studies involving foreign colleagues. A two-center study was conducted at the National Military Medical Clinical Center (MMCC) and at the Catholic Clinical Philippusstift (Essen, Germany) [15]. We examined 79 patients with complaints of chest pain and normal or uninformative ECG and echocardiogram results at rest (difficult to diagnose cases). All patients underwent coronary ventriculography. According to the results of coronary angiography, patients were divided into subgroups with stenosis >70% in at least one of the main coronary arteries (subgroup 1a) and a subgroup of persons without hemodynamically significant stenosis (subgroup 1b). Control group 2 consisted of 30 healthy volunteers close in age. Table 1 shows the indicators of diagnostic value of the complex MCG index to detect significant stenosis of the coronary arteries in difficult to diagnose cases.

An even larger multicenter study was conducted in three leading clinics in Beijing under the guidance of specialists from the main hospital of the Chinese Navy. A total of 133 people were examined

Table 1 Diagnostic value of complex MCG index.

Value indicator	Comparison of subgroup 1a with subgroup 1b	Comparison of subgroup 1a with group 2
Sensitivity (%)	93	93
Specificity (%)	84	94
Positive predictive rate (%)	85	94
Negative predictive rate (%)	93	93

(mean age 59 ± 3.1 years). All surveyed individuals were divided into three groups. The first group (61 people) consisted of patients with severe myocardial ischemia who met the criteria for revascularization: the degree of coronary artery stenosis was $\geq 80\%$ or between 50% and 80%, with a margin of coronary blood flow ≤ 0.8. The second group (13 people) were patients whose myocardial ischemia was confirmed by the "gold standard," i.e., invasive coronary angiography but who had not yet met the criteria for revascularization. The third group (59 people) was the control group.

The percentage of coincidence of MCG results and coronary angiography in each group was as follows: for severe coronary heart disease—85.45%, for mild coronary heart disease—77.78%, in the control group—87.10%.

The study achieved a total sensitivity of 93.75%, a specificity of 87.10%, PPV of 88.24%, and NPV of 93.10%.

Thus, magnetocardiographic examination is a reliable method of diagnosing chronic coronary heart disease, including difficult to diagnose cases.

3.2 Metrics and information technologies of analysis of magnetocardiographic data based on three-dimensional visualization of the solution of the inverse problem

In solving the inverse problem of magnetostatics based on the results of MCS measurements, the first step uses a model of a point source of the magnetic field—a magnetic dipole, the location and vector of the magnetic moment of which must be determined by known (measured) values of magnetic fields [6]. In the subsequent stages of data processing and conversion, other models of the signal source are also used. For example, the source of the magnetic field can be represented as a set of N different magnetic dipoles distributed in the volume of the heart [4]. In this case, it is needed to determine the location of several signal sources distributed as independent in the three-dimensional volume of the human heart by the results of measurements of the magnetic field. A model of a flat system of "currents" (distribution of the CDV) is used for spatial analysis of the MCS and its sources. It is assumed that the plane that is parallel to the plane of measurement, secant with respect to the volume of the heart, and located at a given distance from the plane of measurement is selected. In the proposed [9] algorithm, the coordinate of the plane with the signal sources is a variable, and its value is also determined by the measurements of the magnetic field as the value of the zth coordinate of the dipole source, which was determined at the previous stage of MCG signal processing. The original algorithm for solving the inverse problem for a planar current system is based on the application of the double integral Fourier transform and considers the spatial configuration of the magnetic flux transformer SQUID gradientometer [9]. An algorithm for converting information to solve the inverse problem was developed if the values of CDVs in a given set of slices (layers) were to be determined from the results of MCS [11]. In this case, each of the layers is in a plane parallel to the measurement plane, and the coordinates (depth) of each layer are set either with a given step (uniform distribution) or discretely based on the results of solving the inverse problem obtained in previous stages (nonuniform distribution).

For example, in Figs. 10 and 11, the results of spatial signal analysis for real MCG of a patient with cardiac disorders are shown.

In Figs. 10 and 11, the results of magnetic field measurements are displayed on the monitor screen in the form of a magnetic map in two modes: in the form of isolines of the output signal SQUID gradientometer (upper map) and filling the gaps between the isolines (lower map). The spatial configuration of the

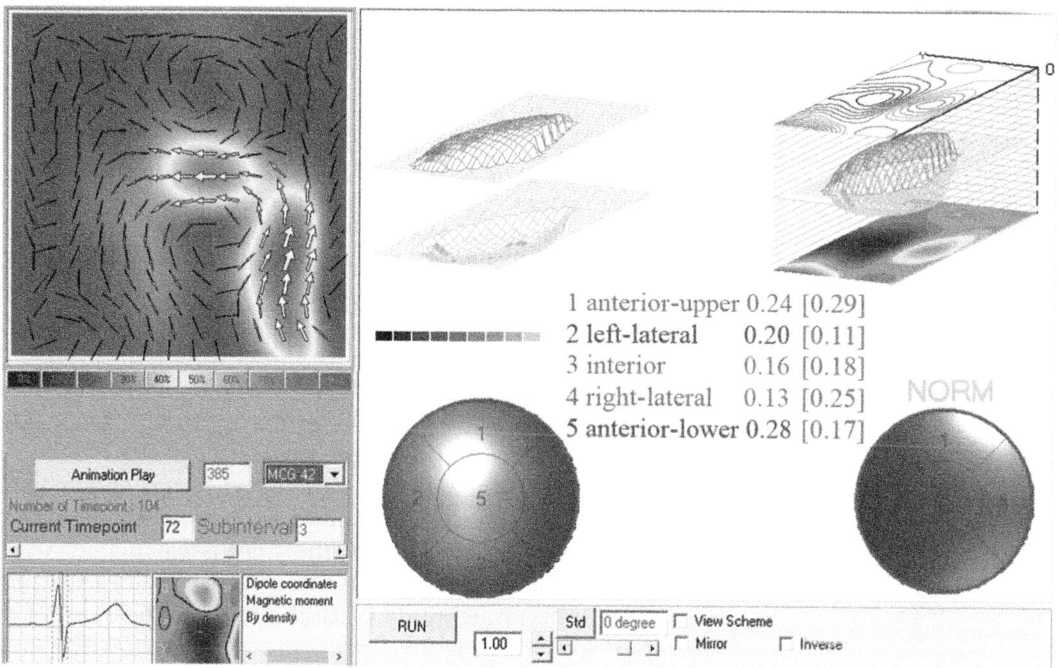

Fig. 10 Display of the solution of the inverse problem for a patient with cardiac disorders.

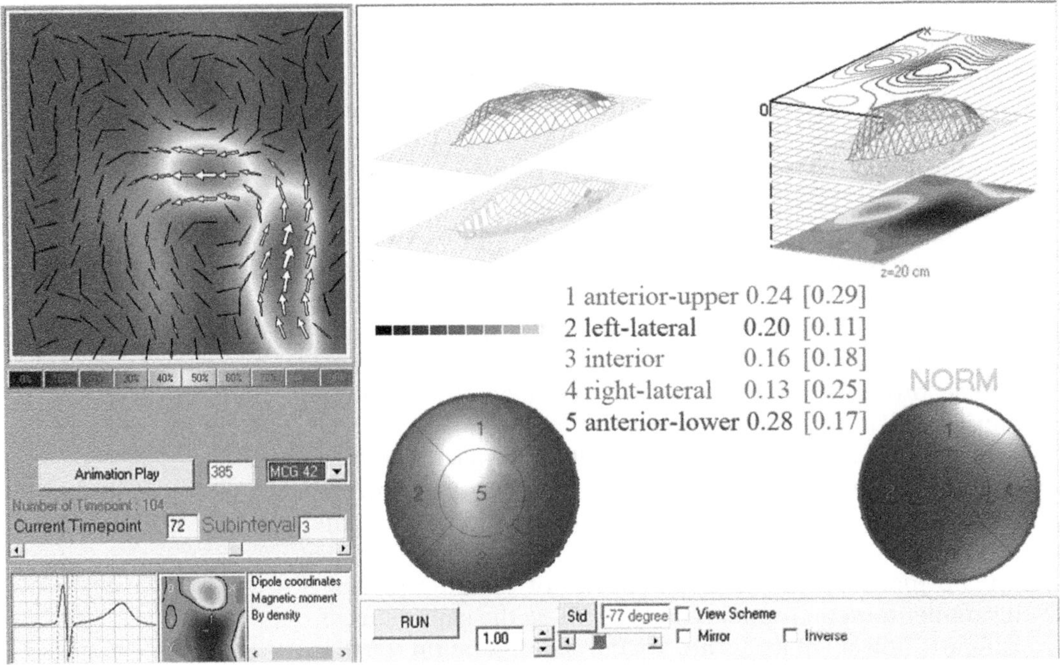

Fig. 11 Display of the solution of the inverse problem for a patient with cardiac disorders; the axis of the ellipsoid is rotated relative to Fig.10.

three-dimensional surface is displayed on the monitor screen as level lines. The points "outside the three-dimensional surface" are highlighted in orange. The spatial configurations of the "lower" and "upper" parts of the ellipsoid, which is a model of the heart, are shown separately.

The power distribution of the CDV is presented in the form of a so-called polar diagram. The principle of charting is based on the segmentation scheme adopted as a standard in the analysis of measurement results in computed tomography and ultrasound of the heart [16]. Software implementation assumes that the three-dimensional surface consists of five segments: 1, anterior; 2, lateral; 3, inferior; 4, septal; and 5, apical.

The relative position and the segments' edges are shown in the diagram (displayed on the monitor screen). For each segment, a continuous power distribution of the CDV is calculated, which is displayed on the monitor screen as a map. Here, the areas most active at the time under study (with the maximum values of the CDV) are displayed in white. Next in intensity follow the areas in red (crimson). Blue is used for areas with minimum power values of the CDV (source is virtually absent). For comparison, the monitor screen (lower right corner of the screen) displays a diagram of the segmentation scheme and the continuous power distribution of the CDV for the corresponding time point of the average "norm." In the next step, for each of the five segments of the three-dimensional surface, the integral value of the power of the CDV is calculated. Then the total value of power throughout the diagram is calculated. The obtained value is used for normalization (the total value of power throughout the diagram is 1). The normalized values of this parameter by segments are displayed in text form on the monitor screen and, for comparison, the corresponding values for the average "norm."

Preliminary quantitative assessment of the spatial configuration of the magnetic field source for the studied MCG record and the average "norm" is calculated using the two-dimensional correlation method. The results of the percentage calculations are displayed on the monitor screen (in full compliance with the average "norm," the coefficient is equal to 100%).

As an additional tool for the spatial analysis of the obtained results, a joint display of the power diagram of the CDV and the scheme of the main arteries of the human heart is used (see Fig. 12).

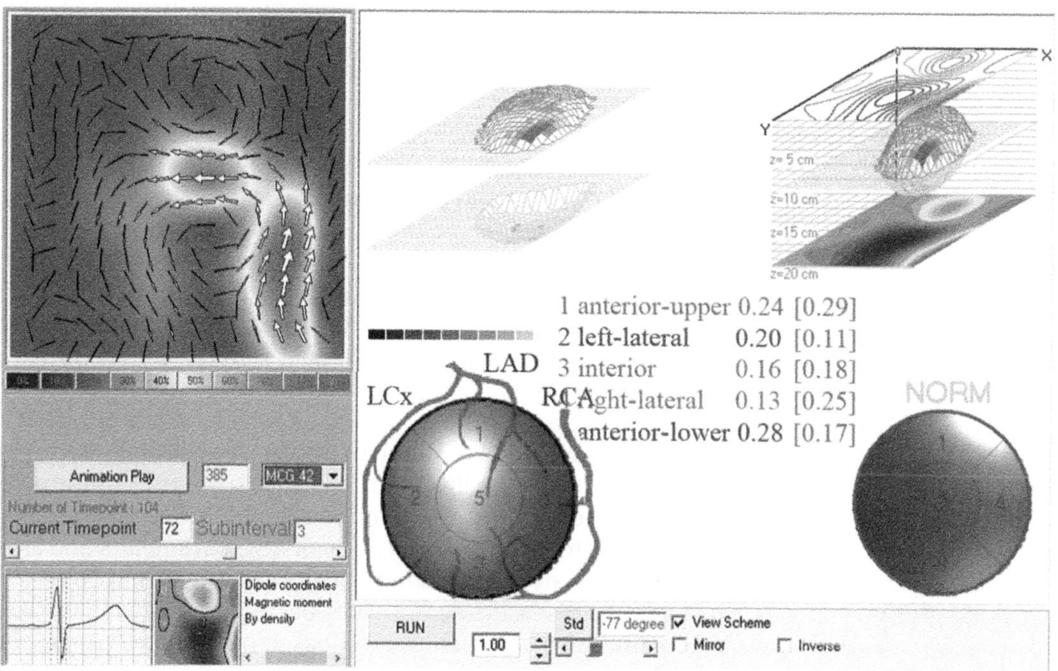

Fig. 12 Model three-dimensional display of the human heart on the monitor screen and the numerical parameters that correspond to a given time of the cardiocycle.

Three-dimensional imaging techniques have been successfully used to solve several important clinical problems, for example, determining the viability of the affected areas of the myocardium in patients with various forms of coronary heart disease. Thus, a high level (74%) of the correspondence between the contractility of the segments of the anterior wall of the left ventricle and the current density in this part of the myocardium in patients with chronic coronary heart disease was found [17].

4. New metrics and information technologies based on computerized electrocardiography

4.1 Principles of the electrocardiogram-scaling technique for detecting subtle changes

The main goal we set for ourselves was to make any electrocardiographic examination informative. Indeed, routine analysis of the electrocardiogram (ECG) is based on the presence of certain electrocardiographic syndromes or phenomena formulated within one of the existing algorithms for visual analysis of the ECG. But in most cases, the analysis of a particular ECG does not show any electrocardiographic syndrome, at least one that clearly indicates the pathology of the heart, i.e., one that belongs to the category of, for example, the Minnesota coding system. At routine analysis, it is necessary to carry all these ECGs to a uniform class: ECGs at which analysis any electrocardiographic syndrome of the major category is not revealed. A question arises: whether all these ECGs are the same in terms of their conditional "distance" to the "reference" ECG of a healthy person. It is clear that they are different. This "distance" may be greater or lesser depending on the state of the myocardium; moreover, it is reasonable to hypothesize that this "distance" reflects the likelihood of serious cardiovascular events. In this sense, routine ECG analysis is uninformative.

We have developed a method (Universal Scoring system) and software for scaling the ECG, which is able to quantify the smallest changes in the electrocardiographic signal. The idea of our technique is, first, to get the biggest array of ECG parameters and alterability of the heart rates; second, the positioning of that data at the axis from the disease-free norm to severe pathology.

Actually, the given technique is based on the well-known theory of Z-scoring [18] where quantitative (usually score) evaluation of test results is provided with a specific scale, which has data-related intragroup scatter of test results. The standard score calculation requires the average test value in the group and its standard deviation.

Here we represent four levels of developed analyzing applications in an ascending order. Each of them is discussed in-depth as follows.

1) The basic level has several independent indicators concerning: (a) the different issues for alterability of the heart rates; (b) typical ECG amplitude and ECG time values, including the ECG wave shape; and (c) changes in heart rhythm.

2) The next level has a set of bound indicators that are approximately equal to the physiological origin.

3) The penultimate level has four integral sets each reflecting various features for the cardiac system functions, which are taken from an ECG, such as different regulation points based on alterability of the heart rates (HRV) assessment, condition of the myocardium based on ECG curves analysis, and malfunctions of cardiac rhythm.

4) The last and most sophisticated level is represented by a main integral index of the cardiac system functional condition.

A significant number of detected analysis-important parameters by the application have their own units like sec, mV, etc., or dimensionless. The study [19] suggests bringing them into small-sized and easy-to-read data crucial for treatment decisions using their no-unit form. It uses an interval axis, typically with 0–100 points, as a scaling function technique to solve this problem. The first has four equal zones: from 0 to 25, from 26 to 50, from 51 to 75, and from 76 to 100, respectively. They are designed to represent four conditions of an organ: normal, having minor changes, having intermediate changes, and having obvious changes. This representation approach uses such zones according to the logics of a body's working state, mostly given by the preclinical diagnosis theory [20].

While so, the average value of the normal range for each indicator in absolute units (for example, in seconds) may be considered to be 100 points of the interval scale. The set of normal values gives quantified borders of the organism functioning, and we can call that a standard. An electric heart generator has been used to run computer simulations, establishing the upper and lower bordering values of the first level indicators in absolute units, which show the gradations of having minor changes, having intermediate changes, and having obvious changes, assured with relevant scientific studies as well. That is why we have adjusted four intervals for each indicator with absolute values, which meet four specific zones by 25 units on the axis of the functional state we used. Further, we should use a procedure within each zone to satisfy the linear bond between the discrete values (in absolute units) and the number of points that satisfy that discrete value. Therefore, we get a linear scale for the bond of absolute values and the number of points on the scale of the functional state for each individual indicator of the first level of analysis. The implemented technique of using this differential axis with 100 marks on it provides us with ECG/AHR slight change analysis convenience and clarity.

Continuing with higher analysis levels, we integrate information from the previous level. It means we average all the acquired figures of all performance parameters at the previous level. In detail, it averages the performance of the first level at the second level, the second at the penultimate level, and the third at the last level. To visualize the gradation of the functional state, the traffic light principles were applied as technique color marking. It establishes the normal zone as green, the minor fluctuation zone as yellow, and the zone for intermediate changes as orange. The last, severe state changes zone is red-colored.

The latter leads to possessing an intuitive interface, based on this easy-to-read green-yellow-orange-red logic. It can be understood, with existing appearance, both by the doctors and by every patient, providing them with priceless opportunity to make correction decisions, for example, about workload and leisure activities, or other common modifications to style of living, etc. (see Fig. 13).

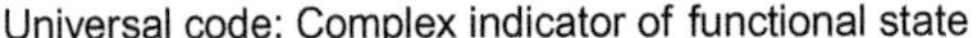
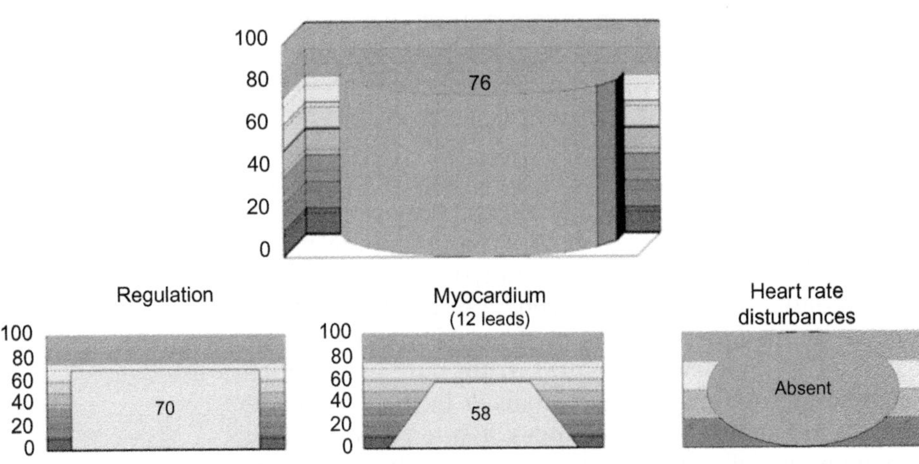

Fig. 13 ECG/HRV universal scoring system with *red* (dark gray in the print version)–*yellow* (light gray in the print version)–*green* (gray in the print version) interface. (For interpretation of the references to color in this figure legend, the reader is referred to the web version of this article.)

4.2 Clinical approbation of new information technologies and metrics of computerized electrocardiography

The proposed scaling method was invented to solve practical problems and is already widely used [21] to solve several different problems in such vital areas as clinical, military, sports, and occupational therapies, including mass-sample research projects.

This led to the cardiac monitoring of more than 20,000 residents of the Ukrainian Khmilnytsky region, mostly from its countryside areas [22]. This ECG and HRV screening included examination of 18 countryside districts of the mentioned region.

Every location had a residents' sample and parameters of more than 100 ECG/ARV tests for each sample item. We got more than 80 digital parameters of social and economic features of those locations. There has also been collected data, which can be named as a comparison (etalon) group of relatively healthy people made up of more than 1000 young volunteers, who went through cardio examination.

The Mahalanobis distance has been gathered for all these districts—between the standard sample and the district residents' one. The degree of mismatch to the standard is represented by this integral indicator. Moreover, we suggested a regression model that looks like:

$$\rho = 1 - \exp\left\{ - \sum_{j=1}^{m} \alpha_j z_j \right\} \tag{16}$$

with the purpose to investigate the impact by social and economic distinctiveness. The resulting variable is the normalized Mahalanobis distance, a crucial component that depends on social and economic indicators and has a correlation matrix spectral analysis in its origin, where m is several crucial items being selected, and {alphas…} are unknown parameters to be determined from statistical data. It has been discovered that nearly 70% of the social and economic environment information is covered by four crucial components.

We assumed that the number of retired workers per area, yearly income cases, and housing estate affordability for the masses as the most important social and economic indicators.

These major indicators can be successfully defined by applying a similar all-around analysis of mass screening results as a very useful approach. The method of ECG scaling we developed is also used in the analysis of a large array of electrocardiographic data in the study of the Institute of Population Health at the University of Oxford [23].

Another field of technology application was to objectively monitor the rehabilitation of military personnel with posttraumatic stress disorder (PTSD), post-concussion syndrome, emotional burnout, and other disorders caused by specific conditions of military service. It is clear that this task is relevant and quite complex. At present, methods for objective monitoring of patients of this type are virtually nonexistent; only appropriate psychological questionnaires are used, which have all the shortcomings inherent in subjective methods and, moreover, are designed to assess only the mental sphere.

In contrast, the technology we have developed allows us to objectively assess both somatic and psychological components. The analysis of the psychoemotional sphere is based on the analysis of heart rate variability (HRV) according to the modified McCraty algorithm (US) based on the model of neurovisceral integration [24].

An analysis of the ECG and HRV of 106 persons was performed. In 79 people, 3-min ECG recordings were performed twice: at the beginning and after spa treatment. The aim of the work was to develop an individual comprehensive indicator of the effectiveness of rehabilitation. It was found that the whole group of studied subjects was divided into two subgroups: subgroup A had a clear improvement in functional status according to the results of in-depth ECG/HRV analysis (51 patients), and subgroup B had no such improvement.

Finally, an automatic decision rule has been developed to determine the individual effectiveness of rehabilitation. This rule includes the six most-informative indicators, of which four indicators were the shape of the ECG and two were indicators of HRV.

The purpose of the next study was to develop an objective assessment of the severity of the physical condition of wounded combatants based on an in-depth analysis of an ECG and HRV. The task of classifying patients by severity of the condition was solved using data mining methods of data analysis. This study proposed a new approach to an objective assessment of the severity of the condition based on the results of an in-depth ECG examination of wounded servicemen who participated in the Anti-Terrorist Operation Zone (ATO) in eastern Ukraine.

The study is based on clinical and instrumental examinations of 141 military persons (men, average age 33 ± 8 years) who participated in the ATO in the East of Ukraine and were hospitalized in the surgical departments of the Main Military Hospital in 2014–15. During their stay at the hospital, doctors determined the severity of each patient's condition in accordance with the classification system of the physical condition of the American Society of

Anesthesiologists (ASAPS) in which 195 records of 12-channel ECGs (5–20 min duration) were analyzed. A multilevel system of indicators was calculated, which determined the functional state of the cardiovascular system of each patient. The final integral assessment of the functional state (FS index) was based on a minimum of 148 quantitative ECG parameters. To develop a classification model for severity, a combination of two data analysis methods was used: clustering (K-means algorithm) and decision tree method (C & RT algorithm). Using the C & RT algorithm, the most informative indicators were selected from the ECG and HRV system of parameters to define regression and classification models of the functional state. A model for classifying the severity of a physical condition by this set of ECG and HRV parameters has been developed. Testing of the models was carried out by the method of 10-fold cross-validation.

The most informative variables were selected, which were included in the model of complex indicators characterizing the regulation of the cardiovascular system and the state of the myocardium. The training sample was 80%, and the test sample was 20%. The results of the regression model of the FS index on the training sample were error 9.1% and correlation coefficient $R=0.94$; on the test sample, error 29%, $R=0.83$. The set of the most informative indicators of ECG predictors of FS, both in regression and classification models, included two indicators for the regulation of the cardiovascular system (an indicator of respiratory arrhythmia and adaptive potential) and five well-known diagnostic markers of myocardial condition (T-wave area, CIIS code, and some others), as well as an indicator of heart rhythm disturbance. The overall accuracy of the classification of severity according to FS predictors was 76.3% [25].

To conclude, a new approach to the classification of the severity of the condition of patients with combat trauma based on a combination of ECG and HRV indicators is proposed. Using data mining methods, we determined the optimal set of predictors of the functional state of the cardiovascular system and developed a classifier for the severity of the condition of patients with combat trauma.

A lookalike method was applied for monitoring of cardiac function with the goal of detecting patients' pathological conditions who had had juvenile idiopathic arthritis to better understand the bond between cardiovascular lesions and the rate of mortality of those patients.

A large number of factors that may be a possible source to early secondary cardiovascular disorders could lead to complexity of clinical interpretation for juvenile idiopathic arthritis patients.

The fact that children are not likely to explain their health complaints makes early diagnosis of these conditions difficult in pediatric practice.

The ECG assessment methods have improved due to the necessity of development of patients' examination hardware.

There were 34 children examined who had had juvenile idiopathic arthritis [26]. In detail, the boys-to-girls ratio was 12:22. Their average age was approximately 10 years old (having an age range from 2 to 17). Each of the diagnosed disease periods had developed from a 3 months to 4 years (making the average 1½ years). Neither instrumental nor laboratory signs of CVS injury (carditis, secondary cardiomyopathy) among the given groups were discovered. Disease presence was measured by means of the Juvenile Arthritis Disease Activity Score (JADAS). The checking of the sixth ECG channel lasted for 5 min each. More than 180 ECG/ARV indicators and the universal ECG scoring system have been processed.

For the purpose of developing an interpretable myocardial damage classifier for further assessing, we suggested a contemporary method that uses the cooperation of clustering (K-means, EM algorithm) and decision tree method (Classification and Regression Trees, CART algorithm).

Disease clinical manifestations analysis for the examined group of children proved that there were almost no complaints raised by the CVS failures; only complaints of a general clinical nature were noticed.

We have revealed the following changes while analyzing data from laboratory checking of those JIA patients. Overall blood test anemia has been observed for four children, typically contributing to the development of myocardium secondary metabolic failures, leading to circulatory hypoxia. The observed erythrocyte sedimentation rate (ESR) was commonly within a normal range (up to 15 mm/h) at the same time, but for several children (up to 10%) it was around 40 mm/h. As for patients' parents, drastic differences from normal biochemical parameters values of them being examined were also not observed. The JADAS-27 consists of four tests: parent/patient global welfare assessment, disease activity from physician global assessment view, active joint count, and ESR or CRP, and was obtained within 9.5 ± 2.04. Immunological parameters of the examined JIA patients satisfied the activity of the inflammatory process as well. Applying standard ECG with 12 channels, no trouble was detected for just three participants (under 10%). Even though detected changes were slight, basically having functional nature, they were not drastically important for a diagnosis of any certain cardiac pathology.

The strong negative correlations of several ECG parameters with JADAS were found, and the five most informative parameters (ST interval and T wave morphology, QRS angle, heart rhythm disturbances) were selected. Then, a CART-based methodology classification algorithm was developed to predict JIA presence. Total classification accuracy was almost 90%. We need to underline that disease activity in the first two grades (i.e., juvenile idiopathic arthritis initial stages) were discovered by four ECG indicators with maximum accuracy.

The next study focused on the treatment of the most common and dangerous heart disease, coronary artery disease (CAD). Every year, mortality from CAD steadily increases. Along with other methods of treatment of severe forms of this disease, one of the most modern and effective is X-ray endovascular plasticity and stenting of coronary arteries. However, X-ray endovascular intervention inevitably causes damage to the coronary vessels and myocardium at least to a minimal degree. Therefore, starting from the first years of widespread coronary vascular surgery, researchers set themselves the task of developing methods for diagnosing the degree of myocardial damage and clarifying the prognostic value of this damage in terms of mortality, revascularization, and myocardial infarction in several years. The aim of our study was to evaluate subtle changes in the ECG immediately after the coronary artery stenting procedure.

Twenty-three patients in the perioperative period of coronary artery stenting were examined. In this study, paired measurements were performed, namely ECG recording for 3 min before and after (several hours) the surgical procedure. A total of 23 pairs of electrocardiographic records were analyzed. In each ECG, 240 primary and calculated indicators were analyzed.

The primary signs of the ECG, which change the most after stenting, were selected. These are mostly indicators that reflect the process of ventricular repolarization. Then, with the help of K-mean cluster analysis, homogeneous groups (clusters) were determined. According to the results of electrocardiography, a cluster with more significant myocardial damage was identified. This group was slightly older than the rest of the patients; the average number of stents in this subgroup was higher and, along with changes in the ECG in patients, showed a deterioration in the HRV index of the psychoemotional state [26].

The electrocardiographic instruments we developed are also used in sports medicine. For example, more than 100 elite ice-hockey youngsters (17-, 18-, and 19-year-olds) have participated in a medical and physiological assessment during NHL Combine. Every one of them had their ECG written in a calm, lying position for 3 min. The analysis of our software implemented these three main points: myocardium state assessment, autonomic nervous system (ANS) assessment, and heart rhythm faults detection. Each point was assigned to a scale of values between 0 and 100 by key physiological parameters, meaning a state between critical pathological (0) and optimal physiology (100), as explained previously. The application has defined a few integrated indices for every point as well as a functional state complex indicator. Optimal values for all three ECG points were shown by 23 sportsmen, with the other 24 proved having mild changes for both myocardium state assessment and INS regulation. The following 36 athletes were detected as having the tiniest cardiac regulation parameters decrease. Only one player was diagnosed with atrial fibrillation, two players with premature ventricular contractions, and the other 98 players tended to show fine ECG rhythm. To conclude, it appears valuable to apply such a differential technique to a group of professional ice-hockey players to obtain important cardiac information from regular ECG screening analysis [27].

The same software and technique were applied for futsal bio and healthcare control as a contemporary methodology. This sport is known for its game plan unpredictability, large variety of performance by players, as well as standard game activities overload.

Playing on an indoor-sized arena means athletes should experience longer intensity phases with much higher anaerobic load in comparison to traditional football and other professional team events, which leads to greater importance of regular medical inspections.

We invited 20 Extra League futsal players to undergo study testing [28].

They represented two teams, 10 from each, and testing was implemented during a friendly game.

The ECG and HRV were taken for five states of body functioning: before the game, having a relatively calm state (warm-up included), just after the game end (match schedule had two halves by 20 min), 10 min and 4 h after the final whistle, and the next day morning. The average main indicators profile was found as having the latter tendencies.

Due to stoppage of the event's stress, there was a decrease of functional state and regulation complex indicator values by 9%; also, there was a decrease of myocardium state indicator by 14%. Meanwhile there was little increase for psychoemotional state indicator value. Summing up the results obtained after a 4-h delay, we saw a total recovery by functional state and myocardium state indicators, but the regulation indicator was still 3.3% under the initial value.

Analyzing the next morning's results, there was an average increase to all parameters but no higher than 1.5% in comparison to the game end data. We estimated that such technology can cut the number of injuries by 30%, giving the teams more opportunities to improve their performance.

A similar design of research was conducted to determine the physiological cost of military officers' activity. Twenty-six officers who took part in the command post exercise at the training ground were examined. Four respondents were teachers at the National University of Defense, and 22 were students. The survey of this group was conducted twice: immediately before the start of command post exercise and 5 days immediately after its end. The duration of ECG recording was 3 min. The physiological cost was determined based on the dynamics of the functional state complex indicator. Thus, an increase of 10% or more of this integral parameter was recognized as a positive trend (i.e., physiological cost is low), a decrease of 10% or more was recognized as negative trend (i.e., physiological cost is high), and changes of less than 10% indicated no significant dynamics (i.e., physiological cost is average).

During the examination, these officers did not complain of any health problems and no pathological changes in the morphology of the ECG were detected, so they were recognized as "practically healthy." According to the functional state complex indicator values, 11 (42%) people did not show significant dynamics (average activity price); 10 (38%) showed positive dynamics, i.e., the body easily adapts to physical and psychological stress (low physiological cost of activity); and 5 (19%) showed negative dynamics (high physiological cost of activity), which indicates reduced compensatory capacity. In our opinion, these officers require dispensary supervision and further assessment of existing workloads.

It should also be noted that. in a subgroup of teachers who were older than students, the high cost of activity was found in 50% of respondents.

At the same time, among the students who performed the functions of unit commanders during the command postexercise, no officer showed a high physiological cost of activity, and in 60% of them, on the contrary, the cost of activity was low. Regarding a separate analysis of the psychoemotional state, in most of the surveyed officers (54%), it improved at the end of the exercise.

Positive dynamics of functional state means improved performance, i.e., the body not only was able to adapt to stress, but its functional state improved due to internal compensatory mechanisms, the body "paid" a relatively low physiological cost, and its physiological reserves were able to adapt to higher levels of stress. On the contrary, negative dynamics of functional state means deterioration of indicators, i.e., the organism was still able to adapt to loadings at the expense of internal compensatory mechanisms, but its physiological condition worsened, the organism "paid" rather high physiological price, and its physiological reserves can appear insufficient at higher load levels.

Note that all examples of the application of the new metric for the analysis of slight changes in the human heart's electromagnetic field are crucial parts of the relevant new diagnostic technologies.

The meaning of the development and implementation of any new diagnostic technology is to solve difficult diagnostic problems that are difficult to solve with existing methods. The previous examples of new metrics fully meet the criteria for solving a complex diagnostic problem in cardiology, and in the first place, there is a wide range of differential diagnosis and low availability and/or high cost of diagnostic methods already included in existing clinical guidelines on this problem. In addition, it should be noted that a key sign of the maturity of the new technology is the presence of certificates of conformity issued by the authorized department of a country, as well as patents confirming its novelty. In this context, it should be noted that the proposed metrics received the relevant international certificates and set of patents for inventions. This is a guarantee of further intensive use of these technologies in medical practice at the international level.

5. New metrics and information technologies based on heart rate variability analysis

5.1 Heart rate variability and pain analysis

The determination of pain syndrome intensity and changes of this intensity over time are important tasks in the practice of extreme conditions medicine, especially military medicine.

The latest techniques on pain or agitation or delirium management for mature patients rely on systematic and thorough pain assessment for severely ill patients, as nobody consistently estimates pain in this population [29]. Even though pain assessment can help to improve patients' comfort and prevent oversedation, this might be a difficult task for severely ill patients. The scale of behavioral pain (BPS), and the tool for critical care pain observation (CPOT) give satisfactory validity and trustworthiness levels and are offered for unspoken pain monitoring. Unfortunately, some limitations are present in such scores, which include variability from expert to expert, inability to apply them for patients receiving neuromuscular-blocking agents, and non-rhythmic pain assessment [30]. Moreover, the scores consider only the physical component of the pain and do not define anxiety and discomfort levels.

For adequate treatment of acute pain syndrome, it is important to prevent a number of complications: thrombotic-embolus, respiratory, ischemic, etc., which reduces the length of hospitalization. Also, qualitative analgesia prevents chronic pain and the development of hyperalgesia.

The individual perception of pain is influenced by demographic factors, gender, age, and ethnicity, as well as the emotional and physical condition of the patient. Existing pain level estimation methods require immediate contact with the patient, as well as the patient being in their right mind.

Finding an objective, reliable, accurate, fast way to determine the intensity of the nociception without the direct involvement of the patient began many decades so. The most promising in this context is the analysis of the autonomic nervous state systems. The physiological basis of the method lies in quite a well-known phenomenon of HRV, which consists of the incidence of intervals between sequences of QRS complexes. It is known that the regulation of cardiac rhythm is the result of the rhythmic activity of the pacemaker cells of the sinus node, modulating the effect of the autonomic and central nervous systems, and humoral and reflexive influences. In particular, HRV reflects the balance between activity of sympathetic and parasympathetic parts of the ANS. It is well-known that the relative parasympathetic tone is a surrogate for antinociception/nociception balance in critically ill patients [31]. However, there are different ways to assess parasympathetic tone using HRV data. It is not clear so far what method of parasympathetic tone analysis is optimal in context of pain intensity assessment.

The aim of this study is to compare different HRV metrics' efficiency for assessment of pain intensity in injured combatants.

Eighteen male combatants (mean age 34 ± 5 years) admitted to intensive care unit for surgical patients of the main military clinical hospital of Ukraine due to mine blast and shrapnel injuries were examined on the second and third days after admission. All patients were conscious, and mechanical ventilation was not used. The ECG records were done by a certified portable ECG device. The duration of each record was 3 min. Immediately after ECG examinations, all patients evaluated pain intensity according to the well-known verbal rating scale (no pain—0 points, weak—1 point, moderate—2 points, strong—3 points, strongest—4 points).

The ECG records were annotated by the PulseWave software developed at the Glushkov Institute of Cybernetics. The annotations, i.e., the sequence of detected ECG fiducial points (P, Q, R, S, T)) were imported into the proprietary HRV Analyzer software package.

Three different HRV metrics were used: Parameters in the time domain are RMSSD (Root mean square of the successive differences) and SDNN (Standard deviation of R-R intervals). The SDNN indicator reflects the effect of both the sympathetic and parasympathetic nervous systems. The RMSSD is an indicator of vagal parasympathetic activity. The RMSSD/SDNN ratio represents the sympathovagal balance of the ANS.

In the frequency domain, the analog of the SDNN indicator is the spectrum power in the low-frequency range from 0.04 to 0.15 Hz, which is denoted as LF (low frequency). The analog of the RMSSD is the spectrum power in the high-frequency range from 0.15 to 0.4 Hz, denoted as HF (high frequency). Accordingly, the HF/LF ratio is analogous to the RMSSD/SDNN ratio.

Research by McCraty et al. [32] showed that negative emotions such as frustration, anger, anxiety, and pain also result in such an incoherent model of the heart rate, that is, the heart rhythm varies greatly and is unpredictable. At the same time, positive emotions, on the contrary, are much more coherent and represent stable harmonic vibrations of the heart rhythm.

In general, negative emotions and pain lead to less synchronization between the parasympathetic and sympathetic nervous system. Thus, the coherence approximates the ratio LF/(VLF + HF), where VLF is very low frequency (0.0033–0.04 Hz).

The HRV metrics were calculated as follows:
- SDNN and RMSSD parameters

The standard deviation of R-R intervals (SDNN) is the integral characteristic of the ANS (ANS) functioning. This parameter depends on the activity of both the sympathetic and parasympathetic links of the ANS; in particular, the increase in SDNN indicates an increase in parasympathetic nerve regulation, while the decrease is due to the growth of sympathetic effects and the suppression of the autonomous circuit activity.

$$\mathrm{SDNN} = \sqrt{\frac{\sum_i (\mathrm{RR}_i - \overline{\mathrm{RR}}\,)^2}{N}} \tag{17}$$

RMSSD (root mean square of the successive differences) is an indicator of vagal-parasympathetic activity.

$$\mathrm{RMSSD} = \sqrt{\frac{1}{n-1} \sum_{i=1}^{n-1} (\mathrm{RR}_{i+1} - \mathrm{RR}_i)^2} \qquad (18)$$

- Spectrum calculation

There are several methods to perform the spectral analysis; most of them are commonly known as nonparametric, for example, FFT, the Fast Fourier Transform, and AR, the autoregressive method (parametric). Low computation costs are one of the yields of the FFT. Meanwhile, there are restrictions to this technique, such as the mean resolution of spectrum, especially having processed frame with short data. Unlike the previously mentioned technique, the AR method creates a much accurate resolution of spectrum for the same frames of short data and allows differentiation of the spectrum on separate components. But the major method issue is the correct prediction of the grade of the optimal model [33].

There are also several algorithms for calculating the autoregressive model. Our software implements Yule-Walker and Burg algorithms. Both give similar results. The optimal order of the model is calculated automatically according to Akaike information criteria (AIC).

- Calculation of coherence ratio

According to McCraty [32], the peak of coherence is the peak on the HRV spectrum in the frequency range from 0.04 to 0.26 Hz. The algorithm for calculating the coherence ration is the following:

To find the largest peak on the spectrum in the frequency range from 0.04 to 0.26 Hz.

To calculate the peak power in a 0.015 Hz window above and below the peak frequency.

To calculate of total spectral power (from 0.033 to 0.4 Hz).

To calculate the coherence ratio using the following equation:

$$\mathrm{Coherence} = \frac{\mathrm{PP}}{\mathrm{TP} - \mathrm{PP}}; \qquad (19)$$

where PP is the power of the peak of coherence, and TP is the total power of the spectrum.

Dependency between HRV parameters and subjectively assessed pain level are shown in Figs. 14–16.

The figures show that the ratio HF/LF correlates with the pain level the best. Correlation coefficients for all three metrics were also calculated:

$$R_{\frac{\mathrm{RMSSD}}{\mathrm{SDNN}}} = 74\%; \quad R_{\frac{\mathrm{HF}}{\mathrm{LF}}} = 76\%; \quad R_{\mathrm{coherence}} = 42\%; \qquad (20)$$

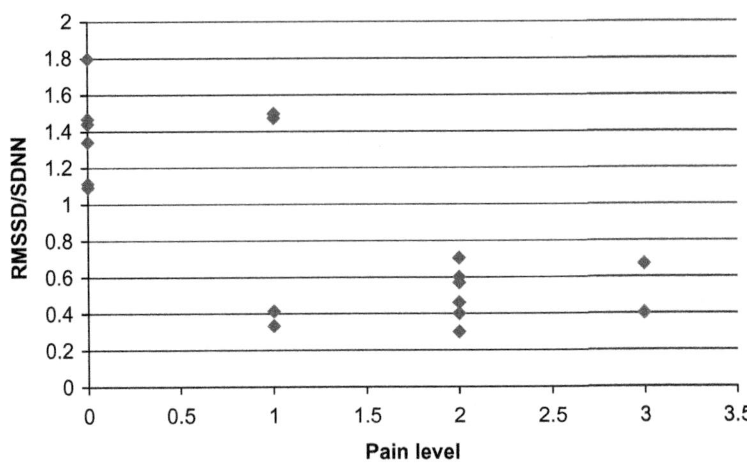

Fig. 14 Dependency between RMSSD/SDNN and pain level.

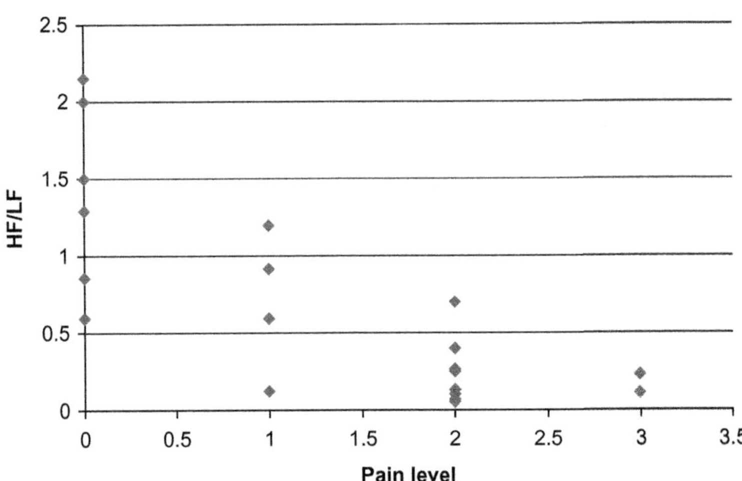

Fig. 15 Dependency between HF/LF ratio and pain level.

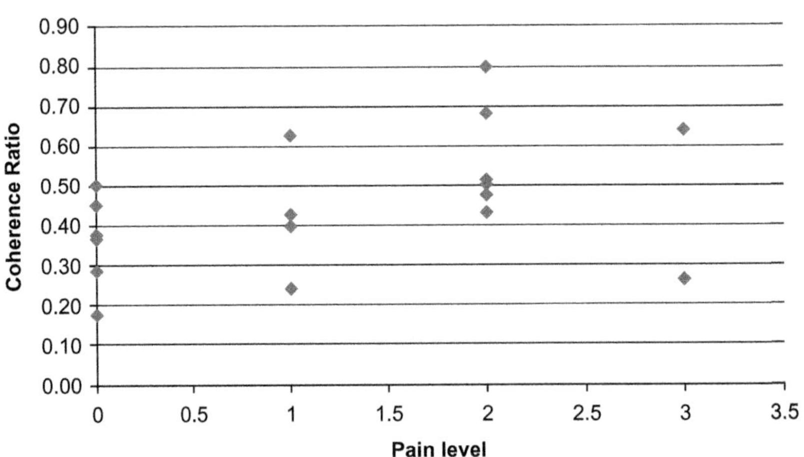

Fig. 16 Dependency between coherence ratio and pain level.

To construct integral index for pain intensity assessment based on HRV metrics, a linear regression model was developed, according to which the pain level can be estimated with the following expression:

$$\text{Pain} = 2.54 - 0.63 \cdot \frac{\text{RMSSD}}{\text{SDNN}} - 0.88 \cdot \frac{\text{HF}}{\text{LF}} \qquad (21)$$
$$- 0.38 \cdot \text{Coh}$$

A correlation coefficient of 77% was achieved with this integral index.

The value of HRV analysis for prediction of mortality and optimization of treatment in the intensive care unit in patients with trauma of different origins are under intensive investigation. Moreover, the value of preadmission sorting of patients with combat trauma using HRV analysis is shown, for example, in a study initiated by Office of Naval Research of Navy and the U.S. Marine Corps [34]. In recent years, the long-time monitoring of HRV has become more and more available even under field conditions as more high-quality miniature optical-based PPG devices emerge.

Thus, the closest correlation with pain intensity was obtained by the HF/LF index, and the RMSSD/SDNN ratio has demonstrated only slightly worse result. In contrast, significant correlation between coherence index and pain intensity was not found.

6. Conclusions

1. The development of new information technologies and metrics for the analysis of small changes in biological signals is a modern technological trend that improves the accuracy of many diagnostic methods, including methods of analysis of electrical activity of the heart.
2. New metrics for the analysis of the spatial structure of 2D magnetocardiographic current density distribution maps allow diagnosing of myocardial ischemia with high accuracy, which has been proven in the course of intercenter studies.
3. Metrics based on three-dimensional visualization (polar diagram) of the electrical activity of the ventricles of the heart based on magnetocardiographic data provide an opportunity to solve important clinical problems, in particular to determine the viability of affected myocardial infarction in patients with various forms of coronary heart disease.

4. A new method of scaling the ECG, designed to detect subtle changes, has found application in various sections of clinical medicine, sports medicine, occupational medicine, as well as in large-scale population studies.

5. An integral HRV index allows for further improvement of the results compared to the results shown by the individual indicators aimed at pain intensity evaluation.

Acknowledgments

The authors truly thank the National Academy of Science of Ukraine, Glushkov Institute of Cybernetics of NAS of Ukraine, National Military Medical Clinical Center as well as hi-tech company Cardiolyse Oy, Finland for their continuous support.

References

[1] E.J. Benjamin, S.S. Virani, C.W. Callaway, A.M. Chamberlain, A.R. Chang, S. Cheng, et al., Heart disease and stroke statistics–2018 update: a report from the American Heart Association, Circulation 137 (12) (2018) 67–492.

[2] M.L. Simoons, P.G. Hugenholtz, Estimation of the probability of exercise induced ischemia by quantitative ECG analysis, Circulation 56 (1977) 552–559.

[3] I.A. Chaikovsky, I.D. Voitovich, Approaches to assessing the degree of maturity of clinical information technologies on the example of technologies for analyzing the electrical activity of the heart, Rep. Natl. Acad. Sci. Ukr. 2 (2014) 160–167 (in Russian).

[4] M. Primin, I. Nedayvoda, Inverse problem solution algorithms in magnetocardiography: new analytical approaches and some results, Int. J. Appl. Electromagn. Mech. 29 (2) (2009) 65–81.

[5] M.A. Primin, V.I. Goumenyuk-Sychevsky, I.V. Nedayvoda, Methods and Algorithms for Localization of Magnetic Field Source, Naukova Dumka, Kyiv, 1992 (in Russian).

[6] M. Primin, I. Nedayvoda, Mathematical model and measurement algorithms for a dipole source location, Int. J. Appl. Electromagn. Mech. 8 (1997) 119–131.

[7] R.L. Fagaly, Superconducting quantum interference device instruments and applications, Rev. Sci. Instrum. 77 (2006) 101101-1–101101-45.

[8] G. Korn, T. Korn, G. Korn, N. Korn, Mathematical Handbook for Scientists and Engineers (Russian Translation), Nauka, Moscow, 1970.

[9] M. Primin, V. Gumeniuk-Sychevskij, I. Nedayvoda, Mathematical models and algorithms of information conversion in spatial analysis of weak magnetic fields, Int. J. Appl. Electromagn. Mech. 5 (1994) 311–319.

[10] I.D. Voitovych, M.A. Primin, V.N. Sosnytskyy, Application of SQUIDs for registration of biomagnetic signals, Low Temp. Phys. 38 (2012) 311–320.

[11] M. Primin, I. Chaikovsky, C. Berndt, I. Nedayvoda, Layer-to-layer heart electrical image based on magnetocardiography data in comparision with perfusion image based on PET, Int. J. Bioelectromagn. 5 (1) (2003) 27–28.

[12] Y.V. Maslennikov, M.A. Primin, I.V. Nedayvoda, The DC-SQUID-based magnetocardiographic systems for clinical use, Phys. Procedia 36 (2012) 88–93.

[13] B. Roth, N. Sepulveda, J. Wikswo Jr., Using a magnetometer to image a two-dimensional current distribution, J. Appl. Phys. 65 (1989) 361–372.

[14] B. Hailer, I. Chaikovsky, S. Auth-Eisernitz, et al., Magnetocardiography in CAD with a new system in an unshielded setting, Clin. Cardiol. 26 (2003) 465–471.

[15] I. Chaikovsky, B. Hailer, V. Sosnytskyy, M. Lutay, G. Mjasnikov, A. Kazmirchuk, M. Budnyk, A. Lomakovskyy, T. Sosnytskaja, Predictive value of the complex magneto-cardiographic index in patients with inter-mediate pretest probability of chronic coronary artery disease: results of a two-center study, Coron. Artery Dis. 25 (6) (2014) 474–484.

[16] M. Cerqueira, et al., Standardized myocardial segmentation and nomenclature for tomographic imaging of the heart. A statement for healthcare professionals from the cardiac imaging Committee of the Council on Clinical Cardiology of the American Heart Association, Circulation 502 (2002) 539–542.

[17] I. Chaikovsky, M. Primin, I. Nedayvoda, et al., Monitoring of myocardial viability in patients with myocardial infarction based on magnetocardiographic analysis of ventricular depolarisation, J. Am. Coll. Cardiol. 72 (Suppl. 16) (2018) C89.

[18] S.D. Colan, Thy way and how of Z-scores, J. Am. Soc. Echocardiogr. 26 (1) (2013) 38–40.

[19] J.A. Vachon, B. Jr, S. Clarke, Validity of the heart rate deflection point as a predictor of lactate threshold during running, J. Appl. Physiol. 87 (1) (1999) 452–459.

[20] R. Chou, B. Arora, Dana, T. et. al., Screening asymptomatic adults with resting or exercise electrocardiography: a review of the evidence for the US Preventive Services Task Force, Ann. Intern. Med. 155 (6) (2011) 375–385.

[21] I. Chaikovsky, Electrocardiogram scoring beyond the routine analysis: subtle changes matters, Expert Rev. Med. Devices 17 (5) (2020) 379–382.

[22] I. Chaikovsky, E. Lebedev, V. Ponomarev, A. Necheporuk, The relationship between ECG/HRV variables and socio-economic factors: results of mass screening in the rural region of Ukraine, Eur. J. Prev. Cardiol. 27 (1_Suppl) (2020) 92.

[23] R. Clarke, I. Chaikovsky, N. Wright, at al., Independent relevance of left ventricular hypertrophy for risk of ischaemic heart disease in 25,000 adults, Eur. Heart J. 41 (2_Suppl) (2020), ehaa946.

[24] R. McCraty, F. Shaffer, Heart rate variability: new perspectives on physiological mechanisms, assessment of self-regulatory capacity, and health risk, Glob. Adv. Health Med. 4 (1) (2015) 46–61.

[25] I. Chaikovsky, O. Kryvova, A. Kazmirchuk, et al., Assessment of the post-traumatic damage of myocardium in patients with combat trauma using a data mining analysis of an electrocardiogram, in: 2019 Signal Processing Symposium (SPSympo), Krakow, Poland, 2019, pp. 34–38.

[26] O.O. Syvoraksha, I. Chaikovsky, Y. Antoniuk, D. Dzuiba, O. Kryvova, O. Loskutov, Assessment of myocardium impairment in coronary stenting according to the results of the analysis of electrocardiogram changes and heart rate variability [in Ukrainian], Emerg. Med. 17 (2) (2021) 87–94.

[27] J.P. Neary, T. Baker, V. Jamnik, at al., Multimodal approach to cardiac screening of elite ice hockey players during the NHL scouting combine, Med. Sci. Sports Exerc. 46 (2014) 742,·.

[28] T. Panchuk, I. Chaikovsky, M. Panchuk, Application of Mobile computer digital devise for current medical and biological control in futsal, in: International Conference on Decision Aid Sciences and Application (DASA), 2020, pp. 427–431.

[29] G. Chanques, A. Pohlman, J.P. Kress, N. Molinari, A. de Jong, S. Jaber, et al., Psychometric comparison of three behavioural scales for the assessment of pain in critically ill patients unable to self-report, Crit. Care 18 (2014) R160.

[30] K. Puntillo, A. Max, J.F. Timsit, L. Vignoud, G. Chanques, G. Robleda, et al., Determinants of procedural pain intensity in the intensive care unit: the Europain1 study, Am. J. Respir. Crit. Care Med. 189 (2014) 39–47.

[31] C. Broucqsault-Dérdian, Measurement of heart rate intensity to assess pain in sedated critical ill patients: a prospective observational study, PLoS One 11 (1) (2016), e0147720.

[32] R. McCraty, The coherent heart heart-brain interactions, psychophysiological coherence, and the emergence of the system-wide order, 2009 induced pain in healthy pupil, Integr. Rev. 5 (2) (2009) 10–115.

[33] E.M. Dantas, M.L. Sant'Anna, R.V. Andreão, C.P. Gonçalves, E.A. Morra, M.P. Baldo, S.L. Rodrigues, J.G. Mill, Spectral analysis of heart rate variability with the autoregressive method: what model order to choose? Comput. Biol. Med. 42 (2) (2012) 164–170.

[34] D. King, M. Ogilvie, B. Pereira, et al., Heart rate variability as a triage tool in patients with trauma during prehospital helicopter transport, J. Trauma 67 (3 Suppl) (2009) 436–440.

Further reading

I. Chaikovsky, O. Oshlianska, A. Artsymovych, at al., Using of data mining methods to evaluate the myocardial damage in children with juvenile idiopathic arthritis, in: 2020 IEEE 40th International Conference on Electronics and Nanotechnology (ELNANO), Kyiv, Ukraine, 2020, pp. 391–395.

12

The role of optimal and modified lead systems in electrocardiogram

N. Prasanna Venkatesh, B. Arya, B. Dhananjay, and J. Sivaraman

Bio-signals and Medical Instrumentation Laboratory, Department of Biotechnology and Medical Engineering, National Institute of Technology Rourkela, Odisha, India

1. Introduction

Atrial fibrillation (AF) is detected using surface electrocardiogram (ECG) as a clinical tool by the widely preferred lead system, standard 12-lead ECG, in resting conditions [1]. Using standard 12-lead system, recording of ECGs for longer durations can cause discomfort to the patients [2]. Therefore, reduced leads set are adequate for prolonged ECG recording to predict cardiovascular diseases, such as detection of silent and undocumented AF prevalent in certain populations with comorbidities (arrhythmia, hypertrophy, diabetes, etc.). To detect myriad of cardiac diseases accurately, researchers developed various reduced lead systems that support and warrant patient feasibility and also increase the diagnostic capability. Although detecting AF is more compatible with reduced lead systems, they are limited due to underlying mechanisms of atrial arrhythmias based on their acquired information. In contrast, comprehensive AF characterization benefits from standard electrode placements, such as detecting wavefront propagation patterns in the atria [3]. Standard lead systems and other lead systems may produce false-positive results in disease detection and arrhythmia classification due to the presence of muscle noise, artifacts in joints, sinus arrhythmias, and ectopic beat in waveforms [4]. On analyzing brief AF episodes, the above shortcomings are evident. The manual reviewing of long-term monitoring of ECG is laborious [5], so improving automated AF detection methods is essential in clinical applications.

Advanced Methods in Biomedical Signal Processing and Analysis. https://doi.org/10.1016/B978-0-323-85955-4.00014-4
Copyright © 2023 Elsevier Inc. All rights reserved.

1.1 Lead theory

The electrical excitation of the heart acts as bioelectric source that produce and spread the electrical conductivity in the surrounding tissues. Therefore, it is possible to acquire time-dependent voltage waveform through the noninvasive surface electrodes known as an ECG. The lead theory defines the liaison between the potential difference generated by ECG leads and cardiac electrical sources. While understanding the liaison, the components to be considered are the cardiac active electrical spot and conductive extracardiac tissues with passive aggregate that make the noninvasive measurement of the heart's electrical conduction using electrophysiological leads.

Einthoven and colleagues [6,7] proposed the classical lead theory that defines the human body as a part of the boundless, uniform conductor in which the electric sources of the heart are characterized by a particular, time-dependent dipole at a static position. Lead I, II, and III are Einthoven's leads formed from the limb electrodes. Wilson eventually developed the augmented unipolar limb leads from Wilson's central terminal, which was later included in Einthoven's theory. Further, the solid angle theory was established by Wilson and colleagues [8] for understanding the potentials in unipolar precordial leads. Instead of a single, stable dipole location, a dual-layered source was presented by this theory. In the middle 1940s and 1950s, a more suitable lead theory, widely mentioned as the volume-conductor theory, was progressed. The human body is a three-dimensional, sporadically shaped, confined, and heterogeneous volume conductor which was first defined by Burger and van Milaan [9–11]. The volume-conductor features that rest on the stable-dipole hypothesis are common with the above theory. According to volume conductor theory, the signals on the human body surface at a specified time, shall be obtained by an electrical heart vector in three-dimensional space. The stable-dipole hypothesis is not much adequate. Studies on body surface potential mapping (BSPM) have determined that the body surface potential dispersions from muscle show characteristics that a particular, stable-position dipole source cannot report. The shortcomings of the stable-dipole hypothesis were overwhelmed by considering the disseminated nature of the electrical impulse of the heart by McFee and Johnston's lead theory [12–14]. It simplifies the lead vector into the lead-field hypothesis and states the source-lead association for every element of the dispersed cardiac impulse.

1.2 BSPM

The conventional ECG has its limitations in AF diagnosis, as it provides limited information on wavefront transmission models in atria. Spatial differences are adequately replicated in a larger number of electrode placements around the body surface. Certainly, restoration of potentials on body surface from the 12-lead ECG fibrillatory waves (f waves) is accompanied by a restoration error of 53%, representing that for more precise demonstration of the f waves, more electrodes are needed [15]. As a result, BSPM is a crucial method for the restoration of f waves [16]. The number of electrodes required for BSPM vary from 56 [3] to 252 [17], with placements in anterior, posterior, and occasionally lateral sites. The electrodes are randomly dispersed [15] or arranged uniformly in a grid around V_1 [3,18]. Wavefront propagation models were established in the initial BSPM studies on AF, denoting either a particular wavefront, a distinct wavefront with losses, or several wavefronts [3]. The recording of electric potentials was made using a customized vest with 56 electrodes in which 40 electrodes in an anterior position and 16 electrodes in the posterior position were fixed around V_1 in a grid with a uniform gap of 2.2 cm. The invented wavefront proliferation maps agreed with those observed using intrusive or optical imaging despite the inferiority of f waves. When comparing the f waves from V_1, recorded using BSPM, they are symbolic by having a single wavefront propagated through the entire atria. In such conditions, the amplitude of f wave and atrial fibrillatory rate (AFR) were identical independents based on the signal recording sites. However, the pattern of f wave varied and relied on the location for a particular wavefront splitting or various concurrent wavefronts that are synchronized.

BSPM was used with 64 electrodes spaced unevenly with 48 electrodes toward anterior and 16 electrodes on posterior position [15]. The cumulative root mean square error (RMSE) of the remodeled signals of the residual leads that are not encompassed in the lead scheme were considered and used to pick the optimum leads. The optimal count of electrodes required for derivation of the AF waves is 23 for producing similar degree of accuracy as the ventricular waves of 12-lead ECG recording with 25% error [15]. According to the finding of same study, for limiting the error down to 10% only 22 electrodes are sufficient for reconstructing ventricular activity. However, 25% error is the most reasonable limit with 23 and 17 leads for AF and P wave detection, respectively.

Assuming that BSPM can effectively identify the form of wavefront propagation, the technique mentioned above can describe the degree of organization of atria. The time-consuming preparation process limits the implementation of BSPM. However, this issue can be reduced by incorporating the electrodes into a smart vest, which will significantly reduce the time needed for the placement of electrodes.

1.3 Modifications in standard ECG lead system

It is more likely to be a clinical advantage for predisposition of AF in the population, if a lead system is developed as a modified standard 12-lead ECG. As a result, numerous such modifications have been suggested [15,19–21]. The conventional ECG can be reconstructed by the restricted design of 10 electrode-modified lead systems. The coordinates of the extremity electrodes aVR, aVL, and aVF should be maintained to sustain Wilson's central terminal, which is made as to the reference for the precordial chest leads. Furthermore, it is preferable to position the electrodes in correlation to traditional recording mainly because improper positioning sites are the most common error while obtaining the standard ECG [22]. The placements of electrodes are calculated heuristically, either by positioning the electrodes near the atria or using a standardization condition. V_3 to V_6 should be placed near V_1 and V_2 as an empirical method for evaluating ECG leads based on amplitude changes in f waves. The precordial electrodes, for example, can be reorganized to form a 2–3 grid arrangement placed on the right side of the torso, with the unchanged position of V_1 and V_2 while V_3 to V_6 replaced by the new electrodes V_{LS}, V_S, V_{RS}, and V_R [19]. One intercostal area above V_1 is the electrode V_S (superior, S). The electrode V_{RS} is placed to the right side of the electrode V_S, while the electrode V_R is placed to the right of V_1 and vertically arranged with V_{RS}. All the placements of the above-discussed electrodes are detailed in Fig. 1a. Preliminary findings using artificial signals of f waves and a physiological model of the thorax and human atria revealed that the leads devised 3 and 17 leads resulted in more detailed information about atrial function than the standard ECG [19,20].

The other derived modifications are aimed on either anterior or posterior leads replacement monitoring [21]. Similar to the lead scheme in [19], V_1 and V_2 remain unchanged, while the four other different leads are reorganized in an anticlockwise direction around V_1 and V_2, as displayed in Fig. 1b. The only difference of lead placement in [19] is that, the lead V_{RS} is placed on the right

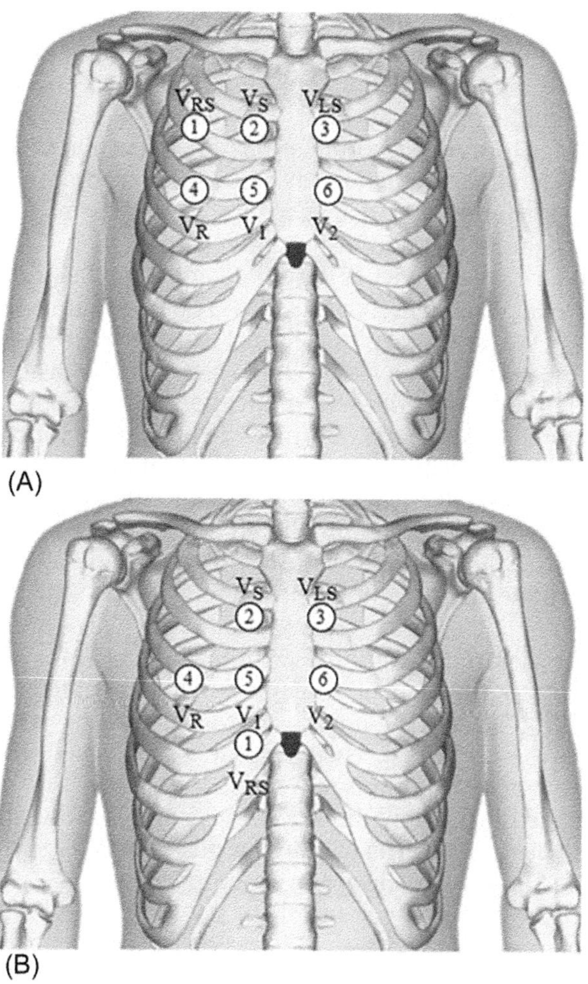

Fig. 1 Modifications derived for electrode placement in anterior part of torso for electrocardiogram in (a) [20] and (b) [22].

upper side of the torso, after one intercostal gap under V_1. Similarly, the posterior electrodes V_{1P} V_{1PS}, V_{2P} and V_{2PS} (posterior superior, PS) are rearranged. Two electrodes are located opposite V_1 and V_2, and the other two are placed in one intercostal space beneath V_1 and V_2. Ensuring the termination of ventricular activity, the utility of the suggested electrode location is investigated in terms of inter-lead dispersion of the AFR was examined. The proximity of V_1 and V_2 resulted in virtually identical AFR, while the dispersion was more significant between the anterior leads.

Moreover the placement of the posterior electrode was correlated with lower frequency dispersion of 35% than the anterior electrode placement, the blending of both approaches may be used to obtain added information. It has been revealed that anterior leads primarily imitate the right atrial AFR [23], while the posterior leads largely reflect the left atrial AFR [24]. The anterior and posterior leads should be equally considered in order to distinguish frequency gradients and the atrial mechanism.

The heuristic approaches described above are helpful in locating electrode placement that provides greater amplitude of f wave; however, it is unable to enhance atrial wave characteristics. Maximizing the ratio of the lowest to the highest singular value of the f wave signal collected from various locations on the body surface is a measurable approach to optimize the positioning of precordial electrodes [20]. According to the heuristic methods, four of the precordial chest electrodes are replaced, although two remain unaltered. V_1 placement is unaltered due to its similarity to the V_4 placement since its f waves are the least correlated to those in V_1. The quest for optimum positioning of the four precordial electrodes in [20] culminated in four different places on the torso, where the electrodes could be positioned to warrant additional atrial knowledge using a physiological model to replicate f waves, as shown in Fig. 2a. One intercostal space above V_1 is where the electrode V_S is mounted. The electrode V_{RS} is placed to the right of the electrode V_S in the same intercostal space. The electrode V_{LS} is located just below the left clavicle, and the electrode V_P is anchored behind the atria at a similar position as V_1. Surprisingly, two of the four current electrode positions, V_S and V_{RS}, were identical to those derived heuristically in [19].

Furthermore, the location of V_S was similar to that of lead S in the EASI lead system, identified by the Frank lead system's E, A, I, and electrode S located over the torso [25]. The simulated f wave signals results revealed that the streamlined and heuristically derived lead systems would extract more information than the traditional electrode placement systems. Nonetheless, the gap in atrial knowledge obtained by the proposed lead schemes was not significant. Given that the electrodes positioned nearer to the atria, resulting in greater f wave amplitudes, optimized placement, which involves electrodes with smaller f waves (V_4 and V_{LS}), is controversial.

Using an iterative lead selection theory, two other adapted 12-lead ECG systems for enhancing the examination of AF were developed. Only leads that increase the details stored in each selected lead set were chosen [26]. In the same way, as the

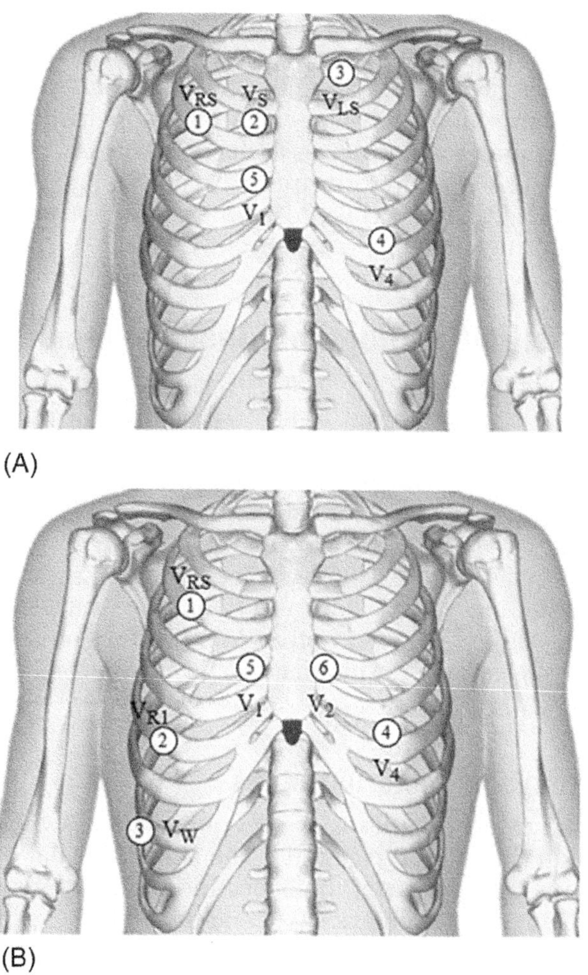

Fig. 2 Modifications derived for electrode placement in anterior part of torso implementing various optimization criteria (a) like the minimum to the maximum singular value ratio of the *f* wave signals and (b) like the restoration error of *f*-wave.

previously mentioned lead systems were repositioned, only four precordial electrodes were replaced by the criterion for selecting leads with added atrial details [15]. Depending on whether V_1 and V_2 or V_1 and V_4 could be held at their traditional locations, the electrode positions were extracted, each of that included the two supplementary electrodes V_{RI} and V_W at right inferior part and another at the waist, as shown in Fig. 2b. Although the electrodes were mounted on distinct areas of the body surface, both lead systems were correlated with a comparable f wave restoration error, which was around 10% lesser than that acquired with the conventional ECG system. A modest reduction in restoration error means that changes to the standard ECG lead system do not result in a significant rise in atrial information. With the added difficulty of electrode positioning, it is unlikely that any changes will be implemented clinically.

2. Modified and optimal lead systems

During ambulatory monitoring in patients with AF, no specified leads are currently used in clinical practice. As a result, regular five-electrode Holter ambulatory recording is usually used to capture six limb leads, namely I, II, III, aVR, aVL, and aVF, in conjunction with any one precordial lead, e.g., V_1 [27]. Standard ambulatory monitors are well used to minimize patient compliance and quality of life [2,28]. As a result, for long-term ambulatory monitoring of AF, single-lead monitors have become a promising choice [29]. To improve AF identification in reduced-lead ECGs, electrode positioning should be designed for f wave analysis.

2.1 Bipolar monitoring leads

Bipolar monitoring leads are developed from two electrodes other than the ground electrode. The simple bipolar recording starts with a minimum of three electrodes. These bipolar leads are configured based on leads I, II, and III as per the requirement of ECG recording. Torso has the advantage of resistance over motion artifacts and supports prolonged monitoring. Bipolar Modified Chest Lead 1 (MCL1) is obtained by fixing the right arm and left arm electrodes in the left infraclavicular region and right fourth intercostal space. The left-arm electrode position is the same as the V_1 location in the standard lead system. The third electrode is the ground electrode placed anywhere away from active electrodes [28]. Simple three-electrode bipolar monitoring was widely used in telemetry applications.

2.2 Modified chest leads

Many modified chest leads are present, and the most common is MCL1 which is configured by changing the lead I position to left infraclavicular and right fourth intercostal space (parasternally in V_1 location). MCL6, a chest lead is configured on V_6 position of the standard lead system. The leads MCL1 and MCL6 generate potentials similar to V_5 and V_6 even in imperfect positions. Popular operating lead CS5 has its right arm electrode below the right clavicle and left arm electrode at V_5. Here, the ground electrode is the left leg electrode [30]. This lead has its application in anterior wall myocardial ischemia detection. CM5, CB5, and CC5 lead differed from CS5 by having the right arm electrode over the manubrium sterni, right scapula, and right anterior axillary line. The remaining electrodes are unchanged as in CS5. CB5 has the advantage of detecting myocardial ischemia and supraventricular tachycardia.

2.3   Minimal monitoring leads

The monitors used for intensive care in recent days have a cable of five electrodes. Four active electrodes are configured over the torso, and fifth electrode is grounded on the right leg position. Among four active electrodes, one is placed at the V_1 position and the rest are nearer to their corresponding limbs. V_1 position is suitable for arrhythmia monitoring and may vary as per the requirement of patient. This standard chest lead position has a clinical value in detecting pacemaker rhythms, bundle branch blocks, and wide QRS tachycardia. This five-electrode system acquires all the limb lead signals with the advantage of one chest lead at a time. They have the capability of better acquisition of ST-segment elevations and rhythm abnormalities. Their application is more in two-channel monitors that simultaneously display a limb lead and a chest lead [28].

2.4   Mason-Likar lead system

The Mason-Likar lead system has its application in exercise stress testing using a treadmill. Mason et al. [5] designed this lead system by siting the limb electrode to the torso and chest electrodes at their original position. This electrode replacement is done to reduce the motion artifacts. The upper limb electrodes are anchored over infraclavicular fossae, 2 cm below the clavicle, medial to the deltoid muscle. The lower limb electrodes are fixed in the anterior axillary line midway between the iliac crest and costal margin. The ground electrode is similar to the standard lead system. The lead system has 12-leads acquired from 10 electrodes. It has its clinical usage in monitoring the ST-segment deviations during thromboembolic therapy [31]. The ECG waveforms recorded using Mason-Likar lead system has morphological variations, obscured Q wave, compared to the standard 12-lead system. Even in post angioplasty cases, the Mason-Likar lead system is significant in monitoring both ischemic and arrhythmic conditions which is possible by unchanged precordial leads. The presence of a large number of chest electrodes hampers the chest X-ray evaluation and defibrillation—also, the stability of chest electrodes is also affected by the hairy chest in both males and females.

2.5 Lund lead system

Lund leads differ from Mason-Likar modification by placing the limb leads in proximal regions of limbs [32]. The changes are made to resist motion artifacts, and the morphology of the ECG is almost the same as obtained in the standard 12-lead ECG. Hence, there are both diagnostic and monitoring applications in the Lund system [17]. The noise level in Lund lead and Mason-Likar lead systems are insignificant and have superior applications than monitoring in the standard lead system [33].

2.6 Derived 12-lead systems

Occasionally, some technical difficulties were encountered in placing all electrodes over the torso. To overcome the drawback in reduced lead systems, automated algorithms were programmed to recreate the missed leads [34]. Rebuilding of leads is either patient-specific or more general templates. Deriving 12-lead ECGs from limb electrodes and two precordial electrodes are technically possible with satisfactory diagnostic accuracy [35].

2.7 Lewis lead

Sir Thomas Lewis developed a lead system during his study on AF and noticed f waves [36]. L_1 is derived from the electrodes between the manubrium and the second intercostal space, L_2 is derived from the electrodes between the second and fourth intercostal space, and L_3 between electrodes in manubrium and left fifth intercostal space, as shown in Fig. 3. Lewis lead is preferred for an accurate diagnosis of wide QRS complex tachycardia [37]. A study was conducted on modifying Lewis lead with all 12 leads to detect ventricular pacing during ventricular conduction [38]. Here, the original Lewis configuration is obtained by transposing the right arm and left arm electrodes.

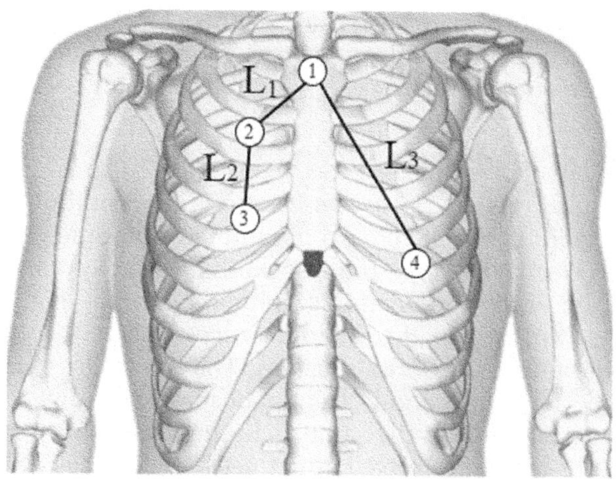

Fig. 3 Lewis lead system.

2.8 Modified Lewis lead

A modified Lewis lead [39] system was proposed exclusively for analyzing atrial activity and atrial-related diseases such as AF, cryptogenic ischemic stroke, etc. The lead L_{M1} is obtained from electrodes between the manubrium and fifth right intercostal space, L_{M2} is obtained from electrodes in the right and left fifth intercostal space as described in Fig. 4. The leads overcome the limitations in Lewis leads like electromyographic noise and ectopic beats. In contrast, a multilead system has an advantage

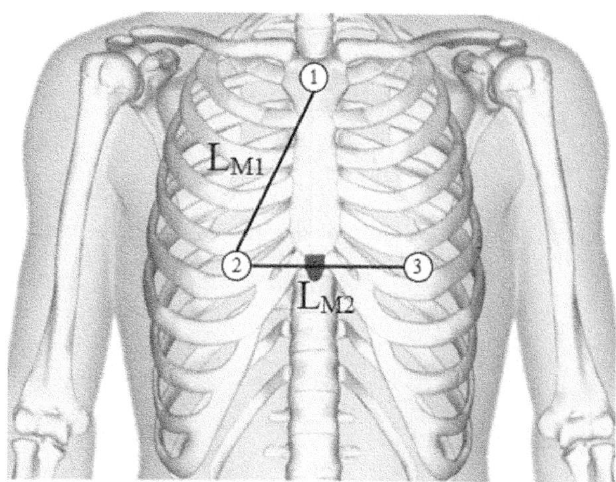

Fig. 4 Modified Lewis lead system.

in atria activation patterns. The modified Lewis lead system is potentially resistant to noise and provides more significant deflection for atrial activity.

2.9 EASI lead system

EASI lead system is a five-electrode system but acquires 12-leads with the help of a programmed computer algorithm [25]. The electrodes A, E, and I of the EASI lead system are also seen in the Frank vectorcardiography system [40]. Fig. 5 shows electrode E placed in the xiphoid process, and S is located in the manubrium part of the sternum. The electrodes A and I are fixed aside across one another along the midaxillary lines. Ground electrode placement is the same as in the Mason-Likar lead system, and 12-leads are derived from the five-electrode EASI system by algebraic transfer method [41]. Excessive artifacts were documented in the EASI lead system while turning from supine position to right [27]. The artifact noise is mostly from electrode I on the midaxillary line. Myoelectric noise is lesser in limb leads than EASI leads. Disease diagnosis like monitoring ischemic episodes is missed in reduced leads, which can be seen by deriving 12-leads. Ischemic events are captured up to 67% from the derived EASI 12-lead monitoring which is not seen in lead II and V_1 [29].

2.10 Fontaine bipolar leads

Arrhythmogenic right ventricular dysplasia (ARVD) shows the epsilon waves while recording Fontaine leads [42]. Fontaine developed it in 1977, which is more sensitive to Epsilon waves

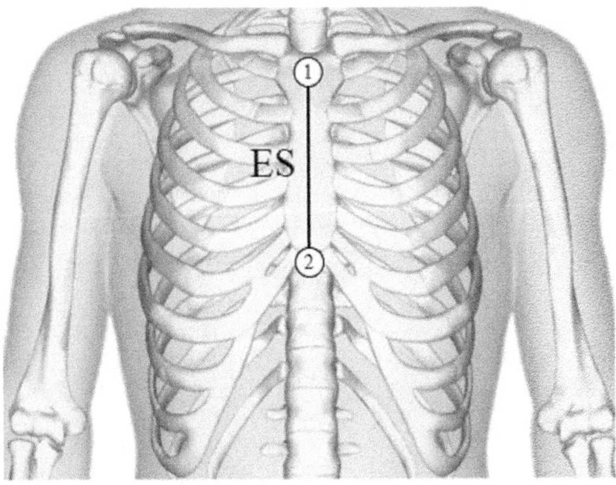

Fig. 5 ES lead of EASI lead system.

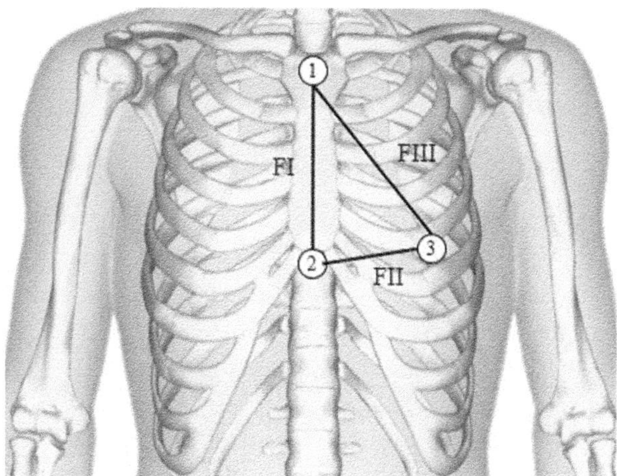

Fig. 6 Fontaine lead system.

during ARVD [43]. The electrodes in Fontaine leads were placed in the upper and lower part of the sternum and also in the V_4 position, as shown in Fig. 6. The Fontaine leads system are F-I formed between the electrodes on sternum, F-II between the electrodes in manubrium and electrode in V_4 position, and F-III between Xiphoid and V_4.

2.11 Modified limb lead system

The dominant ventricular peaks significantly hide the atrial repolarization (Ta wave) phase of ECG. As the Ta wave has clinical advantages in diagnosing atrial diseases, its presence is noticed by depression in the ST segment. Sivaraman et al. [44,45] developed the modified limb lead (MLL) system by modifying the standard limb leads. The right arm electrode is sited in the third right inter-costal space slightly to the left of the mid-clavicular line. Left-arm and left leg electrodes are placed adjacent to one another in the fifth right intercostal space across the mid-clavicular line, as dis-played in Fig. 7. The ground electrode is fixed in a standard posi-tion. Leads I, II, and III are formed as in standard limb leads but with different placement of electrodes and recording characteris-tics. In this lead system, the position of electrodes focuses on the atrial aspects, enhancing the amplitude of the P-wave, which was found equivalent to the amplitude of the R wave of this lead sys-tem. A successive study [46] unmasked the Ta wave and highlighted the significance of Ta wave in atrioventricular block

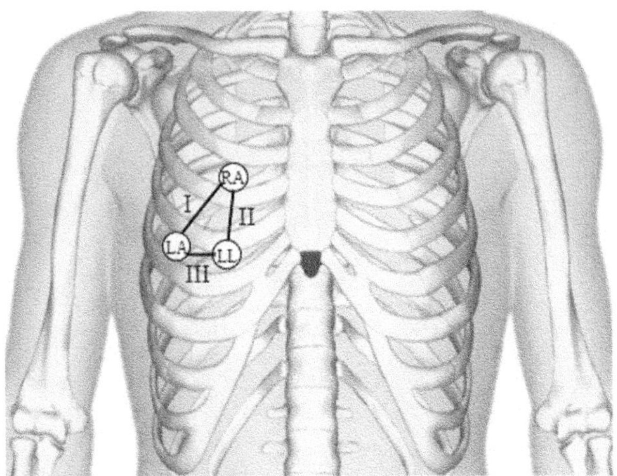

Fig. 7 Modified limb lead system.

(AV block) patients and concluded that Ta wave has longer duration in AV block compared to sinus rhythm.

2.12 Monitoring neonatal and pediatric ECG

Neonatal and pediatric ECG monitoring is complex considering various parameters such as the number of electrodes used to record ECG, and material of electrode that supports prolonged monitoring and prevent any skin related issues due to electrodes and rec. Distinctive leads made of cloth were used to reduce trauma and other damages during procedures.

2.13 P-lead system

The P-lead placement was developed by the BSPM technique to detect the proper electrode placement site for recording P-wave with larger amplitude [47]. Electrode for the P-lead is placed between the right sternal clavicular junction and the left seventh intercostal space in line with the costal margin, as seen in Fig. 8. The study [48] provides three sets of transformation weights based on population by investigating three bipolar leads: P-lead, ES lead, and modified Lewis lead. The leads of the 12-lead ECG are suboptimal in case of atrial activity. In 12-lead ECG, P-wave and atrioventricular (AV) dissociation are not visible, which leads to misdiagnosis of AF and ventricular arrhythmias. Therefore, AV dissociation is challenging to define in 12-lead ECG due to less amplitude or indistinguishable P-waves.

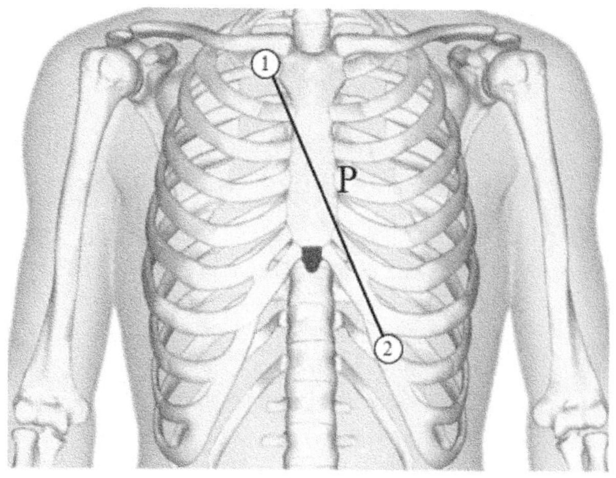

Fig. 8 P-lead system.

3. ECG signal processing

Many researchers have performed studies in various phases of the ECG analysis during the last 2 decades, and few are listed in Table. 1. This chapter offers an in-depth look at the techniques and procedures used to electrodes for analyzing ECG signals. All these works differ in terms of selection criteria and assessment metrics in order to provide researchers in this area with more enhanced perspective and deeper considerations of similar work's assistances. Fig. 9 shows the essential morphological parameters that are considered while performing signal analysis, processing, and classification techniques.

3.1 Data acquisition

The dataset collection is the crucial objective when considering the ECG signal processing, including feature extraction and classification of various arrhythmia conditions. The characteristics reported in analyzing ECG signals aids in determining feature selection for extraction and further examination. The leads considered, the number of leads involved in recording ECG, age, gender, and health status of the patients are all parameters that help in ECG signal analysis and classification. The different ECG data acquisition sources elaborate the design of the data acquisition structure. ECG signal exploration is usually conducted on computer-based software and tested

Table 1 Signal processing approaches for ECG analysis.

Fiducial points [Ref.], Year	Detection method	Performance metrics	Dataset
ST-Segment [49], 2015	Wavelet transform	99% sensitivity	MITDB
QRS, ST-Segment [50], 2015	Wavelet transform	0.009 s QRS duration, 11 s ST duration	MIT, ESCDB
QRS, R-peak [51], 2012	DWT	99.64% sensitivity, 99.91% positive predictive value, 0.54 error	MITDB
QRS-complex [52], 2008	DWT	90.75% sensitivity, 89.2% positive predictive value	ESCDB
QRS, P and T-wave [53], 2009	DWT-based windowing	99.84% sensitivity, 99.8% positive predictive value, 0.0113 error	MITDB, ESCDB, QTDB, and TWADB2008
QRS and R-Peak [54], 2018	Windowing algorithm	94.3% accuracy, 96% sensitivity, 97.3% positive predictive value, 0.3 error	MITDB
R-Peak, ST-Segment [55], 2015	Windowing algorithm	90.1% accuracy	ESCDB
ST-Segment [56], 2016	Time domain	91.37% sensitivity, 45.53% positive predictive value	ESCDB
QRS, ST-Segment [57], 2012	Time domain gradients	[0.04 error] QTDB, [0.06 error] PTDB	QTDB, PTBDB
QRS-Complex [58], 2009	Mathematical morphology	99.81% sensitivity, 99.8% positive predictive value, 99.61% detection rate	MITDB
QRS-Complex [59], 2010	Mathematical morphology	85.76% detection rate	MITDB
QRS-Complex [60], 2012	Mathematical morphology + VLSI detector	99.76% sensitivity, 99.82% positive predictive value, 99.57% detection rate	MITDB
QRS-Complex [61], 2020	Gaussian + SMM	0.17 RMSE	MITDB, QTDB

against publicly accessible datasets. These datasets provide registered electrophysiological parameters of ECG signals. In such recording environments, specific libraries used telehealth sensors to capture ECG signals. Fig. 10 displays the acquired ECG signal of standard lead-II, which needs to be processed further for analysis and disease diagnosis. According to research, the classification of ECG based on single-lead or

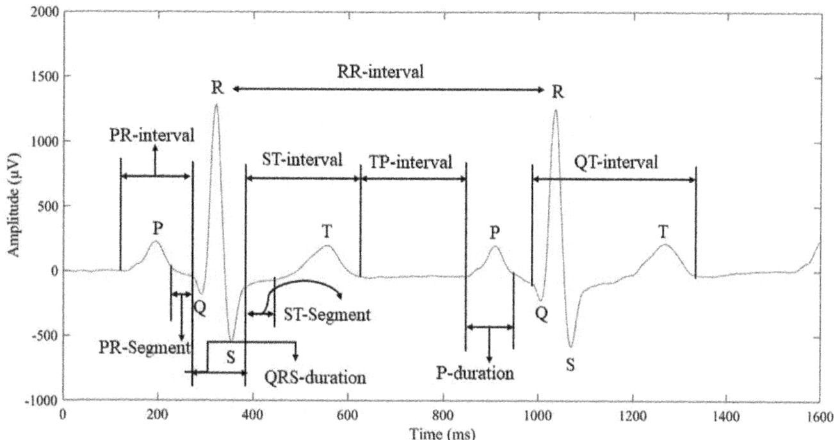

Fig. 9 Electrocardiogram labeled with fiducial markers.

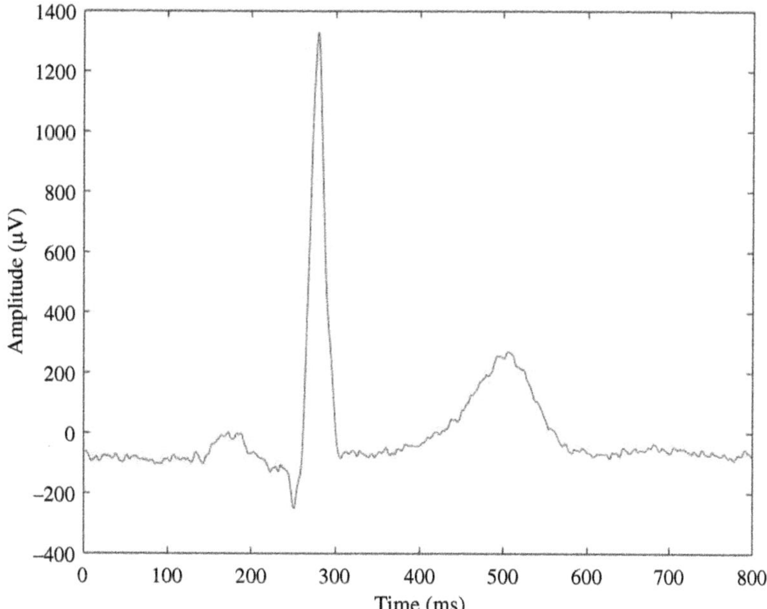

Fig. 10 Standard lead-II ECG waveform.

reduced leads recordings can be as accurate as standard ECG records in some situations. These findings aid researchers in using the ESC-ST-T database widely. Since it contains single limb lead recordings, which may be used to test the efficiency of wearable sensors and devices.

3.2   Denoising techniques

The primary input for the analysis and classification of ECG signals are real-time or recorded ECG signals. ECG data is collected in both situations by connecting surface electrodes and leads over the surface of the body. The noise is bagged along with the ECG during data acquisition, which directly impacts the accuracy in ECG classification. The process of removing noise from the raw signal is known as denoising. Researchers have a goal to eliminate noise from original signals to detect various anomalies reliably. The traditional approach for denoising the ECG signal is designing band-pass filters of range 0.05–45 Hz to validate the quality. Noise can trigger false alarms, which are critical in determining a person's health status. Noise can take several forms; however, it can be broadly divided into external noise and internal embedded noise. The power-line interference or some other forms of noise like white noise are primarily external in nature. Noise is typically eliminated as soon as collecting data from source signals in ECG research. Several techniques to denoise the signal trend are available. The structural similarity matrix (SSIM) [62] can be used to check the consistency of the ECG signal, and metrics like the signal-to-noise ratio (SNR) can be used. Accuracy, mean square error (MSE), RMSE, and convergence rate are other performance metrics identified in the ECG denoising level by researchers.

In recent experiments, researchers have used filters like adaptive notch filter (ANF), finite impulse response (FIR) filter, and other different filtering methods to eliminate noise from the required signal. Any device, either conventional cable leads or a wireless sensor, will inject noise into the ECG signal. The authors of [63] tried to eliminate internal noise from the raw ECG by smoothing technique with FIR filters and achieved an accuracy of 99.3%. Power-line interference (PLI), also called external noise, on the other hand, is the most common disturbance to which the ECG signal is liable. PLI is a common noise source of about 50 to 60 Hz frequency. Studies [64–66] performed the denoising of PLI using the state space recursive least square adaptive filter (SSRLS), a filter-based approach, ANF and fast Fourier transform (FFT), while adaptive control schemes eliminate unknown external disturbances. HDL-based NN-based denoising autoencoders (DAE) and FIR filters [67–69] are used to eliminate other external white noise.

3.3   Feature extraction techniques

ECG classification necessitates the accurate identification of biomarkers in the waveform. A significant QRS complex wave in the waveform expresses the heart's ventricular depolarization.

Its shape provides the foundation for the automatic identification of characteristics and serves as the starting point for various classification methods. Most of the automated algorithms for analyzing ECG rely on QRS complex identification. However, precise QRS detection is difficult due to physiological variations and the inclusion of various noises mixed in the ECG signal. Various approaches focused on derivatives have a more extensive output index for low-frequency noises, though digital filtering systems worked well for high-frequency noise. Many conventional signal processing methods have been suggested in the last decade to detect the fiducial points like QRS complex, R-peak, ST-segment, early repolarization pattern, T wave from ventricular components are considered during feature extraction.

3.4 Signal processing techniques

The first step for marking fiducial points is the QRS complex detection, an essential ventricular component of ECG, and further providing valuable information followed by extracting various other features. Peak detector techniques can detect QRS peak and its wave morphologies, which aids in classifying the ECG signal and detecting multiple types of arrhythmias. After passing through the denoising point, the ECG signal is noise-free and of high quality. The ECG signal is processed into a feature extraction step, which detects fiducial points like the J-point, R-R interval, T-wave, and ST-segment. R-peaks from two ECG cycles determine R-R intervals, and other fiducial points are detected separately from ECG waveforms. Furthermore, the J-point and heart rate functions, which show an essential role in the beat classification of ECG waveform, help to enhance distinguishing ST-segment and its abnormalities. The ST segment is a component of the ECG that provides knowledge about ischemic diseases. Myocardial infarction and angina are also potentially fatal diseases that cause modifications and anomalies in the ST segment. Various algorithms and techniques for detecting the QRS onset and offset, ST-segment, T wave onset and offset have been published in many pieces of literature.

Wavelet transform (WT) is a common technique that researchers have used to detect various points in an ECG signal. Eq. (1) shows the WT representation, here * indicates the complex conjugate.

$$F_{(x,y)} = \int_{-\infty}^{\infty} f(t)\psi^*{}_{(x,y)}(t)\mathrm{d}t \qquad (1)$$

The WT is a common decomposition technique that decomposes and converts a signal into a spatial domain that allows frequency and time parameters to be observed simultaneously. Transformations, like the Fourier Transform and the Wigner distribution, deliver this detail as well. However, WT and its time and frequency representation is helpful, if a specific component needs to be studied. ECG's QRS complex, for example, can deliver knowledge related to different events by understanding its time periods. WT was developed to address certain limitations and substitute for the short-time Fourier transform (STFT).

The knowledge generated by discrete wavelet transform (DWT) for both signal analysis and generation with less processing time and computational efficiency. DWT is simpler to apply, and its roots can be traced back to 1976 when Croiser, Esteban, and Galand developed a technique by making discrete representations of time-domain signals for decomposing. The signal is represented by DWT in both the time and frequency domains. This turn quickly became a common method for analyzing biomedical signals like ECGs. By decomposing the signal, DWT converts the ECG signal into various degrees of resolution. This ascended signal can then be divided into wavelets using filters . A study provides information on WT, DWT, and other variants such as cross wavelet transform (XWT), continuous wavelet transform (CWT), and many more [70]. QRS detection techniques, and heuristic-driven approaches based on various transforms were proposed in [49,50]. The DWT-based windowing system proposed by [51,52] achieves the highest sensitivity of 99.95%. With a sensitivity of 99.84%, a delineation algorithm [53] combined with the DWT-based windowing system improved P, QRS, and T wave identification tested on numerous datasets.

Studies [54,55] suggested various windowing algorithms for detecting fiducial points. These methods show 99.9% accuracy and are equivalent to DWT-based windowing approaches. Time domain-based methods (TD) [56,57], mathematical morphology [58,59] with very large-scale-integration (VLSI) [60], Gaussian filter based synthesized mathematical model (SMM) [61], and derivative-based [71] showed the highest of 99.81% sensitivity, which was slightly lower than DWT. The Karhunen–Loeve transform (KLT) and the legendre polynomials-based transform (LPT) used in [72,73] were helpful in detecting the ST-segment morphology, but they had much lesser sensitivity than [70]. Typically, more than one threshold in the wave is expected to increase the accuracy of QRS detection. However, the R-peaks can be identified using phasor transform (PT) with higher accuracy regardless of amplitude.

Detecting low-amplitude QRS complexes in ECG signals is advantageous [74]. The dyadic wavelet transform (DyWT) is a transformed wavelet transform that takes the ECG convolution and produces dyadically time-scaled wavelets of the signal being evaluated. DyWT is similar to the Hamilton–Tompkins (HT) algorithm, but it has few benefits. The authors of [75,76] used multiwavelet transforms and DyWT to identify the QRS complex but achieved lesser accuracy. The derivative-based algorithm [60] detects the QRS complex by comparing the function to a threshold value computed by heuristically discovered laws. Studies [77,78] suggested the best approach with greater sensitivity for detecting QRS complexes using multilead area curve length (ACL)-based DWT and FIR filters with adaptive thresholds. In contrast, [50] detected the ST-segment with the highest sensitivity using wavelet transforms tested on the MITDB dataset.

3.5 Classification techniques

The ECG signal obtained is then handed out to the denoising and feature extraction processes. Finally, the ECG signal assessment is done to classify the ECG signal depending on the observed fiducial points and the issue of concern in the signal. The classification techniques address both conventional and machine learning approaches for ECG classification. The conventional methods used before the classification of ECG signals are threshold-based methods that have been used to classify ECG beats as regular or abnormal [79,80]. In [81,82], an updated adaptive thresholding-based evaluation method was proposed. As defined in [83], DWT represents ECG signal processing using principal component analysis (PCA) and independent component analysis (ICA).

4. Advantages of optimal and modified leads in ECG signal processing

Optimal and modified leads are mostly application specific. Several optimal and modified leads are discussed in this chapter. The recorded outputs of some of the optimal leads are displayed in Fig. 11. As we know, lead II of the standard lead system is optimal and most commonly used to diagnose several arrhythmias and cardiac disease conditions. Fig. 11a shows the ECG waveform of standard lead II that shows dominant R-peak with elusive P-wave. Fig. 11b shows the ECG waveform of modified limb lead II proposed in [44]. This MLL ECG has reduced R-peak [84], and improves the visualization of P-wave by enhancing its peak amplitude. Also, the MLL and atrial lead system [85] which enhances atrial depolarization wave may aid in improved determination of P wave indices [86] for atrial disease identification. Fig. 11c shows the ECG waveform in Lewis lead which aids in diagnosing arrhythmia, such as QRS tachycardia [37] and other related disorders. So, it shows reduced atrial and ventricular amplitude for healthy controls. Fig 11d displays the modified Lewis lead ECG has three times

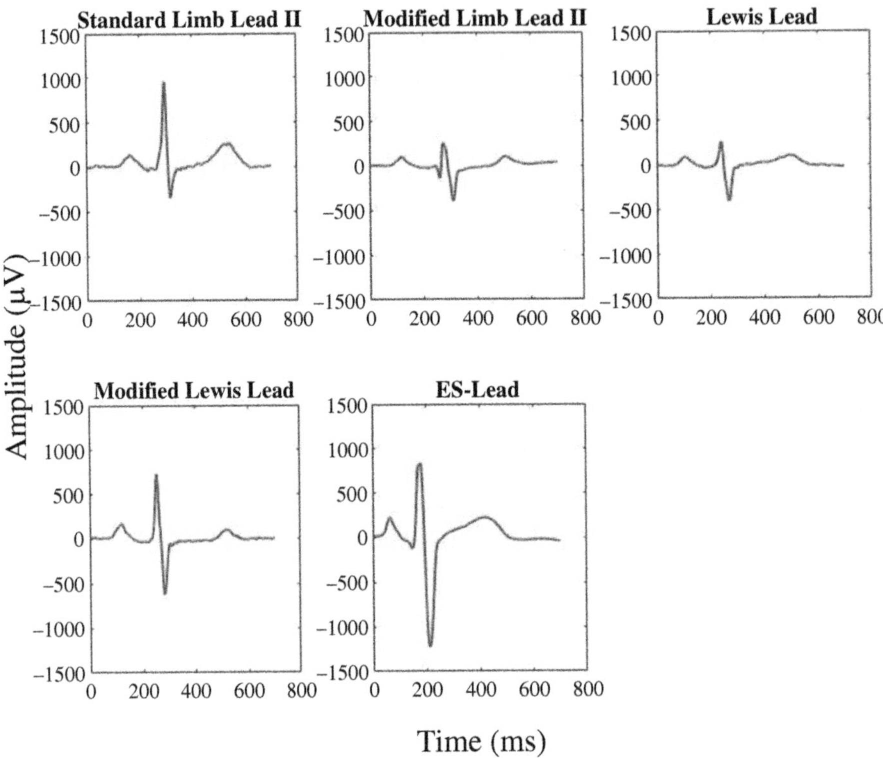

Fig. 11 ECG wave morphology of (a) standard lead-II, (b) MLL-II, (c) Lewis lead, (d) modified Lewis lead, and (e) ES lead.

improved P-wave amplitude than Lewis lead. The wave morphology shows a clear P-wave and QRS complex. ES lead of EASI lead system has prominent P-wave than the standard lead system, which have been proven in different studies [39,47,48]. Fig. 11e shows the wave morphology of ES lead from the EASI lead system.

On applying signal processing techniques like denoising and automatic detection methods, the modified leads show easier detection of wave features than standard leads by reducing computational complexity. For example, the atrial and ventricular depolarization phase analysis in standard lead-II and MLL lead-II were performed using the denoising and fiducial point detection methods. Moving average filter is used to remove the high-frequency noise and to smoothen the signal and an adaptive threshold-based peak detection method is performed. Fig. 12a and b shows the denoised and peak detected ECG waveform of standard lead-II. Fig. 13a and b shows the denoised and peak

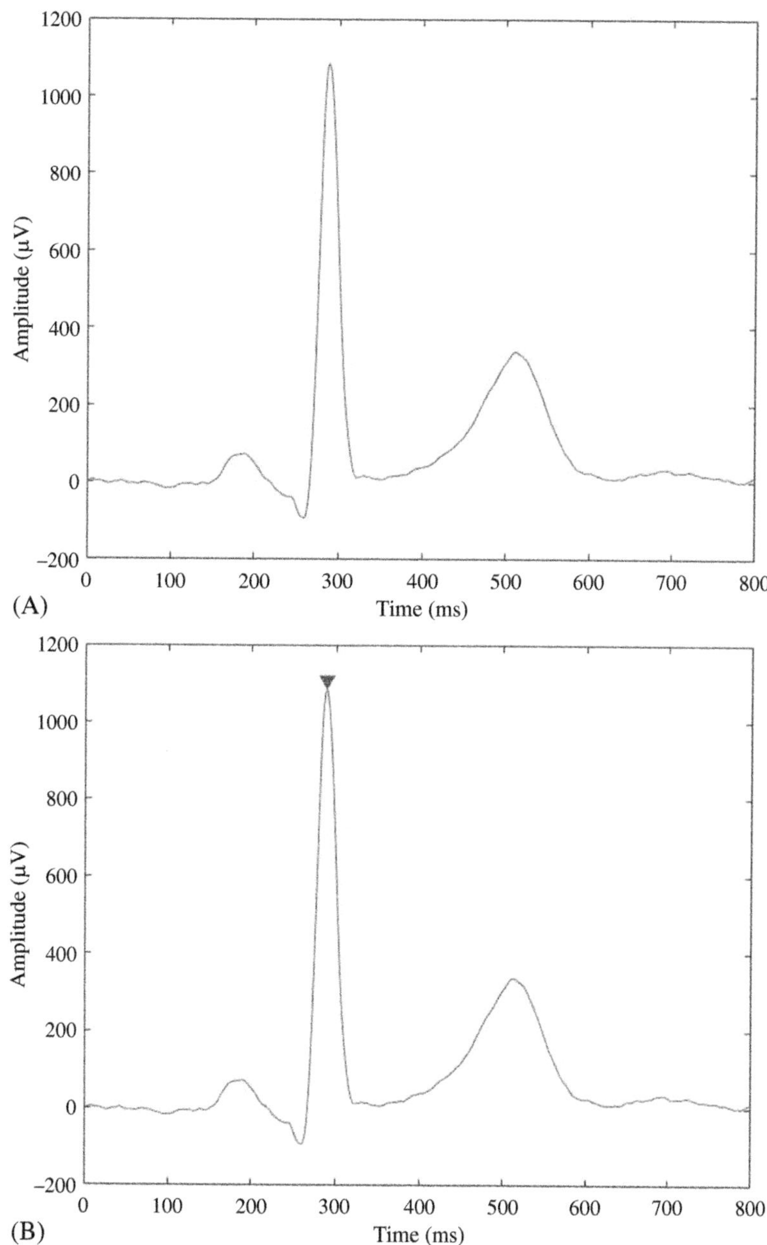

Fig. 12 (a) Denoised standard lead-II single beat ECG. (b) R-peak detected standard lead-II single beat ECG.

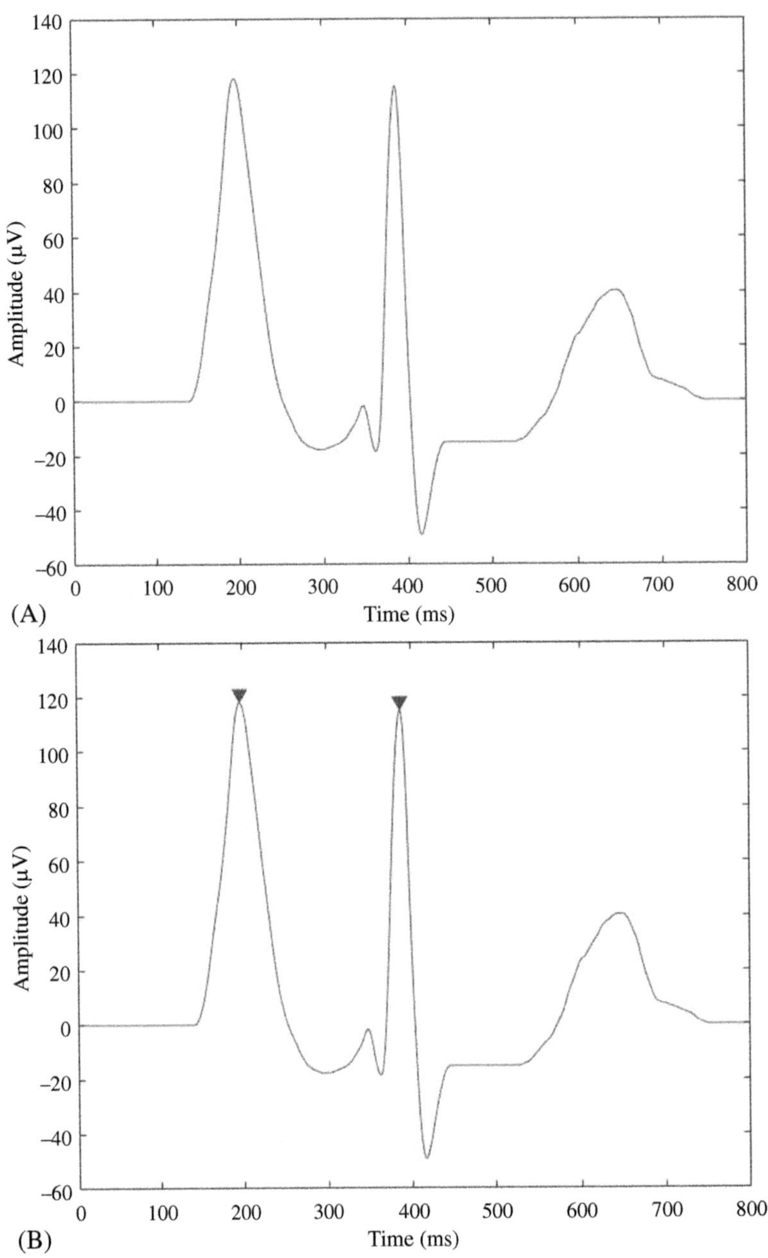

Fig. 13 (a) Denoised MLL-II single beat ECG. (b) P-peak and R-peak detected in MLL-II single beat ECG.

detected ECG waveform of MLL lead-II. It has been noted that only R-peak is detected, and P-wave has a lesser amplitude to recognize and detect. On the other hand, the MLL-II has P-wave greater than $100\,\mu V$ even after signal smoothing and noise removal. Also, it has the advantage of detecting both P and R-peak. Hence, MLL provides an improved atrial diagnostic significance than standard lead-II [87–90].

5. Conclusion

ECG is a valuable tool for diagnosing defects in heart activity. Early detection of cardiac disorders can improve the life expectancy and decrease the mortality and morbidity rate. However, the challenging task is made possible with signal processing and machine learning-based procedures for automatic detection of cardiac disorders. This chapter includes a systematic overview of various signal processing and conventional approaches pre-owned in each level of signal analysis process in ECG, with a focus on ECG analysis approach. Automated and semiautomated methods have been presented to detect R-peaks and QRS complexes and other ECG fiducial points.

Acknowledgments

The authors acknowledge the support from the Ministry of Education, Government of India. The present study was supported by financial grants from the Science and Engineering Research Board (SERB), Department of Science and Technology (DST), Government of India (EEQ/2019/000148).

References

[1] P. Kirchhof, S. Benussi, D. Kotecha, A. Ahlsson, D. Atar, B. Casadei, et al., 2016 ESC guidelines for the management of atrial fibrillation developed in collaboration with EACTS, Eur. Heart J. 37 (38) (2016) 2893–2962.

[2] L. Roten, M. Schilling, A. Häberlin, J. Seiler, N.G. Schwick, J. Fuhrer, et al., Is 7-day event triggered ECG recording equivalent to 7-day Holter ECG recording for atrial fibrillation screening? Heart 98 (8) (2012) 645–649.

[3] M.S. Guillem, A.M. Climent, F. Castells, D. Husser, J. Millet, A. Arya, et al., Non-invasive mapping of human atrial fibrillation, J. Cardiovasc. Electrophysiol. 20 (5) (2009) 507–513.

[4] K. Harris, D. Edwards, J. Mant, How can we best detect atrial fibrillation? J. R. Coll. Physicians. Edinb. 42 (18) (2012) 5–22.

[5] J. Mant, D.A. Fitzmaurice, F.R. Hobbs, S. Jowett, E.T. Murray, R. Holder, et al., Accuracy of diagnosing atrial fibrillation on electrocardiogram by primary care practitioners and interpretative diagnostic software: analysis of data from screening for atrial fibrillation in the elderly (safe) trial, Br. Med. J. 335 (7616) (2007) 1–6.

[6] W. Einthoven, The different forms of the human electrocardiogram and their signification, Lancet 179 (4622) (1912) 853–861.

[7] W. Einthoven, G. Fahr, A. deWaart, Ueber die Richtung und manifeste Groesse der Potentialschwankungen im menschlichen Herzen und ueber den Einfluss der Herzlage auf die Form des Electrokardiogramms, Pfluegers Arch. Ges. Physiol. 150 (6) (1913) 275–315.

[8] F.N. Wilson, F.D. Johnston, F.F. Rosenbaum, P.S. Barker, On Einthoven's triangle, the theory of unipolar electrocardiographic leads, and the interpretation of the precordial electrocardiogram, Am. Heart J. 32 (3) (1946) 277–310.

[9] H.C. Burger, J.B. van Milaan, Heart-vector and leads. Part I, Br. Heart J. 8 (3) (1946) 157–161.

[10] H.C. Burger, J.B. van Milaan, Heart-vector and leads. Part II, Br. Heart J. 9 (3) (1947) 154–160.

[11] H.C. Burger, J.B. van Milaan, Heart-vector and leads. Part III, geometrical representation, Br. Heart J. 10 (4) (1948) 229–233.

[12] R. McFee, F.D. Johnstone, Electrocardiographic leads. I. Introduction, Circulation 8 (4) (1953) 554–568.

[13] R. McFee, F.D. Johnston, Electrocardiographic leads. II. Analysis, Circulation 9 (2) (1954) 255–266.

[14] R. McFee, F.D. Johnston, Electrocardiographic leads. III. Synthesis, Circulation 9 (6) (1954) 868–880.

[15] M.S. Guillem, A. Bollmann, A.M. Climent, D. Husser, J. Millet-Roig, F. Castells, How many leads are necessary for a reliable reconstruction of surface potentials during atrial fibrillation? IEEE Trans. Inf. Technol. Biomed. 13 (3) (2009) 330–340.

[16] M.S. Guillem, A.V. Sahakian, S. Swiryn, Derivation of orthogonal leads from the 12-lead electrocardiogram. Performance of an atrial-based transform for the derivation of P loops, J. Electrocardiol. 41 (1) (2008) 19–25.

[17] M. Haissaguerre, M. Hocini, A.J. Shah, N. Derval, F. Sacher, P. Jais, et al., Noninvasive panoramic mapping of human atrial fibrillation mechanisms: a feasibility report, J. Cardiovasc. Electrophysiol. 24 (6) (2013) 711–717.

[18] M.S. Guillem, A.M. Climent, J. Millet, Á. Arenal, F. Fernández-Avilés, J. Jalife, et al., Noninvasive localization of maximal frequency sites of atrial fibrillation by body surface potential mapping, Circ. Arrhythm. Electrophysiol. 6 (2) (2013) 294–301.

[19] Z. Ihara, V. Jacquemet, J.M. Vesin, A. van Oosterom, Adaption of the standard 12-lead ECG system focusing on atrial electrical activity, Comput. Cardiol. 32 (2005) 203–205.

[20] Z. Ihara, A. van Oosterom, V. Jacquemet, R. Hoekema, Adaptation of the 12-lead electrocardiogram system dedicated to the analysis of atrial fibrillation, J. Electrocardiol. 40 (1) (2007), 68.e1–e8.

[21] D. Husser, M. Strigh, L. Sörnmo, I. Toepffer, H.U. Klein, S.B. Olsson, et al., Electroatriography–time-frequency analysis of atrial fibrillation from modified 12-lead ECG configurations for improved diagnosis and therapy, Med. Hypotheses 68 (3) (2007) 568–573.

[22] W. Wenger, P. Kligfield, Variability of precordial electrode placement during routine electrocardiography, J. Electrocardiol. 29 (3) (1996) 179–184.

[23] A. Bollmann, N. Kanuru, K. McTeague, P. Walter, D. DeLurgio, J. Langberg, Frequency analysis of human atrial fibrillation using the surface electrocardiogram and its response to ibutilide, Am. J. Cardiol. 81 (12) (1998) 1439–1445.

[24] S. Petrutiu, A.V. Sahakian, W.B. Fisher, S. Swiryn, Manifestation of left atrial events in the surface electrocardiogram, Comput. Cardiol. 33 (2006) 1–4.

[25] G.E. Dower, A. Yakush, S.B. Nazzal, R.V. Jutzy, C.E. Ruiz, Deriving the 12-lead electrocardiogram from four (EASI) electrodes, J. Electrocardiol. 21 (Suppl) (1988) S182–S187.

[26] R.L. Lux, C.R. Smith, R.F. Wyatt, J.A. Abildskov, Limited lead selection for estimation of body surface potential maps in electrocardiography, IEEE Trans. Biomed. Eng. 25 (3) (1978) 270–276.

[27] A. Welinder, L. Sornmo, D.Q. Field, C.L. Feldman, J. Petttersson, G.S. Wagner, et al., Comparison of signal quality between EASI and Mason-Likar 12-lead electrocardiograms during physical activity, Am. J. Crit. Care 13 (3) (2004) 228–234.

[28] B.J. Drew, R.M. Califf, M. Funk, E.S. Kaufman, M.W. Krucoff, M.M. Laks, et al., Councils on cardiovascular nursing, clinical cardiology, and cardiovascular disease in the young. Practice standards for electrocardiographic monitoring in hospital settings: an American Heart Association scientific statement from the councils on cardiovascular nursing, clinical cardiology, and cardiovascular disease in the young: endorsed by the international society of computerized electrocardiology and the American Association of critical-care nurses, Circulation 110 (17) (2004) 2721–2746.

[29] B.J. Drew, M.M. Pelter, M.G. Adams, S.F. Wung, 12-Lead ST-segment monitoring vs single-lead maximum ST-segment monitoring for detecting ongoing ischemia in patients with unstable coronary syndromes, Am. J. Crit. Care 7 (5) (1998) 355–363.

[30] P.K. Dash, Electrocardiogram monitoring, Indian J. Anaesth. 46 (4) (2002) 251–260.

[31] P. Johanson, J. Rossberg, M. Dellborg, Continuous ST monitoring: a bedside instrument? A report from the assessment of the safety of a new thrombolytic (ASSENT 2) ST monitoring substudy, Am. Heart J. 142 (1) (2001) 58–62.

[32] O. Pahlm, G.S. Wagner, Proximal placement of limb electrodes: a potential solution for acquiring standard electrocardiogram waveforms from monitoring electrode positions, J. Electrocardiol. 41 (6) (2008) 454 457.

[33] A. Welinder, G.S. Wagner, C. Maynard, O. Pahlm, Differences in QRS axis measurements, classification of inferior myocardial infarction, and noise tolerance for 12-lead electrocardiograms acquired from monitoring electrode positions compared to standard locations, Am. J. Cardiol. 106 (4) (2010) 581–586.

[34] S.P. Nelwan, J.A. Kors, S.H. Meij, J.H. van Bemmel, M.L. Simoons, Reconstruction of the 12-lead electrocardiogram from reduced lead sets, J. Electrocardiol. 37 (1) (2004) 11–18.

[35] S.P. Nelwan, S.W. Crater, C.L. Green, P. Johanson, T.B. van Dam, S.H. Meij, et al., Assessment of derived 12-lead electrocardiograms using general and patient specific reconstruction strategies at rest and during transient myocardial ischemia, Am. J. Cardiol. 94 (12) (2004) 1529–1533.

[36] T. Lewis, Auricular fibrillation, in: Clinical Electrocardiography, fifth ed., Shaw and Sons, London, UK, 1931.

[37] A.L.M. Bakker, G. Nijkerk, B.E. Groenemeijer, R.A. Waalewijin, E.M. Koomen, R.L. Braam, et al., The Lewis lead: making recognition of P waves easy during wide QRS complex tachycardia, Circulation 119 (24) (2009) 592–593.

[38] M. Huemer, H. Meloh, P. Attanasio, A. Wuzler, A.S. Parwani, H. Matsuda, et al., The Lewis lead for detection of ventriculoatrial conduction type, Clin. Cardiol. 39 (2) (2016) 126–131.

[39] A. Petrėnas, V. Marozas, G. Jaruševičius, L. Sörnmo, Modified Lewis ECG lead system for ambulatory monitoring of atrial arrhythmias, J. Electrocardiol. 48 (2) (2015) 157–163.

[40] E. Frank, An accurate, clinically practical system for spatial vectorcardiography, Circulation 13 (5) (1956) 737–749.

[41] D.Q. Feild, C.L. Feldman, B.M. Horacek, Improved EASI coefficients: their derivation, values and performance, J. Electrocardiol. 35 (Suppl. 4) (2002) 23–33.

[42] G. Fontaine, Stimulation studies and epicardial mapping in ventricular tachycardia: study of mechanisms and selection for surgery, in: H.E. Kulbertus (Ed.), Re-Entrant Arrhythmias: Mechanisms and Treatment, University Park Press, Baltimore, 1977, pp. 334–350.

[43] B. Gottschalk, M. Gysel, R. Barbosa-Barros, R.P. De Sousa Rocha, A.R. Pérez-Riera, L. Zhang, et al., The use of Fontaine leads in the diagnosis of arrhythmogenic right ventricular dysplasia, Ann. Noninvasive Electrocardiol. 19 (3) (2014) 279–284.

[44] J. Sivaraman, G. Uma, S. Venkatesan, M. Umapathy, V.E. Dhandapani, A novel approach to determine atrial repolarization in electrocardiograms, J. Electrocardiol. 46 (4) (2013), e1.

[45] J. Sivaraman, G. Uma, S. Venkatesan, M. Umapathy, V.E. Dhandapani, Normal limits of ECG measurements related to atrial activity using a modified limb lead system, Anatol. J. Cardiol. 15 (1) (2015) 2–6.

[46] S. Jayaraman, U. Gandhi, V. Sangareddi, U. Mangalanathan, R.M. Shanmugam, Unmasking of atrial repolarization waves using a simple modified limb lead system, Anatol. J. Cardiol. 15 (8) (2015) 605–610.

[47] A. Kennedy, D.D. Finlay, D. Guldenring, R.R. Bond, J. McLaughlin, Detecting the elusive P-wave: a new ECG lead to improve the recording of atrial activity, IEEE Trans. Biomed. Eng. 63 (2) (2016) 243–249.

[48] A. Kennedy, D.D. Finlay, D. Guldenring, R.R. Bond, D.J. McEneaney, A. Peace, et al., Improved recording of atrial activity by modified bipolar leads derived from the 12-lead electrocardiogram, J. Electrocardiol. 48 (6) (2015) 1017–1021.

[49] N. Fujita, A. Sato, M. Kawarasaki, Performance study of wavelet based ECG analysis for ST-segment detection, in: 2015 38th International Conference on Telecommunications and Signal Processing (TSP), Prague, Czech Republic, July 9–11, 2015, pp. 430–434.

[50] T.T. Khan, N. Sultana, R.B. Reza, R. Mostafa, ECG feature extraction in temporal domain and detection of various heart conditions, in: 2015 International Conference on Electrical Engineering and Information Communication Technology (ICEEICT), Savar, Bangladesh, May 21–23, 2015, pp. 1–6.

[51] Z. Zidelmal, A. Amirou, M. Adnane, A. Belouchrani, QRS detection based on wavelet coefficients, Comput. Methods Prog. Biomed. 107 (3) (2012) 490–496.

[52] F.A. Afsar, M. Arif, J. Yang, Detection of ST segment deviation episodes in ECG using KLT with an ensemble neural classifier, Physiol. Meas. 29 (7) (2008) 747–760.

[53] A. Ghaffari, M.R. Homaeinezhad, M. Akraminia, M. Atarod, M. Daevaeiha, A robust wavelet-based multi-lead electrocardiogram delineation algorithm, Med. Eng. Phys. 31 (10) (2009) 1219–1227.

[54] A.E. Curtin, K.V. Burns, A.J. Bank, T.I. Netoff, QRS complex detection and measurement algorithms for multichannel ECGs in cardiac resynchronization therapy patients, IEEE J. Transl. Eng. Health Med. 6 (2018) 1–11.

[55] M. Xu, S. Wei, X. Qin, Y. Zhang, C. Liu, Rule-based method for morphological classification of ST segment in ECG signals, J. Med. Biol. Eng. 35 (6) (2015) 816–823.

[56] N. Uchaipichat, C. Thanawattano, A. Buakhamsri, The development of ST-episode detection in Holter monitoring for myocardial ischemia, Proc. Comput. Sci. 86 (2016) 188–191.

[57] E.B. Mazomenos, T. Chen, A. Acharyya, A. Bhattacharya, J. Rosengarten, K. Maharatna, A time-domain morphology and gradient based algorithm for ECG feature extraction, in: 2012 IEEE International Conference on Industrial Technology, Athens, Greece, March 19–21, 2012, pp. 117–122.

[58] F. Zhang, Y. Lian, QRS detection based on multiscale mathematical morphology for wearable ECG devices in body area networks, IEEE Trans. Biomed. Circuits Syst. 3 (4) (2009) 220–228.

[59] J.L. Hu, S.D. Bao, An approach to QRS complex detection based on multiscale mathematical morphology, in: 2010 3rd International Conference on Biomedical Engineering and Informatics, Yantai, China, October 16–18, 2010, pp. 725–729.

[60] C.F. Zhang, T.W. Bae, VLSI friendly ECG QRS complex detector for body sensor networks, IEEE J. Emerg. Sel. Topics Circuits Syst. 2 (1) (2012) 52–59.

[61] J.P. do Vale Madeiro, J.A.L. Marques, T. Han, R.C. Pedrosa, Evaluation of mathematical models for QRS feature extraction and QRS morphology classification in ECG signals, Measurement 156 (2020), 107580.

[62] Y. Shahriari, R. Fidler, M.M. Pelter, Y. Bai, A. Villaroman, X. Hu, Electrocardiogram signal quality assessment based on structural image similarity metric, IEEE Trans. Biomed. Eng. 65 (4) (2018) 745–753.

[63] C. Lastre-Dominguez, Y.S. Shmaliy, O. Ibarra-Manzano, M. Vazquez-Olguin, Denoising and features extraction of ECG signals in state space using unbiased FIR smoothing, IEEE Access 7 (2019) 152166–152178.

[64] N. Razzaq, S.A.A. Sheikh, M. Salman, T. Zaidi, An intelligent adaptive filter for elimination of power line interference from high resolution electrocardiogram, IEEE Access 4 (2016) 1676–1688.

[65] F. Shirbani, S.K. Setarehdan, ECG power line interference removal using combination of FFT and adaptive non-linear noise estimator, in: 2013 21st Iranian Conference on Electrical Engineering (ICEE), Mashhad, Iran, May 14–16, 2013, pp. 1–5.

[66] G.S. Furno, W.J. Tompkins, A learning filter for removing noise interference, IEEE Trans. Biomed. Eng. 30 (4) (1983) 234–235.

[67] S. Al-Khammasi, K.A.I. Aboalayon, M. Daneshzand, M. Faezipour, M. Faezipour, Hardware-based FIR filter implementations for ECG signal denoising: A monitoring framework from industrial electronics perspective, in: 2016 Annual Connecticut Conference on Industrial Electronics, Technology & Automation (CT-IETA), Bridgeport, CT, USA, October 14–15, 2016, pp. 1–6.

[68] M. Faezipour, T.M. Tiwari, A. Saeed, M. Nourani, L.S. Tamil, Wavelet-based denoising and beat detection of ECG signal, in: 2009 IEEE/NIH Life Science Systems and Applications Workshop, Bethesda, MD, USA, April 9–10, 2009, pp. 100–103.

[69] H.T. Chiang, Y.Y. Hsieh, S.W. Fu, K.H. Hung, Y. Tsao, S.Y. Chien, Noise reduction in ECG signals using fully convolutional denoising autoencoders, IEEE Access 7 (2019) 60806–60813.

[70] A.N. Akansu, P.A. Haddad, R.A. Haddad, P.R. Haddad, Multiresolution signal decomposition, in: Transforms, Subbands, and Wavelets, Academic, New Jersey Institute of Technology, Newark, NJ, 2001.

[71] D. Sadhukhan, M. Mitra, R-peak detection algorithm for ECG using double difference and RR interval processing, Proc. Technol. 4 (2012) 873–877.

[72] M. Amon, F. Jager, Electrocardiogram ST-segment morphology delineation method using orthogonal transformations, PLoS One 11 (2) (2016), e0148814.

[73] A. Smrdel, F. Jager, Automated detection of transient ST-segment episodes in 24h electrocardiograms, Med. Biol. Eng. Comput. 42 (3) (2004) 303–311.

[74] A. Martínez, R. Alcaraz, J.J. Rieta, Application of the phasor transform for automatic delineation of single-lead ECG fiducial points, Physiol. Meas. 31 (11) (2010) 1467–1485.

[75] R. Gautam, A.K. Sharma, Detection of QRS complexes of ECG recording based on wavelet transform using Matlab, Int. J. Eng. Sci. Technol. 2 (7) (2010) 3038–3044.

[76] B. Subramanian, ECG signal classification and parameter estimation using multiwavelet transform, Biomed. Res. 28 (7) (2017) 3187–3193.

[77] A. Ghaffari, M.R. Homaeinezhad, M.M. Daevaeiha, High resolution ambulatory holter ECG events detection-delineation via modified multi-lead wavelet-based features analysis: detection and quantification of heart rate turbulence, Expert Syst. Appl. 38 (5) (2011) 5299–5310.

[78] D.B. Saadi, G. Tanev, M. Flintrup, A. Osmanagic, K. Egstrup, K. Hoppe, et al., Automatic real-time embedded QRS complex detection for a novel patch-type electrocardiogram recorder, IEEE J. Transl. Eng. Health Med. 3 (2015) 1–12.

[79] S. Banerjee, M. Mitra, Application of cross wavelet transform for ECG pattern analysis and classification, IEEE Trans. Instrum. Meas. 63 (2) (2014) 326–333.

[80] A. Kumar, M. Singh, Ischemia detection using isoelectric energy function, Comput. Biol. Med. 68 (2016) 76–83.

[81] M. Faezipour, A. Saeed, S.C. Bulusu, M. Nourani, H. Minn, L. Tamil, A patient-adaptive profiling scheme for ECG beat classification, IEEE Trans. Inf. Technol. Biomed. 14 (5) (2010) 1153–1165.

[82] J. Pan, W.J. Tompkins, A real-time QRS detection algorithm, IEEE Trans. Biomed. Eng. 32 (3) (1985) 230–236.

[83] R.J. Martis, U.R. Acharya, L.C. Min, ECG beat classification using PCA, LDA, ICA and discrete wavelet transform, Biomed. Signal Process. Control 8 (5) (2013) 437–448.

[84] J. Sivaraman, G. Uma, M. Umapathy, A modified chest leads for minimization of ventricular activity in electrocardiograms, in: 2012 International Conference on Biomedical Engineering (ICoBE), Penang, Malaysia, February 27–28, 2012, pp. 79–82.

[85] N.P. Venkatesh, A. Bhardwaj, J. Sivaraman, B. Dhananjay, A new lead system for improved recording of P-wave amplitude and its significance with existing optimal leads, in: 2021 Seventh International Conference on Bio Signals, Images, and Instrumentation (ICBSII), Chennai, India, March 25–27, 2021, pp. 1–5.

[86] A. Bhardwaj, J. Sivaraman, Study of P wave indices in sinus rhythm and tachycardia, in: 2021 Seventh International Conference on Bio Signals, Images, and Instrumentation (ICBSII), Chennai, India, March 25–27, 2021, pp. 1–5.

[87] J. Sivaraman, G. Uma, S. Venkatesan, M. Umapathy, N. Keshavkumar, A study on atrial ta wave morphology in healthy subjects: an approach using P-wave signal-averaging method, J. Med. Imaging Health Inform. 4 (5) (2014) 1–6.

[88] R. John, J. Sivaraman, Effects of sinus rhythm on atrial ECG components using a modified limb lead system, in: 2017 4th International Conference on Signal Processing, Computing and Control (ISPCC), Solan, India, September 21–23, 2017, pp. 527–530.

[89] A. Jyothsana, B. Arya, J. Sivaraman, Stability analysis on the effects of heart rate variability and premature activation of atrial ECG dynamics using ARMAX model, Phys. Eng. Sci. Med. 43 (4) (2020) 1361–1370.

[90] J. Sivaraman, G. Uma, P. Langley, M. Umapathy, S. Venkatesan, G. Palanikumar, A study on stability analysis of atrial repolarization variability using ARX model in sinus rhythm and atrial tachycardia ECGs, Comput. Methods Prog. Biomed. 137 (2016) 341–351.

13

Adaptive rate EEG processing and machine learning-based efficient recognition of epilepsy

Saeed Mian Qaisar[a,b]

[a]*Electrical and Computer Engineering Department, Effat University, Jeddah, Saudi Arabia.* [b]*Communication and Signal Processing Lab, Energy and Technology Research Center, Effat University, Jeddah, Saudi Arabia*

1. Introduction

Mobile healthcare is a trend and technology that is still developing. As a result, a lot of progress is being made in the mobile device industry, including smart sensors and smartphones. Wearable sensors have an effect on smart sensor data used to detect biomedical signals. Clinically connected wearables involved stethoscopes, blood pressure sensors, electrocardiogram (ECG) recorders, and portable EEG systems. Wearable design firms have developed groundbreaking instruments and methods for capturing and analyzing body signals. As a result, biomedical signals obtained from wearable sensors allow real-time mobile monitoring of patients with chronic diseases. Furthermore, the majority of these biomedical signs have therapeutic effects in terms of illness or condition management [1].

The technological advancements in sensors development have evolved the domain of wearable biomedical gadgets. Most of modern wearable biomedical implants are kept wireless and are based on the concepts of wireless sensing nodes and internet of things. They permit to attain a remote and mobile healthcare tracking. This approach is particularly beneficial for senior citizens. This improvement in sensors domain with advancement in signal processing and analysis side has revolutionized the modern healthcare system. Modern gadgets and tools are frequently deployed to monitor, facilitate and support the medical practitioners [2,3]. In this sense, several fields and domains are evolving such as medicated fabrics and wears which have built in wearable

Advanced Methods in Biomedical Signal Processing and Analysis. https://doi.org/10.1016/B978-0-323-85955-4.00013-2
Copyright © 2023 Elsevier Inc. All rights reserved.

wireless sensors for continuous health monitoring of patients with serious illness [1].

The valuable advancements in surgical devices and pharmaceutical systems have recently been made to meet the demands of modern clinical diagnosis and treatment. In fact, the advanced medical equipment in healthcare centers provides rapid and accurate analysis. The elderly patients, including those with chronic disorders, need constant real-time patient surveillance. Patient tracking and study of captured biomedical signals rely heavily on cloud-based electronic healthcare monitoring devices. People's health data is regularly collected by a real-time patient management framework, and is used to investigate the risk involved in sensitive health situations. Sensor-based electronic patient monitoring equipment has risen to a new level of popularity in personalized healthcare frameworks. It is particularly developed in recent years as a result of the connectivity of cloud servers and sensing devices via advancements in internet of things technology [4]. The use of a cell phone's networks, Bluetooth technologies, the global positioning system are all part of mobile health [5].

Epilepsy is one of the major cerebral diseases. According to statistical data, presented in [6], globally millions of people are affected by epilepsy. Brief electrical disruptions in the cerebral system generate epileptic seizures. It disconnects certain neurons from the cerebral network and can cause damage. This may be the result of partial or generalized seizures [7]. Patients with untreated epilepsy may suffer serious consequences [8]. At least 20% of all epilepsy patients had seizures as a result of the medication's ineffectiveness [8]. Many studies have been inspired by this to develop novel methods of epileptic seizure control, such as medicine injection and patient alert [9]. This form of seizure management provides patients with early alarms and prevents them from taking too much medicine [9]. As a result, accurate and predictive seizure detection will improve not just the effectiveness of diagnosis but also the patients' quality of life.

Examining EEG signs can help identify epileptic symptoms [10]. In this sense, various wireless EEG implants have been launched [11,12]. Nonetheless, detecting EEG-based seizures is difficult. Since EEG signals are derived from several scalp electrodes, it necessitates a significant amount of data to address [13]. The EEG signal is also affected by noise and physiological artifacts. It lowers recognition and diagnostic efficiency [14–16]. Fig. 1 depicts the concept of automatic epileptic seizure categorization schemes. The incoming EEG signals are first digitized using suitable analog to digital converters, as can be seen in diagram. These signals are then fragmented and the noise is reduced using an appropriate denoising process. After that, classifiable features are derived and passed

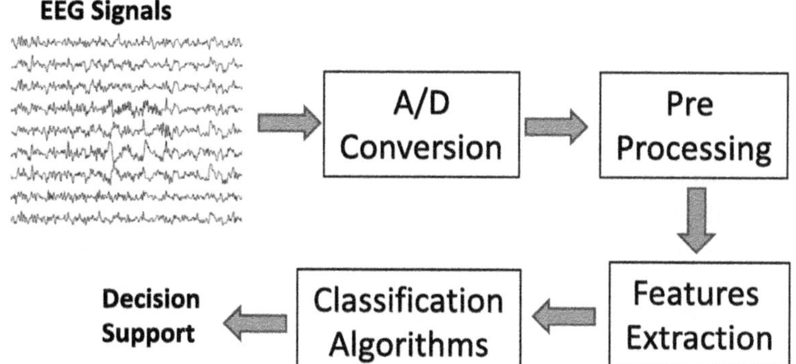

Fig. 1 The block diagram of a typical automated epileptic seizure classification system.

on to the classification module. The learned classifier is used to categorize the incoming sample, and a decision is taken and conveyed to the health server.

Kalman filtering [17], orthogonal wavelet transformation, adaptive filters [18,19] and principal component analysis [20] are frequently used preprocessing techniques which are proposed in the literature. After preprocessing stage the conditioned signal is analyzed by robust methods. Certain famous methods are wavelet-based decomposition, short time Fourier transformation and auto regression [15,21–28].

The discriminative features mined during the features extraction stage are used to carry out the automatic diagnosis of epileptic seizures. For the classification of EEG signals, various machine learning algorithms such as neural networks, support vector machines (SVMs), and random forest have been studied in the literature [21–28].

The early detection of epileptic seizures will lead to a stable diagnosis of epilepsy. For successful healthcare, precise and timely reporting to doctors is critical. In this sense, mobile healthcare services have the potential to expand chronic disease management [15,29,30]. Epileptic patients need close monitoring. In this case, wearable EEG implants are the most effective instruments [15,29,30]. They register and process the EEG signals and send information about the patient's condition to the healthcare server. In case of urgency an alarming notification is sent to the healthcare emergency ward [30].

The EEG encoding plays a key role in cloud-based mobile healthcare frameworks [15,29,30]. This lowers the system's cost, usage, and processing latency while also improving its efficiency. It's crucial to efficiently reduce the dimension of multichannel EEG signals while keeping the diagnostic details [15,29–34].

The conventional EEG processing methods are based on uniform fix rate sampling process [21–28]. Regardless of the incoming

EEG signal variations, the device runs at a constant tempo. As a result, a massive amount of redundant samples are collected, analyzed, and maintained [14–16,35]. The use of event-driven analog to digital converters [36–39] will solve these limitations. They allow the acquisition and processing activities to be adjusted in response to incoming signal time variations. In comparison to traditional methods, this gives the proposed solution a significant numerical advantage [36–38].

In the framework of cloud-based mobile healthcare, this chapter focuses on the advancement of successful automatic epileptic seizure detection. An effective method is proposed which attains a precise epileptic seizure automatic identification by compressing data in real time and effectively manipulating and distributing it. It is accomplished by combining event-driven acquisition, adaptive rate processing and interpretation, statistical attribute extraction from subbands and machine learning techniques.

2. The electroencephalogram (EEG) for healthcare

In the world of medicine, there was a need for brain scans. It inspired medical doctors to learn more about how brains function from the perspective of epilepsy (an abnormality of electrical brain activity). The first attempt was made in 1895 by physicist Wilhelm Roentgen, who used clinical X-ray equipment. Ionizing radiation is used to create images of the body in clinical X-ray. However, X-ray can be harmful to one's health; additionally, the brain tissues are not visible on X-ray. Electroencephalography and magnetoencephalography, for example, have been proposed as alternatives to X-ray in this framework.

The electrical activity of the cerebral system could be monitored in a noninvasive manner by using the EEG. The first EEG recording machine was invented by Hans Berger. He suggested that brain impulses change based on the brain's functioning state. A variety of electrodes are placed in various locations on the scalp during the EEG acquisition procedure. An amplifier connects each electrode to an EEG recording unit. Finally, for visualization purpose the EEG signals are processed via computer and also displayed on a monitor screen which is connected with computer. These visuals permit the medical practitioners to analyze the cerebral condition of the concerned patient by visualizing the displayed EEG graphs. EEG is widely used in social psychology, cognitive science, psychiatry, and psycho physiological analysis for a variety of reasons. Since EEG signals provide a large volume of data, computer-assisted EEG signal analysis should be created for a deeper understanding of mental states. An electrode cap is mounted on the scalp to collect EEG signals. EEG wave signals for various brain states are analyzed and recognized by computers [40].

The EEG is recorder by deploying particular category of electrodes on the intended patient head. It could be in the form of a cap or helmet. These electrodes are commonly placed on the scalp of the head via a headset; however, there are other methods in which can be partially or fully invasive through surgery implants of such electrodes inside the human skull. Other tests are less common than the EEG because of their high sensitivity to the ambient environment, lack of portability, bulkiness in size, and high cost. Additionally, EEG allows to explore the electrical activity of brain directly. It permits to rapidly diagnose any abnormalities in the functionality of the cerebral system. This feature is not available in the blood flow estimation-based techniques. Positron emission tomography measures metabolic activities. In comparison to an EEG-based approach, these are tacit facts about the electrical stimulation of the brain which can result in a slower detection of improvements in neuronal activity of the brain.

According to [41], the valuable spectral content of the EEG signal exists between 0.5 and up to 60 Hz. As a function of the spectral band, the signal is classified as Delta [0.5, 4] Hz, Theta [4, 8] Hz, Alpha [8, 13] Hz, Beta [13, 30] Hz, and Gamma [30, 60]. Fig. 2 is a visual representation of the categorized waves.

Epileptic systems are defined according to the ability of the system to detect, extract, and translate pulses produced by the cerebral system, as well as it is a system that acts on the EEG waveforms [41].

An important thing to note about how epileptic systems work is that the subject using the system must go through a training period, where the system "trains" to detect and analyze the signals in order to operate correctly and more efficiently [41].

There are two main types of collecting data for epileptic systems: invasive and noninvasive. The noninvasive approach involves placing sensors on the scalp of the subject and the brain pulses are collected through them. This is called an electroencephalograph (EEG). This technique follows specific protocols, where these sensors are placed intelligently in particular areas of the brain according to the data the researchers need to acquire. This technique is also reasonably inexpensive and safe; however, because the pulses are passing through the skull they can be attenuated, and a number of factors add noise to them, which means that some data might be compromised [41].

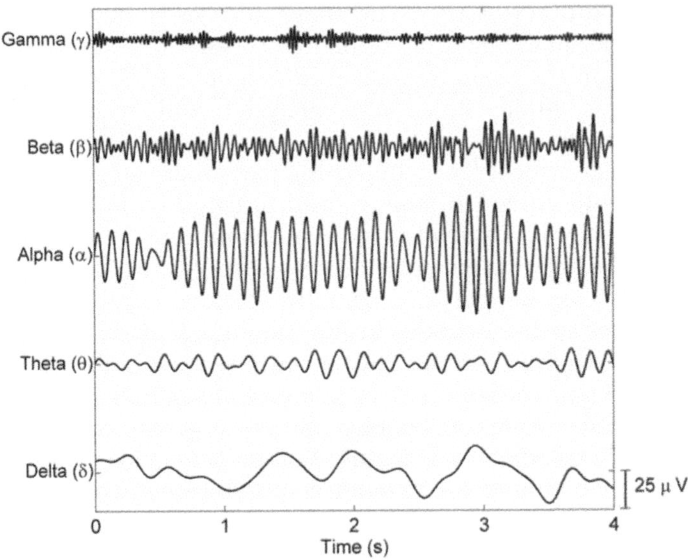

Fig. 2 Example of EEG signals.

The invasive process, on the other hand, involves inserting electrodes directly in brain tissue to read brain pulses. This technique might result in cleaner pulses (less noise) but is more dangerous and ethically ambiguous. In addition, since surgery is needed to accomplish this technique of data acquisition, costs are higher [41]. To contend with these trade-offs, researchers must balance the benefits and drawbacks of each approach against one another.

The motivation behind this investigation is to enable epileptic systems to function in real-time. It will allow providing adequate assistance to intended patients in a timely manner.

From the perspective of essential signal evaluation, EEG signal analysis is significant because it can be used to identify and diagnose a variety of cerebral diseases. In reality, for healthy people who want to monitor their mental activity and stress levels, a wearable helmet could be used [1,3]. Cloud-based healthcare systems, which combine mobile devices, massive computing ability, and resource scalability, are critical in the growth of mobile health services. A cloud-based mobile healthcare framework allows for real-time analysis of sensor data generated by various patients in multiple regions [42]. A paradigm based on wireless sensor networks, cell phones, and cloud computing is proposed to achieve these goals. This architecture is made up of two interconnected modules: a front-end module and a back-end module. The front-end module collects EEG signals from the patient's scalp using body sensors and sends the information to the cloud [43].

Neurological disease control is the most difficult in terms of brain wave characteristics. Since the electrodes used to collect brain impulses with many touch points generate a large volume of data. Moreover, the analysis must be done for a long period and in an uninterrupted fashion. In [44]. The authors created a handheld EEG processing solution that can aid in detecting drowsy driving caused by fatigue in order to prevent possible traffic accidents. In [45] authors suggested an approach for helping drivers. It employs a noninvasive wireless EEG sensor with front-end processor and facilitate driver in making augmented decisions. In Askamp and van Putten [46], authors have devised an EEG automated system for epileptic seizure identification. In [47], a mobile EEG signals processing solution is devised by authors. It uses sensors with a smartphone-based application for monitoring the cerebral system functioning. In Stopczynski et al. [48], a smartphone and smart wireless sensors-based EEG signal processing solution is proposed. It monitors the activity of cerebral system of intended patients. In [43], authors suggested a cloud computing and smartphone-based automatic processing system for EEG signals. The EEG signals recording and preprocessing is carried out in the cell phone. Onward, the cell phone communicates with the cloud service using the necessary protocols. The data management, feature mining, machine learning–based categorization are all part of the cloud computing-based application. In Ranganathan et al. [49], a comprehensive review of EEG processing-based epilepsy detection methods is presented. In [50], authors suggested an appealing and beneficial approach of biomedical signal analysis-based health monitoring infrastructure. It is suitable for continuous monitoring of patients with critical diseases. They also introduced a user interface scheme, which is critical for the consistency and acceptability of the monitoring mechanism, as well as taking advantage of the proposed remote monitoring system's benefits. They also introduced a scenario that could be used to track epileptic seizures. A control mechanism may be programmed to warn the patient in advance about a potential seizure attack. It can allow the patient to avoid potentially hazardous environments such as swimming pools and streets while still taking a preventative medication. Furthermore, this allows them to take as less medication as possible rather than doing it on a regular basis [51]. Researchers have developed a system for epileptic treatment that allows for constant patient surveillance, the collection of EEG recordings, the detection of epileptic cases, and the storage of data for analysis by a clinician. The research goal is to contribute in the evolution mobile healthcare systems. It can be done by developing the smart sensing technologies and building a computing engine that can automatically predict epileptic seizures by processing the EEG signals, received from the headset. This framework is beneficial for long-term mobile tracking of the concerned epileptic patients [52]. The framework, on the other hand, would not be dependent on spike identification, which is not always indicative of an impending seizure [53].

3. Signal acquisition, preprocessing, and features extraction

Many kinds of artifacts, such as movement of eyes, arms, and other muscles with interfering noises, can be found in biomedical signals, and these artifacts can be removed and treated by variety of techniques. Several methods could be used to clear these artifacts. Many artifacts and noise can be filtered out by the hardware filters used in biomedical equipment [54]. To discern a variety of patient's health conditions and patterns, biomedical signals are acquired and analyzed. Preprocessing, attributes mining, and selection of discriminative features and automated machine learning-based categorization are the three major elements of biomedical signal analysis and processing. A measure of preprocessing stage performance is carried out in terms of signal-to-noise ratio (SNR). With a lower SNR, biomedical signal characteristics are suppressed in the remainder of the signal, making similar patterns difficult to detect. However, a higher SNR makes differentiation easier. By transforming signals, researchers use a variety of approaches to remove or at least minimize unnecessary signal components. These techniques can help to improve the SNR [55].

The idea of proposed scheme is represented with the aid of block diagram seen in Fig. 3. The suggested structure as shown in Fig. 3 has a front-end processing module that includes stages for preconditioning, time-frequency analysis, and function extraction. Onward the mined discriminative features are conveyed toward the cloud where the classification process is carried out for automated diagnosis of epileptic seizure.

3.1 Dataset

The EEG recordings in the Neurology & Sleep Centre, Hauz Khas dataset, were obtained using the uniform 10–20-electrode positioning scheme [56]. The data is collected with 12-bit resolution ADCs and a 200 Hz sampling rate. The records in question are

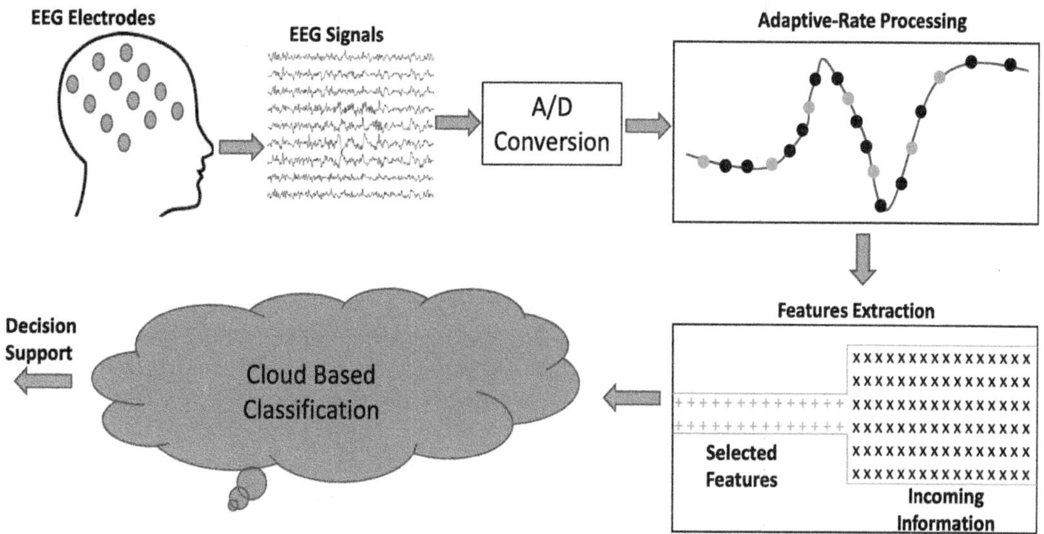

Fig. 3 The proposed EEG processing framework.

divided into 5.12-s fragments, each with 1024 measurements. Each fragment is regarded as a separate instance. A total of 150 instants are taken into account. These instants belong to one of the three expected classes: ictal, interictal, and preictal.

3.2 Reconstruction

Analog signals are translated to digital signals, A/D conversion, in a variety of applications using sampling and quantization operations. The circuit is named as analog to digital converter (ADC) [37]. After that, use digital signal processors to process the digital signals. Following that, the interpreted signals are converted from digital to analog using DACs.

Using Fourier analysis, the sampling process can be described from a frequency domain perspective, analyze its causes, and discuss the reconstruction phenomenon [37]. Let $x_a(t)$ be an analog signal. Its spectral representation is achievable by using Eq. (1):

$$x_a(j\Omega) \triangleq \int_{-\infty}^{\infty} x_a(t)e^{-j\Omega t}\,dt \tag{1}$$

Ω is the frequency. Inverse of Eq. (1) inverse is given by Eq. (2).

$$x_a(t) = \frac{1}{2\pi} \int_{-\infty}^{\infty} x_a(j\Omega)e^{j\Omega t}\,d\Omega \tag{2}$$

To find (n) we have to sample $x_a(t)$ at sampling interval Ts. The process can be described as: $x(n) \triangleq x_a(nT_s)$. Let $X(e^{jw_n})$ is the frequency domain transformed version of $x(n)$. According to [57] the aliasing formula is:

$$X\left(e^{j\omega}\right) = \frac{1}{T_s} \sum_{t=-\infty}^{\infty} x_a\left[j\left(\frac{\omega}{T_s} - \frac{2\pi}{T_s}l\right)\right] \tag{3}$$

$$\omega = \Omega T.$$

Therefore, the discrete signal could an aliased version of the identical analog signal because there will be overlap if the higher frequencies are not properly sampled, and they overlap with lower frequencies. The phenomenon is further described with the help of Fig. 4.

The used EEG dataset waveforms are up-sampled with a factor of 100 to evaluate the event-driven analog to digital converter module. A specifically designed array of cascaded cubic-spline interpolators is used for up-sampling [57].

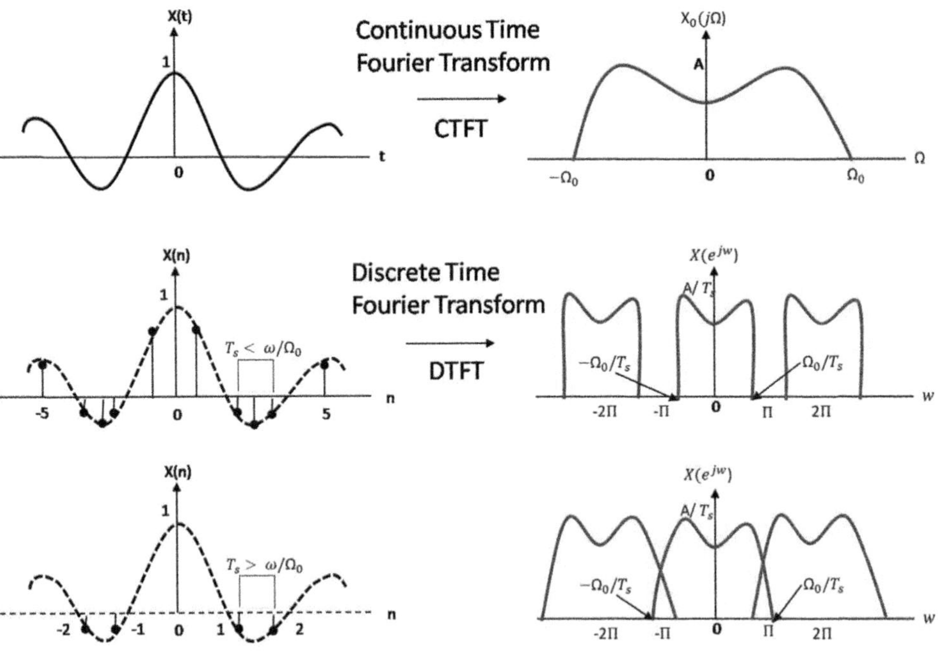

Fig. 4 The impact of sampling in the time and frequency domains.

3.3   Adaptive rate acquisition

The reconstructed signal $x(t)$ is conveyed to EDADC. The existing EEG processing systems are founded on the basis of conventional ADCs. On the other hand, the designed EEG However, the acquisition process is time-varying and adjustable in accordance with the changes in the incoming signal [41]. This process is depicted in Figs. 5–7.

The concept behind the event-driven sampling is only to obtain the sample if the reconstructed input signal $x(t)$ intersects with one of the thresholds. These thresholds are tactfully placed alongside the amplitude dynamics, $\Delta x(t)$, of the incoming EEG signals. To keep the quantum, q, unique, the step among consecutive thresholds is kept constant. It renders a uniform distribution schemes of thresholds [39]. For clarification of the difference between the acquisition principles of ADCs and EDADCs, the following example is considered.

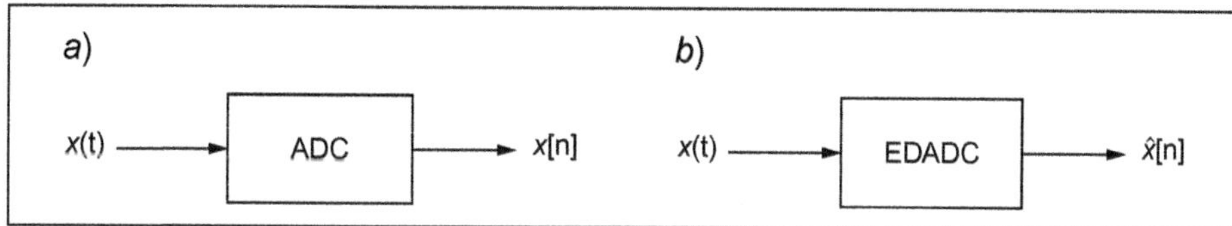

Fig. 5 ADC (A) and EDADC (B).

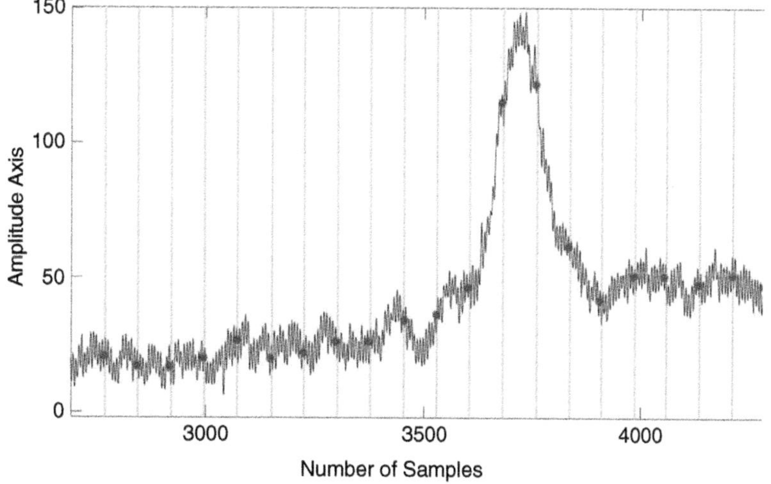

Fig. 6 The acquisition principle of ADC.

In the case of ADC samples are taken at constant intervals. Let us consider the EEG signal, $x(t)$, shown in Fig. 6. The acquisition process is performed at a steady rate. In this way, not many samples are recorded around the valuable peak of the incoming signal. On the other hand, several unwanted and redundant samples are gathered around the baseline of incoming signal. The red dots in Fig. 6 represent the samples taken at regular time intervals.

In the case of EDADC, samples are not taken at constant intervals. Let us consider the EEG signal, $x(t)$, shown in Fig. 7. An EDADC is used, and the samples are taken only where there is an activity in the signal. This allows for more efficient sampling such that the samples represent the valuable information. This technique is better than time-invariant ADC because it requires a lower number of samples and does a better job of getting samples that contain data. The red dots in Fig. 7 represent the samples taken at the peak of activity in the signal.

The variation in the count of samples, collected from the incoming signal by utilizing the conventional ADC and the EDADC is evident from Figs. 6 and 7. For the classical ADC to be able to extract as much of the vital information, acquired by the EDADC, the sampling frequency must be multiple times higher than the one shown in Fig. 6.

The majority of existing EEG processing methods are developed by using the concept fix rate uniform sampling [15]. Regardless of the types of translation in the input signal, the system's computing load and processing operation remain constant. As a result, they are limited, particularly while processing the nonstationary and intermittent biomedical signals such as ECG. They collect and store a large amount of duplicate information. It reaffirms the value of adapting the device acquisition and processing

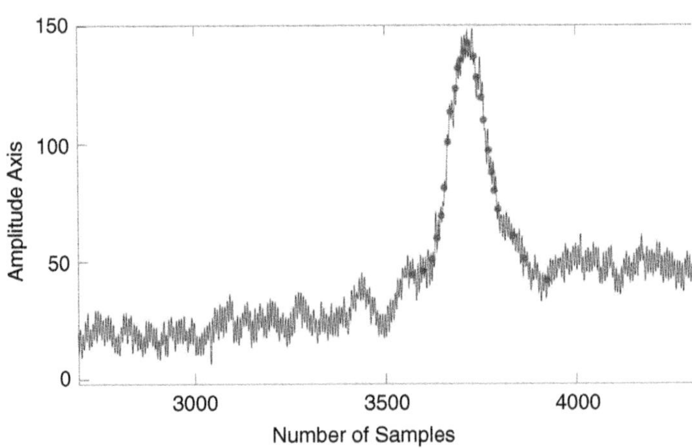

Fig. 7 The acquisition principle of EDADC.

rate in response to temporal fluctuations in the incoming signal. It ensures that the proposed approach has a significant computational advantage over traditional methods [58,59].

In this research, the analog conditioned EEG signals, coming from electrodes, are recorded by using appropriate Event Driven A/D converters (EDADC). The conventional uniform sampling and processing theory governs the functionality of majority of existing ADCs. Therefore, in conventional schemes, regardless of its transient nature, the signal is acquired at a steady rate, i.e., without taking advantage of signal local variations [57]. As a result, these fix rate solutions can be inefficient, particularly when dealing with random biomedical signals. In [60], the EDADCs are used to address this flaw. They use a method called nonuniform threshold crossing sampling. The sampling operation's density is modified in response to the incoming signal's temporal variations [61]. The approach is favorable in case of intermittent EEG like signals and can allow to attain a significant compression and processing effectiveness.

3.4 Adaptive rate segmentation

The data obtained from EDADC does not have an equal distance between them in time. So, using classical techniques cannot be used to process or analyze the data [32,35,58]. The windowing is an essential operation, and it is required for the limited time data acquisition to fulfill the practical system implementation specifications [57]. To obtain the windowed version of a sampled signal x_n, the picked N sample segment must be centered on τ, as given by following equation:

$$xw_n = \sum_{n=\tau+\frac{L}{2}}^{\tau+\frac{L}{2}} x_n.w_{n-\tau} \tag{4}$$

xw_n is the windowed version of x_n, L is the length in seconds, τ is the central time of w_n, F_S is the sampling frequency, N can be calculated by:

$$N = LxF_S \tag{5}$$

Performing digital signal processing and analysis required a finite set of data. Windowing functions are applied to capture a limited frame of data [59] (Fig. 8).

The segmentation of the EDADC output is realized by using the Activity Selection Algorithm (ASA) [32,58]. This is built on the sampling nonuniformity and permits the realization of adaptive rate hybrid features extraction.

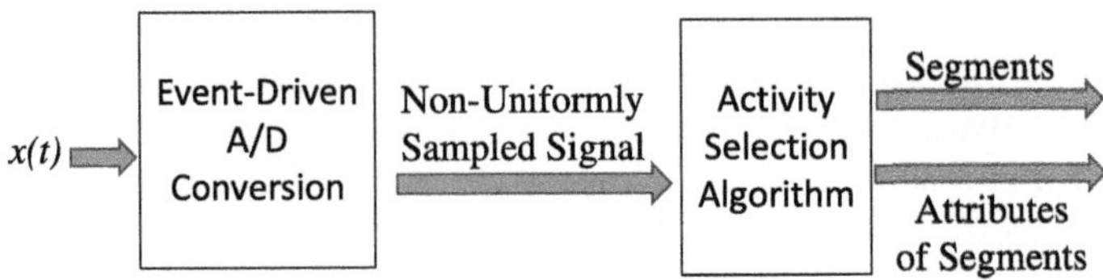

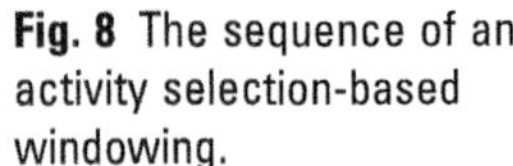
Fig. 8 The sequence of an activity selection-based windowing.

3.5 Adaptive rate interpolation

Interpolation is needed during the resampling phase, which adds artifacts in the resampled signal as compared to the original. The error of this process is determined by the characteristics of interpolator which is used to resample the segmented signal. Additionally this error is also dependent on the selected amplitude dynamics and resolution of the EDADC. Methods to compute the error of resampling in the proposed case as a function of the convert's resolution and dynamics and interpolator attributes is presented in [62].

3.6 Adaptive rate filtering

For the de-noising of biomedical signals, digital filters are widely used. The traditional filtering methods are inherently time-invariant. The device is designed to handle the worst-case scenario. A fixed sampling frequency is used to collect the signal, which is then analyzed by a fixed order filter. It may lead to an unnecessarily high rise in the computing load and processing operation of the device. In this context, multirate processing strategies are proposed [63–65]. Adaptive rate filtering methods are devised based on multirate processing approaches [32,59].

The reference filter bank is constructed with acceptable requirements for a range of reference sampling frequencies $Fref$. The, elements of $Fref$ are selected according to the method described in [32].

An effective reference filter is chosen during the online computation. The online comparison is carried out between $Fref$ and the average sampling frequency of segment W^i, named as Fs^i. Based on this comparison a suitable filter is selected from the predesigned filters bank for filtering the segment W^i. Before filtering the intended segment W^i is resampled uniformly by using the simplified linear interpolation approach at a rate of Frs^i [32]. This Frs^i adaptation allows us to resample W^i at Nyquist rates or sub-Nyquist rates. As a result, it avoids unnecessary resampling and noise removal operations during the postadaptive rate data resampling and denoising procedures. As a result, the proposed solution's computational complexity and power usage effectiveness is assured.

The adaptation method in the proposed techniques necessitates additional operations for each chosen segment. The selection of a reference filter is the first step. Onward, an efficient interpolator is used to execute the data resampling process online. As a result, the numerical complexity of the interpolator should be considered. For the intended use, the interpolation method should be carefully chosen to offer an attractive tradeoff between computational complexity and resampling accuracy. The program determines which interpolator to use as a function of the intended application. A simplified linear interpolator is used in this analysis. Once a segment of EEG signal is uniformly resampled then in next stage it is conditioned by removing unwanted noise. The proposed adaptive processing strategies are expected to significantly improve the computing performance and resource consumption of advanced cloud-based health tracking systems if they are successfully and smartly integrated in the solution.

3.7 Feature extraction method

The signal processing domain has lot of wavelet transform applications. It is frequently used to deal with both stationary and nonstationary signals. Certain famous application examples are the reduction of electrical noise from signals, the identification of sudden discontinuities and the compression of huge quantities of data. Similar to the Fourier transform, which represents a signal with sine and cosine functions of infinite length, the wavelet transform will decompose a signal into a set of constituent signals known as wavelets, each with a well described, dominant frequency. The wavelet transform breaks the incoming signal in wavelets. Wavelets are transient functions of short duration centered on a given time. The problem with the Fourier transform is that knowledge on what occurs in time is lost by transferring from the time domain to the frequency domain. It is easy to gauge the frequency content of the signal being studied by looking at the frequency spectrum, obtained using the Fourier transform. However, it is impossible to predict when the signal's corresponding elements, in the expected frequency spectrum, will appear or disappear. The wavelet transform, on the other hand, performs analysis in both the time and frequency domains. It provides information regarding the change of the frequency content of signal with respect to time. In this sense, following the work, presented in [41], the wavelet transform is used for decomposing the considered EEG signals in subbands. Eq. (6) describes the procedure. The scaling and translation parameters are represented by s and u, respectively.

$$W_x^\psi(u, s) = \frac{1}{\sqrt{S}} \int_{-\infty}^{+\infty} x(t)\psi \times \left(\frac{(t-u)}{s}\right) dt. \tag{6}$$

A discrete time version of the wavelet transform is used to process the digitized version of EEG signals. It is based on the Daubechies algorithm. Half-band finite impulse response filters are used to obtain subbands decomposition. These are made up of a cascaded network of subsampling lows pass and high pass filters. At each stage of half-band filtering, the approximation, a_m^i, and detail, d_m^i, coefficients are computed. The processes is mathematically given in Eqs. (7) and (8). In Eqs. (7) and (8), the levels of decomposition are indicated by using, m. The half-band low pass and high pass subsampling filters are respectively denoted as h_{2n-k}^i and g_{2n-k}^i. The used disctere time wavelet analysis scheme is depicted in Fig. 9.

$$a_m^i = \sum_{k=1}^{K_g^i} xf_n^i \cdot g_{2n-k}^i \tag{7}$$

$$d_m^i = \sum_{k=1}^{K_g^i} xf_n^i \cdot h_{2n-k}^i. \tag{8}$$

The classifiable attributes are extracted by using the wavelet coefficients which are obtained for each considered subband. The subbands d_1, d_2, d_3, d_4, and a_4 are included in this analysis. The 12 statistical features are derived for each sub-band. As a consequence, each denoised segment is presented with 60 attributes, reducing the dataset dimension from 150×1024 to 150×60 and

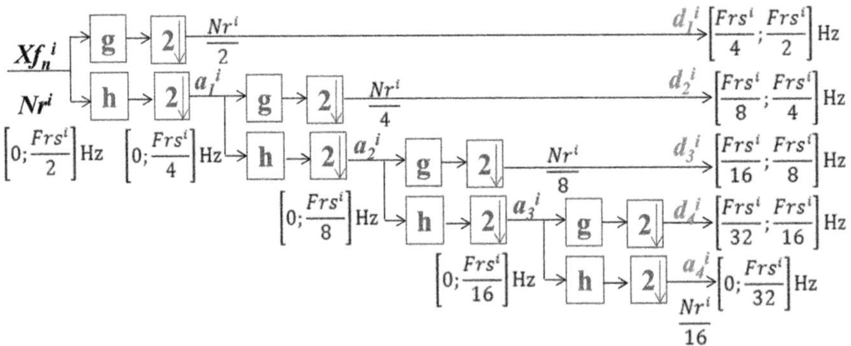

Fig. 9 The proposed DWT scheme.

naming it P. The extracted subbands features are described as follow.

Signal Power Spectrum (SPS): The power spectrum is computed using the average of the absolute values of the spectral beans.

Mean Absolute Value (MAV): The mean absolute value of a signal is computed by averaging over all coefficients using their absolute values.

Standard Deviation (STD): The standard deviation is in fact the square root of the variance. It is computed by finding the deviation of each subband coefficient from the mean value of all coefficients of the considered subband.

Mean Ratio (MR): The mean ratio of a signal is given as the ratio between the mean values of d^i (detailed signal) to a^i (approximate signal). If both signals have similar mean, the value will be 1.

Zero Crossings (ZC): The number of times a signal changes its polarity is known as zero crossings, i.e., from positive to negative or vice versa.

Entropy (ENT): The entropy of a signal is the measure of distortion in the signal computed using Shannon's entropy. The entropy is computed after normalization such that the maximum amplitude is scaled to 1.

Peak Positive Value (PPV): The peak positive value of a signal is its largest amplitude (in the positive direction) for the coefficient under consideration.

Second Peak Positive Value (SPP): The second peak positive value is the second largest positive amplitude of the signal coefficient under consideration.

Peak Positive Index (PPI): The peak positive index is the index along the signal where the peak positive value (PPV) is observed.

Peak Negative Value (PNV): The peak negative value of a signal is its lowest amplitude (in the negative direction) for the coefficient under consideration.

Second Peak Negative Value (SPN): The second highest negative magnitude of the considered subband coefficients is the second peak negative value.

Peak Negative Index (PNI): The peak negative index value is the location along the signal where the PNV is observed.

3.8   Machine learning methods

Machine learning algorithms for identification, detection, and diagnosis of biomedical signals have sparked a lot of interest in the scientific community recently. Heart disease diagnosis, coronary hypertrophy, myocardial ischemia, and epileptic seizure prediction and identification are also forms of life-threatening cases. The importance of early and accurate diagnosis and identifications is critical in order to prescribe the necessary prevention precautions or treatments.

In this aim, medical practitioners employ several diagnosis procedures and techniques such as tomographic scans, EEG and magnetic resonance imaging [66].

The signal processing and machine learning tools and techniques can be effectively incorporated to attain first level diagnosis and decisions. It can facilitate the task of medical practitioners. Moreover, a long term and continuous clinical supervision and tracking of patients with serious illness can be effectively realized by using the automated biomedical signals processing and machine learning techniques [66]. Since biomedical signals provide a large volume of data, the main classification challenge is determining how to classify biomedical signal recordings. Important features must first be separated from the obtained biomedical signals, then their dimensions must be shortened, and the reduced features must finally be used for classification. In simple words, an algorithm that can automatically categorize the incoming data into one or more categories can be called a classifier. An educational example is the email spam identifier. It tries to label an incoming email as a spam or not and onward places it in the spam or inbox folders. The classifier is based on certain well defined mathematical rules. It employs these rules with training dataset to develop a model for the considered application. Onward this model is used to label the incoming samples and to automatically categorize them. In the classification process, class tags are applied to the derived features of a collection of data during classification. A classifier is a type of algorithm that performs classification. EEG signals have been classified using a variety of machine learning–based classifiers. In this paper, we look at a few of the more common ones, which are described below. We use a 10-fold cross validation in both situations, which was also used to set the parameters.

3.8.1 K-nearest neighbors (K-*NN*)

The k-NN algorithm [67] is a popular classifier that finds the distance of the test data to the k nearest neighbors in the training data to decide its category label. Let v_j represents a sample and $\langle v_j, l_j \rangle$ represents the pair of the data vector along with its label, $l_j \in [1, C]$ where C denotes the maximum classes in the dataset. Then, the k-NN process to classify a new vector z, is given in Eq. (9).

$$\operatorname*{argmin}_{j} \operatorname{dist}(\boldsymbol{v}_j, z)\forall j = 1..N \tag{9}$$

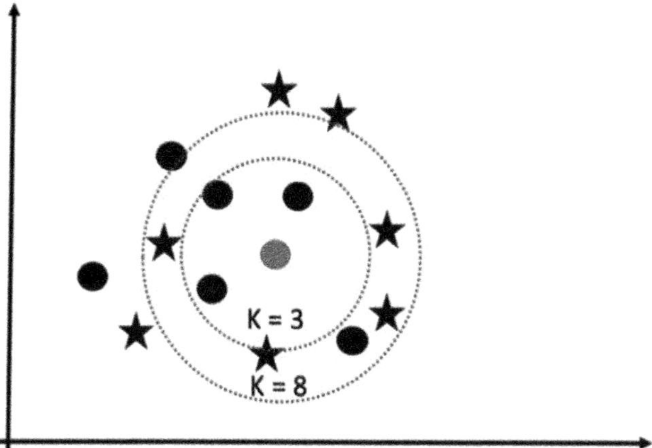

Fig. 10 KNN algorithm concept.

where $dist(,)$ is a distance measure. The value of k is usually set to a small odd number to ensure a majority consensus. Similarly, any distance metric can be used including classical metrics such as Manhattan, Euclidean, Chebyshev, Hamming, Minkowski, etc., or advanced metrics such as the χ-Sim, Cosine similarity, etc. [67].

Fig. 10 explains the k-NN algorithm in a basic form. In this example, the dataset is the same set of data as in the SVM, also composed of stars and circles. The red circle represents the test sample to be classified. The k-NN algorithm takes the test sample as a center of the circle and the diameter of the circle depends on the variable "k." "k" represents the number of neighbors inside the circle. When "k" is three the red circle is classified as belonging to the circle class. However, when "k" is increased to eight then the classification becomes less accurate.

3.8.2 Artificial neural network (ANN)

The ANNs can be named as the artificial adaptive systems. These are developed by getting inspired from the functionality and operation of the human brain [68]. In simple words, these are structures that can change their internal configuration in response to a feature goal. They are typically suited for solving the nonlinear problems. They follow the fuzzy laws and can tune their attributes to obtain the best solution of a targeted problem. The nodes, also known as processing elements, and the linkage between processing elements basically form the ANN. Each processing element has its own feature for transforming its input to an output. Each element has its specific input, used to receive information from other elements or environment. Similarly each element has its specific output, used to convey information to

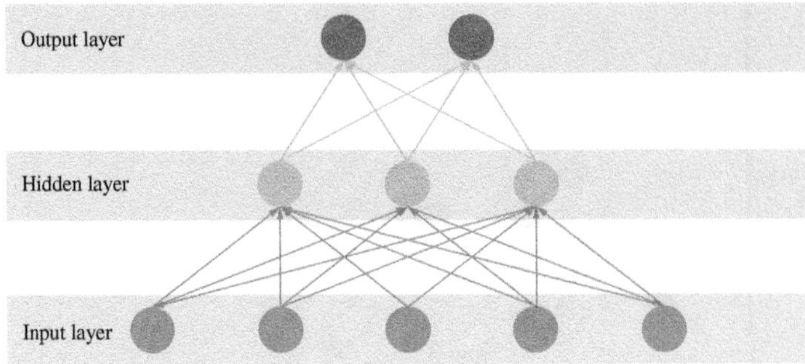

Fig. 11 ANN algorithm concept.

other elements or environment. The processing elements are grouped in layers as shown in Fig. 11. Weights of the processing elements can be tuned by using training data. It prepares the model for targeted application. Onward, this model can be used to classify the incoming samples among different categories.

3.8.3 Support vector machines (SVM)

In SVM, the first task is to find those samples that represent the boundary conditions. These are known as support vectors. Onward these are utilized to search for the optimal hyperplane that separates these vectors from the contrary classes [67]. We enhance the distance between the adjacent points, i.e., the points closest to the boundary, to do this. This is done by optimally separating the hyperplane that divides the data of the two classes described in Eq. (10) where x represents the data vector ($x=[x_1, x_2, ..., x_p]$) having attributes. The weight vector is given by $w=[w_1, w_2, ..., w_p]$, and the scalar bias is b.

$$h(x) = \text{sign}(w \cdot x^{\mathrm{T}} + b). \tag{10}$$

For the case of SVM, the weights w are adjusted in a manner that a test sample x renders either a positive outcome of the classifier h for class one or a negative result of the classifier h for class two. Other parameters are also involved, such as the c parameter (called regularization parameter), which determines the penalty for misclassification during training, and the slack variables.

When the two classes are not linearly separable, a Kernel function [67] is used to that transforms samples into a higher dimension where they may be detachable. Moreover, for classifying data with more than two classes, multiple approaches can be used. For instance, we can keep it as a two-class problem by keeping the label of one class (positive class) and relabeling all other classes with the same label (negative class). This may be repeated for each class during classification to identify samples of that particular class. It is known as the One-vs-All approach. Another widely used technique is to consider samples of only two categories at a time and to classify the data using a round-robin fashion. That is known as the One-vs-One approach [67].

Fig. 12 explains how the SVM algorithms work in a straightforward way. In this example, the dataset is composed of stars and circles. The end-goal is to divide them into two classes: the star class and the circle class. The two diagonal lines both accomplish the task of separating the dataset into the two categories. One is, though, superior to the other. The line with the greatest distance from the closest point in each set, according to SVM, is the best. Fig. 9 illustrates that the gap between the blue line to the nearest data point is Z2. However, the distance between the green line to the closest data point is Z1 because Z2 is superior to Z1. As a result, the blue line is the smarter splitter according to SVM, and it will be used to identify the results.

Data is not usually this easy to classify. SVM, as mentioned before, uses kernel functions to determine the hyperplane that will classify the data in the most optimal way. The following diagrams demonstrate how the kernel function can transform the data from the input space to the feature space. This is done because the data can be classified in a much easier and clearer way.

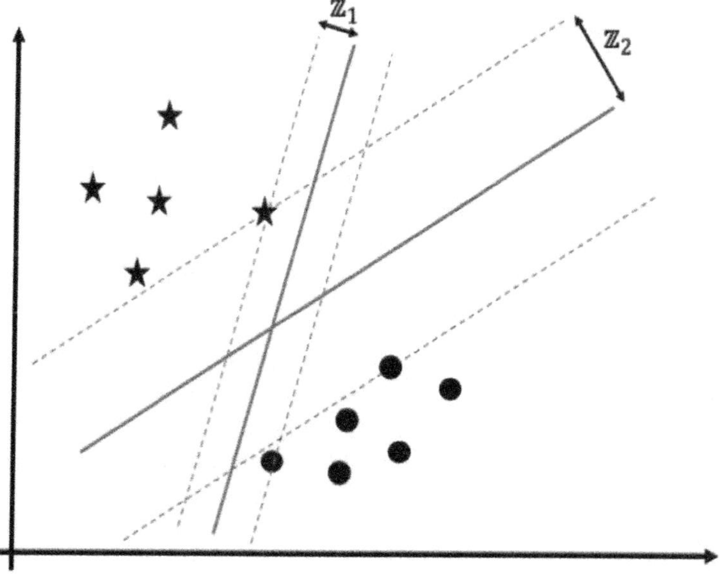

Fig. 12 SVM algorithm concept.

3.9 The performance evaluation measures

The following evaluation measures are used.

3.9.1 Samples ratio

It is given in Eq. (11). Where SR^i is the samples ratio for W^i. N_r and N_{LC}^i are, respectively, the number of samples exist in W^i for the classical and the proposed cases

$$SR^i = \frac{N_r}{N_{LC}^i}. \tag{11}$$

3.9.2 Compression ratio

It tests the suggested method performance in diminishing the size of data that must be conveyed to the post classification stage. The comparison is rendered with the traditional method of sending received EEG signals to the cloud without any attribute extraction or dimension reduction. The process is given in Eq. (12). Where R_{COMP} is the compression ratio and it is computed as a ration between N_r and P. N_r and P are the datasets, respectively, conveyed to the cloud-based classifier stage in the traditional and the suggested approaches. Each element in N_r and P is presented with 12-bit of resolution.

$$R_{COMP} = \frac{N_r}{P}. \tag{12}$$

The method used in this study has numerous advantages in terms of hardware efficiency, compression, encoding, and transmission. However, there is a slight loss of consistency as it operated at adaptive rates. Therefore, we assess the overall framework in terms of performance of classification so that we can rely on how and compare it with existing fix rate solutions. To avoid any biasness and manipulation, the cross-validation technique is employed. This aid in minimizing any abnormal effects on the dataset, the specific training–testing break on the dataset, parameter, or classifier could raise the problem of bias [67]. Many of the algorithms were tested on the same dataset using 10-fold cross-validation. We save the indices of the training and test sets for each training-test in each fold and ensure that the same indices are used for all algorithms. Furthermore, we choose to measure the outcomes using various measurement criteria, as seen below, to minimize metric bias.

3.9.3 Accuracy (ACC)

The algorithm's results are compared to the actual ones by using the measure of accuracy. It is also defined as the number of test dataset labels that were correctly predicted. These are used to calculate classification accuracy. Eq. (13) describes the procedure. In Eq. (13), true positives, true negatives, false positives, and false negatives are represented by TP, TN, FP, and FN.

$$\text{Accuracy} = \frac{\text{TP} + \text{TN}}{\text{TP} + \text{TN} + \text{FP} + \text{FN}}. \tag{13}$$

3.9.4 Specificity (SP)

It is a metric that calculates the amount of correctly labeled TN as a percentage of all negatives (i.e., negatives that were classified as negations and negatives that were wrong classified as positives). Consequently, the specificity is also known as the "absolute negative" limit. It is given in Eq. (14).

$$Sp = \frac{\text{TN}}{\text{TN} + \text{FP}}. \tag{14}$$

3.9.5 F-measure (F1)

It is a commonly used score that combines precision and recall. Mathematically, the $F1$ is given using Eq. (15) where $\text{precision} = \frac{\text{TP}}{\text{TP} + \text{FP}}$ and $\text{recall} = \frac{\text{TP}}{\text{TP} + \text{FN}}$.

$$F1 = \frac{2 \times \text{precision} \times \text{recall}}{\text{precision} + \text{recall}}. \tag{15}$$

3.9.6 Kappa index (kappa)

It is used to determine how often two clusterings agree. It is a mathematical calculation that takes into account the probability of such an arrangement occurring by chance, and it is considered more reliable than simple accuracy measure. We use the Cohen's kappa scale, which is commonly used to assess clustering outcomes and can be expressed using Eq. (16). In Eq. (16), p_0 denotes the probability of agreement between the predicted and desired tags, and thus, p_e denotes the probability of such agreement occurring by chance.

$$\text{kappa} = 1 - \frac{1 - p_0}{1 - p_e}. \tag{16}$$

4.　Results

The proposed method's performance is assessed by using the EEG signals, obtained from the Hauz Khas dataset. Fig. 13 shows examples of EEG time series from the different considered groups.

The EEG signals in this study were acquired using a 4-bit resolution EDADC. Examples of EEG waveforms, acquired with 4-bit resolution EDADC are shown in Fig. 14.

The EDADC concentrates only on the related signal parts and adjusts the sampling rate in response to temporal variations in the signal [57]. Its performance is calculated in terms of compression gain and the number of captured samples The Activity Selection Algorithm (ASA) adjusts the window function length based on the nonuniformly time partitioned EEG signal's characteristics. For each W^i, it often adjusts the resampling frequency. As a result, its efficiency is compared to the time-invariant classical windowing method in terms of adjusting the window length and number of samples per window. The adaptive rate interpolation technique is used to resample the segmented signal uniformly. The data resampling is done using simplified linear interpolation.

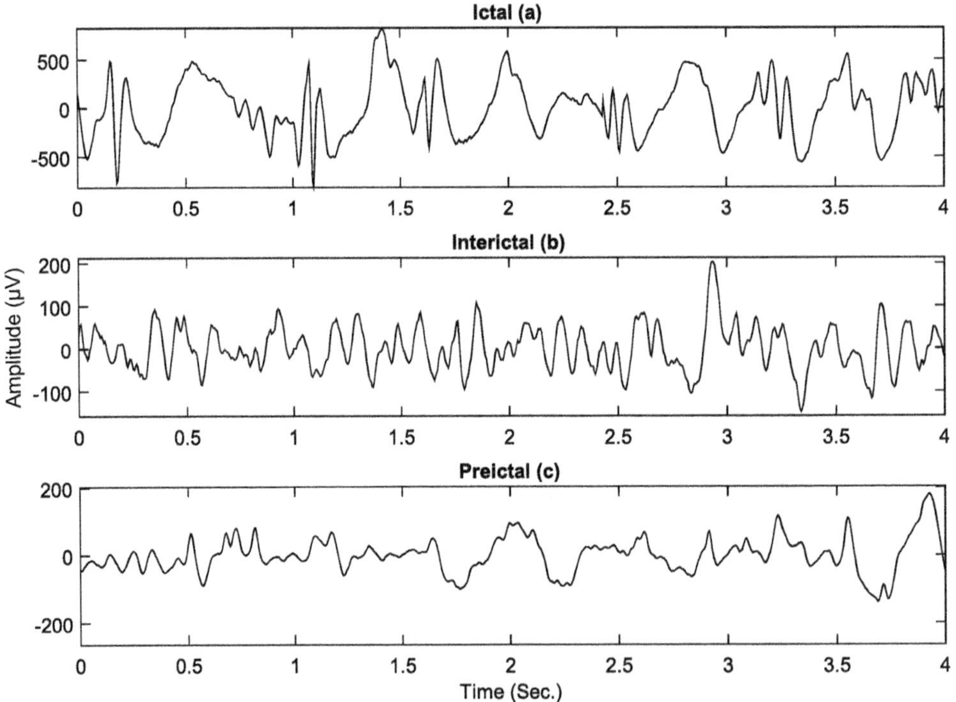

Fig. 13 Examples of EEG time series.

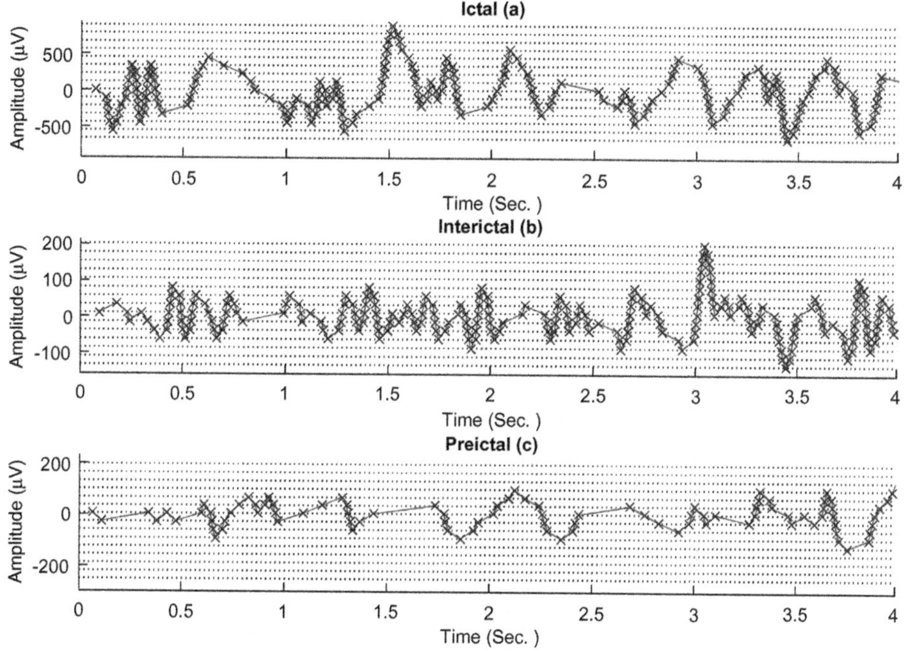

Fig. 14 Examples of EEG waveforms, acquired with 4-bit EDADCs.

The ARFIR technique is used to de-noise the resampled signal. It begins with a significant decrease in the noise removal operation's processing effectiveness. The adaptive rate subbands decomposition is used to derive the de-noised signal discriminative parameters. Subbands are used to extract statistical characteristics. In order to make classification decisions, some robust classification algorithms use these extracted parameters. The overall system's success is investigated in recognition rate. It also represents the accuracy of the proposed system's results.

Each instance in the classic case is made up of 1024 samples. The digital representation of the analog EEG signal $y(t)$ is y_n. y_n's spectral material is restricted to [$FC_{min} = 0.5$; $FC_{max} = 40$] Hz. The restored variant of y_n is $\tilde{x}(t)$, which is onward digitized with obtained with a 4-bit resolution EDADC.

The continuous incoming signal, after digitization, is segmented by the ASA. It tunes the resampling frequency of each segment by analyzing its local parameters. In this fashion, it permits the adaptive rate and efficient noise removal and subbands decomposition of the incoming signal instants.

All instances of each class are considered while calculating the samples ratios. For all 50 instants of ictal the average samples ratio of 2.6-fold is attained. For all 50 instants of interictal the samples ration of 2.8-fold is secured and for 50 instances of preictal category an average samples ration of 2.7-fold is obtained. As a result, the overall average mean decrease, for all 150 instances of three considered categories, in samples collection is 2.7 times.

Adaptive rate simplified linear interpolation is used to uniformly resample the chosen segments at the output of ASA. The resampled segments are subjected to adaptive rate filtering techniques to remove unnecessary noise [59].

Low energy noise is present at frequencies greater than $30\,\mathrm{Hz}$ and can be removed for successful epilepsy detection [15]. In this case, an offline bank of band-pass filters is constructed. Every filter's cut-off frequencies are chosen from a range of $[F_{Cmin}=0.5;\ F_{Cmax}=30]$ Hz. It allows you to concentrate on the appropriate EEG band while reducing background noise [32]. As a result, classification accuracy has improved [15]. The filters bank is programmed to deal with an array of sampling frequencies, $Fref$, between $Fs_{min}=63.7\,\mathrm{Hz}>2.\ F_{Cmax}$ to $F_r=200\,\mathrm{Hz}.\ \Delta=5.8\,\mathrm{Hz}$ is chosen. It results in 24 filters in the bank. Table 1 shows a list of the used filters orders in the designed bank of filters. It demonstrates how a lower order filter benefits from a reduction in sampling frequency, and vice versa.

Adaptive rate DWT is used to examine the filtered instances. After applying the proposed features mining approach, each EEG instance is presented with 60 features. On the other hand,

Table 1 The reference filters bank orders.

hc_k	$h1_k$	$h2_k$	$h3_k$	$h4_k$	$h5_k$	$h6_k$
$Fref_c$ (Hz)	63.7	69.5	75.3	81.1	86.9	92.7
K^i	19	21	23	25	27	29
hc_k	$h7_k$	$h8_k$	$h9_k$	$h10_k$	$h11_k$	$h12_k$
$Fref_c$ (Hz)	98.5	104.3	110.1	115.9	121.7	127.5
K^i	31	33	35	37	39	41
hc_k	$H13_k$	$h14_k$	$h15_k$	$h16_k$	$h17_k$	$h18_k$
$Fref_c$ (Hz)	133.3	139.1	144.9	150.7	156.5	162.3
K^i	43	45	47	49	51	53
hc_k	$h19_k$	$h20_k$	$h21_k$	$h22_k$	$h23_k$	$h24_k$
$Fref_c$ (Hz)	168.1	173.9	179.7	185.5	191.3	197.1
K^i	54	56	58	60	62	64

each EEG instance is originally made up of 1024 samples. Therefore, $R_{COMP} = 17.1$ is attained.

This promises that the data transfer process, bandwidth, and power usage are all reduced by the same amount.

For classification, we used the data matrix P. To prevent bias, we use a 10-fold cross-validation approach. The previously defined and listed evaluation metrics are used for each experiment. Table 2 summarizes the findings. If there are not enough samples, cross validation is a successful test technique. It divides the available dataset in k equal-sized subsets at random and then iterates over them. Following the completion of all k iterations, the model constructed without individual instances in the training set is used to create a projected class mark for each instance in the dataset. Using one or more output tests, the predicted class labels are compared to the actual class labels. The testing and validation or test sets were successfully partitioned using the k-fold cross-validation methodology. The set's usable instances can be used for both model development and assessment, but not at the same time [69].

Results from Table 2 describe that for the studied case the best accuracy score of 95% is secured by the ANN. The k-NN follows with 89% accuracy score and SVM is at the last with 85% accuracy score.

For the conducted study, the ANN attains the best F-measure value of 0.94. The k-NN follows with 0.87 F-measure value and SVM attains the third best F-measure value of 0.81.

The ANN also secures the best Kappa index value of 0.92 for this conducted study. The k-NN attains 0.73 Kappa index value and follows the ANN. The SVM attains the third best Kappa index value of 0.71.

For the conducted study, the ANN attains the best specificity value of 0.98. The k-NN follows with 0.93 specificity value and SVM attains the third best specificity value of 0.91.

It confirms that for the studied case, the ANN outperformance the k-NN and SVM algorithms. It shows a higher robustness and

Table 2 Performance of different classifiers using four evaluation metrics.

Classifier	ACC	F1	Kappa	Sp
ANN	0.95	0.94	0.92	0.98
k-NN	0.89	0.87	0.73	0.93
SVM	0.85	0.81	0.71	0.91

lesser chances of getting bias of the ANN as compared to the k-NN and SVM classifiers for the studied case. While achieving an effective reduction in the count of collected samples the suggested method also attains the best accuracy score of 95%.

5. Discussion and conclusion

The recent developments in smart sensor systems are booming in the wearable industry. It permits the scientists to refine wearable models for a variety of uses. The cloud-based mobile health management is an evolving field of study. It has a lot of potential and benefits. This is the reason that it has drawn interest from a wide range of healthcare technology experts. As a result of these advancements, the growing understanding of cloud-based mobile health tracking in various fields suggests that incorporating wearable devices into healthcare applications and medical home monitoring would be appealing. Innovations in smart application and sensor technologies provide creative tools for improving the quality of treatment for chronic disease patients. Biomedical signal monitoring for adverse circumstance diagnosis is a novel approach that has the potential to revolutionize healthcare. The aim is to use a cloud-based electronic healthcare device to monitor any critical situation, such as an epileptic seizure.

One of the objectives of this chapter is to reflect most of these advancements while also identifying certain critical research issues. Using smart signal sensing, synthesis and machine learning software, a platform for cloud-based healthcare applications is developed. Patients with chronic conditions, such as epilepsy, require constant and accurate remote control. In this sense, this chapter presents a cloud-based mobile healthcare surveillance framework for predicting and detecting epileptic seizures by interpreting and analyzing EEG signals. The key contribution of this book chapter is to describe that how the intelligent use of wireless biomedical gadgets with signal processing and machine learning methods can render an automated and configurable mobile healthcare solution. This solution can be used for an effective surveillance of remote patients with chronic disorders.

The key benefit of the suggested method as compared to the conventional fix rate counterparts is the diminishing of redundant samples for processing and the addition of real-time compression gain. It aptitudes for a notable processing effectiveness with significant data transmission activity reduction and power efficiency. It shows that an intelligent incorporation of these methods can enhance the performance of traditional fix rate processing bases solutions. The performance of system is tested by using the Hauz Khas epilepsy database. The process proved to be realistic, accurate, and efficient in measuring and analyzing EEG signals, according to the results.

To reduce the signal transmission rate, the invented approach utilizes the adaptive rate EEG signal processing with machine learning algorithms. The feature extraction is done with the aid of a wavelet analysis scheme. Each subband's statistical features are extracted for further analysis. These derived features are sent to a cloud-based classification module for automatic epileptic seizure diagnosis and identification. It leads to a substantial reduction in the number of obtained samples, as well as a significant compression advantage for the device.

The system attains average sampling ratios of 2.6-, 2.8-, and 2.7-fold, respectively, for ictal, interictal, and preictal categories. The overall average sampling ratio of 2.7-fold is achieved for all considered categories of the EEG signals for Hauz Khas dataset. The system also secures a compression gain of 17.1-fold for the studied case with a best classification accuracy score of 95%. It guarantees that the designed adaptive rate EEG processing and classification techniques secures a good classification performance, comparable to current classical fixed rate counterparts, while ensuring a major computational advantage and compression gain over them. The proposed technique is effective, and it has the ability to aid in the advancement of modern mobile healthcare solutions.

In the future, the success of the proposed method will be investigated using a different epilepsy dataset and expanded groups of EEG signals. Other feature extraction techniques, such as Autoregressive Berg and Cosine Transform, will be investigated in the future, as well as their effect on system performance.

In future the performance of suggested approach can be studied for another epilepsy dataset while considering extended classes of the EEG signals. Another future work is to explore other features extraction techniques and their impact on the performance of system such as Autoregressive Berg and Round Cosine Transform. Other possibilities include miniaturization, optimization, and embedded applications of the proposed solutions.

Acknowledgments

The Effat University funds this work under grant number Decision No. UC#9/29 April.2020/7.1-22(2)1. The author is thankful to Dr. A. Subasi and Dr. S.F. Hussain for fruitful discussions.

References

[1] Y. Athavale, S. Krishnan, Biosignal monitoring using wearables: observations and opportunities, Biomed. Signal Process. Control 38 (2017) 22–33.

[2] B.G. Celler, R.S. Sparks, Home telemonitoring of vital signs—technical challenges and future directions, IEEE J. Biomed. Health Inform. 19 (1) (2015) 82–91.

[3] V. Mihajlović, B. Grundlehner, R. Vullers, J. Penders, Wearable, wireless EEG solutions in daily life applications: what are we missing? IEEE J. Biomed. Health Inform. 19 (1) (2015) 6–21.

[4] M. Kay, J. Santos, M. Takane, mHealth: new horizons for health through mobile technologies, World Health Organ. 64 (7) (2011) 66–71.

[5] P. Guzik, M. Malik, ECG by mobile technologies, J. Electrocardiol. 49 (6) (2016) 894–901.

[6] E. Trinka, P. Kwan, B. Lee, A. Dash, Epilepsy in Asia: disease burden, management barriers, and challenges, Epilepsia 60 (2019) 7–21.

[7] V.N. Vakharia, J.S. Duncan, J. Witt, C.E. Elger, R. Staba, J. Engel Jr., Getting the best outcomes from epilepsy surgery, Ann. Neurol. 83 (4) (2018) 676–690.

[8] C. Harden, T. Tomson, D. Gloss, J. Buchhalter, J.H. Cross, E. Donner, J.A. French, A. Gil-Nagel, D.C. Hesdorffer, W.H. Smithson, Practice guideline summary: sudden unexpected death in epilepsy incidence rates and risk factors: report of the Guideline Development, Dissemination, and Implementation Subcommittee of the American Academy of Neurology and the American Epilepsy Society, Epilepsy Curr. 17 (3) (2017) 180–187.

[9] P. Klein, I. Tyrlikova, Prevention of epilepsy: should we be avoiding clinical trials? Epilepsy Behav. 72 (2017) 188–194.

[10] R. San-Segundo, M. Gil-Martín, L.F. D'Haro-Enriquez, J.M. Pardo, Classification of epileptic EEG recordings using signal transforms and convolutional neural networks, Comput. Biol. Med. 109 (2019) 148–158.

[11] M.A. Sayeed, S.P. Mohanty, E. Kougianos, H.P. Zaveri, eSeiz: an edge-device for accurate seizure detection for smart healthcare, IEEE Trans. Consum. Electron. 65 (3) (2019) 379–387.

[12] M. Tohidi, J.K. Madsen, F. Moradi, A low-power, low-noise, high-accurate epileptic-seizure detection system for wearable applications, Microelectron. J. 92 (2019) 104600.

[13] A.L. Schröder, H. Ombao, Fresped: frequency-specific change-point detection in epileptic seizure multi-channel EEG data, J. Am. Stat. Assoc. 114 (525) (2019) 115–128.

[14] S.M. Qaisar, A. Subasi, Efficient epileptic seizure detection based on the event driven processing, Procedia Comput. Sci. 163 (2019) 30–34.

[15] S.M. Qaisar, A. Subasi, Effective epileptic seizure detection based on the event-driven processing and machine learning for mobile healthcare, J. Ambient. Intell. Humaniz. Comput. (2020) 1–13.

[16] S.M. Qaisar, A. Subasi, Adaptive rate EEG signal processing for epileptic seizure detection, Presented in 2019 13th International Conference on Sampling Theory and Applications (SampTA), IEEE, Bordeaux, France, 2019, pp. 1–3.

[17] K. Baskar, C. Karthikeyan, Epilepsy seizure detection using akima spline interpolation based ensemble empirical mode Kalman filter decomposition by EEG signals, J. Med. Imaging Health Inform. 9 (6) (2019) 1320–1328.

[18] A.G. Correa, L.L. Orosco, P. Diez, E.L. Leber, Adaptive filtering for epileptic event detection in the EEG, J. Med. Biol. Eng. 39 (6) (2019) 912–918.

[19] M. Sharma, S. Shah, P. Achuth, A novel approach for epilepsy detection using time–frequency localized bi-orthogonal wavelet filter, J. Mech. Med. Biol. 19 (01) (2019) 1940007.

[20] G. Chen, W. Xie, T.D. Bui, A. Krzyżak, Automatic epileptic seizure detection in EEG using nonsubsampled wavelet–Fourier features, J. Med. Biol. Eng. 37 (1) (2017) 123–131.

[21] A. Achmamad, A. Jbari, A comparative study of wavelet families for electromyography signal classification based on discrete wavelet transform, Bull. Electr. Eng. Inform. 9 (4) (2020) 1420–1429.

[22] E. Alickovic, J. Kevric, A. Subasi, Performance evaluation of empirical mode decomposition, discrete wavelet transform, and wavelet packed decomposition for automated epileptic seizure detection and prediction, Biomed. Signal Process. Control 39 (2018) 94–102.

[23] A. Bhattacharyya, R.B. Pachori, A. Upadhyay, U.R. Acharya, Tunable-Q wavelet transform based multiscale entropy measure for automated classification of epileptic EEG signals, Appl. Sci. 7 (4) (2017) 385.

[24] A. Nishad, R.B. Pachori, Classification of epileptic electroencephalogram signals using tunable-Q wavelet transform based filter-bank, J. Ambient. Intell. Humaniz. Comput. (2020) 1–15.

[25] M. Sharma, R.B. Pachori, U.R. Acharya, A new approach to characterize epileptic seizures using analytic time-frequency flexible wavelet transform and fractal dimension, Pattern Recogn. Lett. 94 (2017) 172–179.

[26] K. Singh, J. Malhotra, IoT and cloud computing based automatic epileptic seizure detection using HOS features based random forest classification, J. Ambient. Intell. Humaniz. Comput. (2019) 1–16.

[27] I. Ullah, M. Hussain, H. Aboalsamh, An automated system for epilepsy detection using EEG brain signals based on deep learning approach, Expert Syst. Appl. 107 (2018) 61–71.

[28] X. Zhao, R. Zhang, Z. Mei, C. Chen, W. Chen, Identification of epileptic seizures by characterizing instantaneous energy behavior of EEG, IEEE Access 7 (2019) 70059–70076.

[29] M.E. Bayrakdar, Priority based health data monitoring with IEEE 802.11 AF technology in wireless medical sensor networks, Med. Biol. Eng. Comput. 57 (12) (2019) 2757–2769.

[30] M.-P. Hosseini, T.X. Tran, D. Pompili, K. Elisevich, H. Soltanian-Zadeh, Multimodal data analysis of epileptic EEG and rs-fMRI via deep learning and edge computing, Artif. Intell. Med. 104 (2020) 101813.

[31] D. Gurve, D. Delisle-Rodriguez, T. Bastos-Filho, S. Krishnan, Trends in compressive sensing for EEG signal processing applications, Sensors 20 (13) (2020) 3703.

[32] S.M. Qaisar, Efficient mobile systems based on adaptive rate signal processing, Comput. Electr. Eng. 79 (2019) 106462.

[33] S.M. Qaisar, A computationally efficient EEG signals segmentation and de-noising based on an adaptive rate acquisition and processing, Presented in 2018 IEEE 3rd International Conference on Signal and Image Processing (ICSIP), IEEE, Shenzhen Research Institute, Southeast University, China, 2018, pp. 182–186.

[34] M. Tohidi, J.K. Madsen, F. Moradi, Low-power high-input-impedance EEG signal acquisition SoC with fully integrated IA and signal-specific ADC for wearable applications, IEEE Trans. Biomed. Circuits Syst. 13 (6) (2019) 1437–1450.

[35] S.M. Qaisar, A. Mihoub, M. Krichen, H. Nisar, Multirate processing with selective subbands and machine learning for efficient arrhythmia classification, Sensors 21 (4) (2021) 1511.

[36] Y. Hou, J. Qu, Z. Tian, M. Atef, K. Yousef, Y. Lian, G. Wang, A 61-nW level-crossing ADC with adaptive sampling for biomedical applications, IEEE Trans. Circuits Syst. Express Briefs 66 (1) (2018) 56–60.

[37] S.M. Qaisar, A. Subasi, Cloud-based ECG monitoring using event-driven ECG acquisition and machine learning techniques, Phys. Eng. Sci. Med. 43 (2) (2020) 623–634.

[38] N. Ravanshad, H. Rezaee-Dehsorkh, Level-crossing sampling: principles, circuits, and processing for healthcare applications, in: Compressive Sensing in Healthcare, Elsevier, 2020, pp. 223–246.

[39] A. Sabo, S.M. Qaisar, The event-driven power efficient wireless sensor nodes for monitoring of insects and health of plants, Presented in 2018 IEEE 3rd International Conference on Signal and Image Processing (ICSIP), IEEE, Shenzhen Research Institute, Southeast University, China, 2018, pp. 478–483.

[40] S. Siuly, Y. Li, Y. Zhang, EEG Signal Analysis and Classification, Springer, 2016.

[41] S.M. Qaisar, S.F. Hussain, Effective epileptic seizure detection by using level-crossing EEG sampling sub-bands statistical features selection and machine learning for mobile healthcare, Comput. Methods Prog. Biomed. 203 (2021) 106034.

[42] Y.-L. Zheng, X.-R. Ding, C.C.Y. Poon, B.P.L. Lo, H. Zhang, X.-L. Zhou, G.-Z. Yang, N. Zhao, Y.-T. Zhang, Unobtrusive sensing and wearable devices for health informatics, IEEE Trans. Biomed. Eng. 61 (5) (2014) 1538–1554.

[43] S. Sareen, S.K. Sood, S.K. Gupta, An automatic prediction of epileptic seizures using cloud computing and wireless sensor networks, J. Med. Syst. 40 (11) (2016) 226.

[44] B.-G. Lee, B.-L. Lee, W.-Y. Chung, Mobile healthcare for automatic driving sleep-onset detection using wavelet-based EEG and respiration signals, Sensors 14 (10) (2014) 17915–17936.

[45] C.-C. Lin, P.-Y. Lin, P.-K. Lu, G.-Y. Hsieh, W.-L. Lee, R.-G. Lee, A healthcare integration system for disease assessment and safety monitoring of dementia patients, IEEE Trans. Inf. Technol. Biomed. 12 (5) (2008) 579–586.

[46] J. Askamp, M.J. van Putten, Mobile EEG in epilepsy, Int. J. Psychophysiol. 91 (1) (2014) 30–35.

[47] K. Honda, S.N. Kudoh, Air brain: The easy telemetric system with smartphone for EEG signal and human behavior, Proceedings of the 8th International Conference on Body Area Networks, ICST, 2013, pp. 343–346.

[48] A. Stopczynski, C. Stahlhut, J.E. Larsen, M.K. Petersen, L.K. Hansen, The smartphone brain scanner: a portable real-time neuroimaging system, PLoS One 9 (2) (2014), e86733.

[49] L.N. Ranganathan, S.A. Chinnadurai, B. Samivel, B. Kesavamurthy, M.M. Mehndiratta, Application of mobile phones in epilepsy care, Int. J. Epilepsy 2 (1) (2015) 28–37.

[50] M.A. Serhani, M. El Menshawy, A. Benharref, SME2EM: smart mobile end-to-end monitoring architecture for life-long diseases, Comput. Biol. Med. 68 (2016) 137–154.

[51] X. Li, X. Yao, Application of fuzzy similarity to prediction of epileptic seizures using EEG signals, Presented in International Conference on Fuzzy Systems and Knowledge Discovery, Springer, Berlin, Heidelberg, 2005, pp. 645–652.

[52] D. Callegari, E. Conte, T. Ferreto, D. Fernandes, F. Moraes, F. Burmeister, R. Severino, EpiCare—A Home Care Platform Based on Mobile Cloud Computing to Assist Epilepsy Diagnosis, 2014, pp. 148–151.

[53] E. Džaferović, S. Vrtagić, L. Bandić, J. Kevric, A. Subasi, S.M. Qaisar, Cloud-based mobile platform for EEG signal analysis, Presented in 2016 5th International Conference on Electronic Devices, Systems and Applications (ICEDSA), IEEE, Ras Al Khaimah, UAE, 2016, pp. 1–4.

[54] S. Sanei, Adaptive Processing of Brain Signals, John Wiley & Sons, 2013.

[55] B. Graimann, B. Allison, G. Pfurtscheller, Brain–computer interfaces: a gentle introduction, in: Brain-Computer Interfaces, Springer, 2009, pp. 1–27.

[56] P. Swami, T.K. Gandhi, B.K. Panigrahi, M. Tripathi, S. Anand, A novel robust diagnostic model to detect seizures in electroencephalography, Expert Syst. Appl. 56 (2016) 116–130.

[57] S.M. Qaisar, Échantillonnage et Traitement Conditionnés par le Signal: Une Approche Prometteuse pour des Traitements Efficaces à pas Adaptatifs, in: PhD Dissertation, Grenoble Intitute of Technology, University of Grenoble Alpes, Grenoble, France, 2009.

[58] S. Mian Qaisar, F. Alsharif, Signal piloted processing of the smart meter data for effective appliances recognition, J. Electr. Eng. Technol. 15 (2020) 2279–2285.

[59] S.M. Qaisar, L. Fesquet, M. Renaudin, Adaptive rate filtering a computationally efficient signal processing approach, Signal Process. 94 (2014) 620–630.

[60] S. Mian Qaisar, S. Fawad Hussain, Arrhythmia diagnosis by using level-crossing ECG sampling and sub-bands features extraction for mobile healthcare, Sensors 20 (8) (2020) 2252.

[61] L. Jambi, S. Alsubaie, S.M. Qaisar, An event-driven power efficient surveillance and lighting system in the Saudi Arabia perspective, Presented in 2018 IEEE 3rd International Conference on Signal and Image Processing (ICSIP), IEEE, Shenzhen Research Institute, Southeast University, China, 2018, pp. 423–427.

[62] S.M. Qaisar, M. Akbar, T. Beyrouthy, W. Al-Habib, M. Asmatulah, An error measurement for resampled level crossing signal, Presented in 2016 Second International Conference on Event-Based Control, Communication, and Signal Processing (EBCCSP), IEEE, Krakow, Poland, 2016, pp. 1–4.

[63] Z. Duan, J. Zhang, C. Zhang, E. Mosca, A simple design method of reduced-order filters and its applications to multirate filter bank design, Signal Process. 86 (5) (2006) 1061–1075.

[64] D. Noh, T. Katsianos, Multi-Rate System for Audio Processing, U.S. Patent and Trademark Office, Washington, DC, USA, 2018. U.S. Patent No. 9,609,451.

[65] M. Vetterli, A theory of multirate filter banks, IEEE Trans. Acoust. Speech Signal Process. 35 (3) (1987) 356–372.

[66] R. Begg, D.T. Lai, M. Palaniswami, Computational Intelligence in Biomedical Engineering, CRC Press, 2007.

[67] G. Bonaccorso, Machine Learning Algorithms, Packt Publishing Ltd, 2017.

[68] J.S. Hallinan, Chapter 1—computational intelligence in the design of synthetic microbial genetic systems, in: C. Harwood, A. Wipat (Eds.), Methods in Microbiology, 40, Academic Press, 2013, pp. 1–37, https://doi.org/10.1016/B978-0-12-417029-2.00001-7.

[69] P. Cichosz, Data Mining Algorithms: Explained Using R, John Wiley & Sons, 2014.

14

Development of a novel low-cost multimodal microscope for food and biological applications

Chavali Ravikanth[a,*], Bikash K. Pradhan[a,*], Deepti Bharti[a], Angana Sarkar[a], Ananya Barui[b], Preetam Sarkar[a], Satyapriya Mohanty[c], and Kunal Pal[a]

[a]Department of Biotechnology and Medical Engineering, National Institute of Technology, Rourkela, India. [b]Center of Healthcare Science and Technology, Indian Institute of Engineering Science and Technology, Shibpur, India. [c]Department of Cardiothoracic and Vascular Surgery, All India Institute of Medical Sciences (AIIMS), Bhubaneswar, India

1.   Introduction

The analysis of the matter at its true size is a fascinating and challenging task for researchers. However, the discovery of object magnification using glass lenses allowed researchers to explore previously existing but unseen systems around us quickly. Among the different glass lenses-based object magnification systems, the compound microscope has received special attention from hobbyists to researchers across different domains. Since its development, the compound microscope has become an essential tool, especially in bioscience. The compound microscope is most commonly used to visualize and study the structures of the microorganisms, plant/animal cells, and their inter/intracellular interactions within the living organisms. However, these microscopes cannot capture images for future reference and analysis. With the advent of digital imaging systems, it is now possible to convert a compound microscope into a digital microscope by

*Authors contributed equally.

Advanced Methods in Biomedical Signal Processing and Analysis. https://doi.org/10.1016/B978-0-323-85955-4.00016-8

Copyright © 2023 Elsevier Inc. All rights reserved.

attaching a digital imaging system to the eyepiece lens. This change has significantly upgraded the capability of traditional compound microscopes. Such systems have been explored in biomedical applications (e.g., cell counting [1], tumor cell detection [2], pathogen detection [3], tissue engineering [4], etc.), and food industries (e.g., microstructure analysis [4], detection of contaminants [5]).

The imaging through a digital microscope is usually carried out in a single modality. Common modalities include bright-field, dark-field, oblique, polarization, phase contrast, differential interference contrast, Rheinberg, etc. There are specific systems wherein a combination of multiple modalities is being performed. Utilizing the advancements and breakthroughs made in optics and optical devices, it is now possible to create motorized digital microscopes with multimodal imaging capabilities at a lower cost. The inclusion of multiple imaging modalities into a single digital microscope allows overall contrast enhancement of the microstructures of the objects under test [6,7]. Further, highlighting the microstructures in the region of interest is also possible using such a system. Along with multimodal imaging, simultaneous run of multiple modalities will further enhance the details and contrast of the acquired magnified digital image. However, the development of digital microscopes that offer simultaneous multimodal imaging is costly and challenging to manufacture. Due to this, such microscopes are a rare tool in the hands of bioscience researchers. Hence, tapping the unutilized potential of simultaneous multimodal microscopic imaging using digital microscopes can benefit the scientific community.

In the present study, we report developing a fully functional, easy-to-build, and affordable digital microscope capable of performing multiple simultaneous microscopic imaging modalities. The proposed microscope uses conventional optical hardware components of a traditional digital compound microscope in conjunction with the specifically designed hardware filter set. The filter set designed for the proposed device intercepts the illumination pathway. It allows modulating the path and nature of the light waves that are striking the specimen and consequently alters its properties such as angle of incidence, luminous intensity, polarization direction, aperture, and bandwidth. By doing so, the proposed device can perform imaging not only in bright-field, dark-field, oblique, polarization, and Rheinberg illumination modes but also in combination of illumination modes such as dark-field and oblique, dark-field and polarization, Rheinberg and oblique, and Rheinberg and polarization, simultaneously. With simultaneous multimodal imaging, the proposed device subdues the limitations of a single modality by other modalities. It results in overall contrast enhancement of the specimen under investigation. Also, overlooked details in the region of interest can be highlighted using the proposed device, which a single imaging modality cannot enhance. The device's proper functioning was finally tested by analyzing various food samples to microorganisms (collected from the nearby pond).

2. Literature review

A microscope is an essential tool to analyze materials/microbes that are unseen by the human eye. These devices are helpful for biological studies, including anatomy and morphology, and have also been used in the industry for quality control. The recent advancements in the said field have combined the traditional microscopic system with various state-of-the-art technology. Researchers nowadays are looking for a more simple, easy-to-use, and cost-effective microscopic system that increases the acceptability and usability of the device. Further, the improvement in the design has also achieved substantial growth in the last few years. Kent and Bacon (2017) have demonstrated a simple and affordable digital microscope developed using Raspberry Pi, Raspberry Pi camera, and off-the-shelf readily available components [8]. As per their survey, the authors reported that around 70% of the school could not afford a microscope, which hampers the quality of lab studies. Hence, they tried to eliminate the issue with the development of a low-cost microscopy system. In a similar study, Gurkan et al. (2011) developed a cost-effective microscope that could be specially applied for point-of-care medical diagnostics [9] that was achieved using lensless imaging technology which enabled the device to make a rapid and affordable diagnostic decision. Fernandez et al. (2018) have reported an automated microscope that efficiently helps in urine analysis. The device used a microcontroller, which captured the images of four different urine constituents including red blood cells (RBC), white blood cells (WBC), calcium oxalate, and bacteria [10]. An automated microscope has also been reported in the literature to detect a fungal infection that analyses the skin, hair, and nail samples [11]. Rawat et al. (2017) have developed a low-cost, field-portable microscope integrated with a cell phone sensor. The device can be used as a low-cost alternative in disease diagnosis in countries with limited access to healthcare facilities [12]. Along with the aforesaid biological applications, several studies have also emphasized the design of microscopic systems. In

[13], the author has improved their microscope's resolution to better morphological analysis of the smallest colloids based on their shape, size, porosity, elemental composition, etc. Pacheco et al. (2017) have developed a novel microscopic system that provides high-resolution images with a large field of view. The device also captured images from multiple regions and focal points [14]. The authors used a 0.5 numerical aperture (NA) confocal fluorescence microscope that was prototyped with a 3 mm × 3 mm field of view and 12 mm working distance. Further, an array of nine beams was scanned over the field of view in nine different regions to speed up the acquisition time by a factor of nine. In [15], the authors have developed an optical microscope with adaptive stage adjustment. The device helped in eliminating human error that is associated with the manual adjustment of the traditional devices. Here, the authors have employed an adaptive regulator that controls the stage movement effectively to reach the desired position.

Despite the evolutionary changes in the build, design, and application in the field of microscopy, the cost of these devices is still a major constrain in their usability and acceptability. Additionally, it is not possible to afford sample-specific microscopes used to analyze sample of a particular type. Further, developing a microscopic system in different imaging modalities will enhance its applicability and provide more imaging data at a lower cost. In [16], a single-chip scanning probe microscope has been reported that has a provision to perform both atomic force microscopy and scanning thermal microscopy. Herein, a thermal-piezoresistive resonant sensor was used that holds the tip-sample interaction force constant, whereas the local heat transfer effect was measured using a bolometer-style probe. A single-chip scanning probe was used to measure the local electro-thermal signals. Mehta et al. (2021) have developed a field-portable multimodal microscopic system that can perform imaging in fluorescence, bright field, and quantitative phase mode [17]. Herein, fluorescence microscopy gives molecular information, whereas phase microscopy gives the texture, morphology, etc. The components of the device were fabricated using a 3D printer and then assembled into a single unit that makes the system compact and portable. In their recent study, Watanabe et al. (2021) reported a direction-dependent multimodal optical microscope [6]. The device can be operated using Raspberry Pi, LED lights, and a Raspberry Pi camera module. Using the proposed device, multimodal imaging, including bright-field, dark-field, polarization, and differential phase-contrast, is possible. The authors also produced direction-dependent dark-field as well as differential phase-contrast images. Further, the structure in the dark-field and differential phase-contrast images was enhanced using a pair of opposite line or rectangular illumination. In a similar study [7], the authors reported wide-field multimodal imaging using a smartphone. The system used the in-built camera for imaging and the LED flashlight of the smartphone as the optical source. The device also uses a compact plastic optical setup, fabricated using a 3D printer containing the specimen holder. The proposed system allows imaging in three dynamically adaptable modes such as bright-field, oblique illumination, dark-field, and total internal reflection dark-field on a single platform.

A comprehensive literature search suggests that though many studies have attempted to design a low-cost device, only a few showed possible results. In contrast, others fit only either for a specific application or imaging modality. For example, the device reported in [18–20] were used to analyze red blood cells, lunar soil, and collagen fibers, respectively. However, when it comes to multimodal imaging, the higher cost restricts its wider use. The current study challenges eliminating these two issues and proposes a cost-efficient device and can perform imaging in nine dual modes.

3. Materials and methods

3.1 Material and software

The objective lenses of the microscope ($10\times$ magnification; DIN semiplan achromatic) and microscope condenser with adjustable slit diameter slider were procured from the local microscope shop. The microscope eyepiece camera (Model: MD500; CMOS 5-megapixel camera module; AmScope, USA) was procured from AmScope.com. Marine-grade plywood sheets (thickness: 6 mm and 22 mm), PVC foam sheet (thickness: 4 mm), double-sided tape (length: 50 cm and width: 2.5 cm), adhesive (Fevicol), stainless steel bolts (Ø: 6 mm and size: 6 in.), stainless steel nuts (Ø: 6 mm), and white decorative laminate sheet (thickness: 1 mm) were procured from the wood supplies shop. Black paper sheets (thickness: 100 GSM) and clear transparent plastic sheets (size: A4, thickness: 80 GSM) were procured from a local stationery supplies shop. 1-W white LED (3.3 V–350 mA) with aluminum heat sink, connecting wires (22 AWG), LM2596 buck converter, CA-1235 adjustable power supply modules, single-side laminated FR4 copper clad PCB board, and SPST electronic switches were procured from a local electronics vendor. Dilute methylene blue solution (1.875%; 1.875 g for 125 mL), ferric chloride, microscope slides ($75\,mm \times 25\,mm \times 1.35\,mm$), injection syringes, toothpicks, fingerpricks, and coverslips ($18\,mm \times 18\,mm \times 0.17\,mm$) were procured from MEI lab. The matte black vinyl sticker sheet, smooth chrome-plated stainless steel rods (diameter: $6\,mm$), rust-free stainless steel threaded rods (diameter: $6\,mm$; thread-pitch: $1\,mm$), flanged brass nut inserts (inner diameter: $6\,mm$), Raspberry Pi CSI camera cable (15 pins; length: $60\,cm$), Samsung EVO micro-SD card (32-GB; Class 10), Arduino Mega (ATmega2560 microcontroller; clock speed: $16\,MHz$; flash memory: $256\,Kb$; analog I/O pins: 14; digital I/O pins: 54), gooseneck mobile phone holder, and USB-A to USB-B cable were procured from the online store (Amazon Pvt. Ltd., India). Linear motion ball bearings (inner diameter: $6\,mm$), brass shaft couplers (for shaft diameter: $6\,mm$), HDMI to micro-HDMI (HDMI Version 1.4) cable, Multiturn precision potentiometer ($1\,k\Omega$), Raspberry Pi 4 Model B (RBP; 64-bit; $1.4\,GHz$ Quadcore ARM processor; $2\,GB$ RAM), switched-mode power supply (SMPS; $12\,V$–$10\,A$), Step-down dual USB output power supply module (input: 6–$40\,V$; output: $5\,V$–$3\,A$), USB-A to USB-C wire with ON/OFF button ($3\,A$–$5\,V$), Single pole double throw AC switch ($250\,V$–$10\,A$), RepRap Arduino Mega Polulu Shield (RAMPS; Version: 1.4), Analog dual-axis breakout joystick modules, NEMA17 stepper motors (4 lead hybrid motor; holding torque: $0.412\,Nm$; step angle: 1.8 degree; current: $1.2\,A$ per phase), DRV8825 stepper motor drivers and NEMA17 mounting brackets were procured from the "Robu.in" online store. Flanged type linear motion ball bearings ($6\,mm$ inner diameter) and self-drilling screws (diameter: $3.5\,mm$) were procured from the "IndiaLocalShop.com," an online store. Peripheral devices like the mouse (Logitech M90; Wired), keyboard (Logitech K480; Bluetooth), an LCD screen (Sony Bravia Full HD TV), required for the functioning of the RBP, were procured from the local market. Color laser printer (HP; wireless) was procured from a local computer supplies shop. Linux-based RBP OS (Version 1.4) was downloaded from raspberrypi.org. Python programming language (Version: 3.8.5), PyQt5 libraries, Qt Designer application, OpenCV libraries, Arduino IDE application, and their respective dependencies were downloaded from websites, namely, "python.org," "pypi.org," "build-system.fman.io," "opencv.org," and "Arduino.cc."

3.2 Development of the microscope

The proposed microscope has been made up of five assemblies, namely, sample magnification and imaging assembly (SMIA), sample illuminator assembly (SIA), filter holder assembly

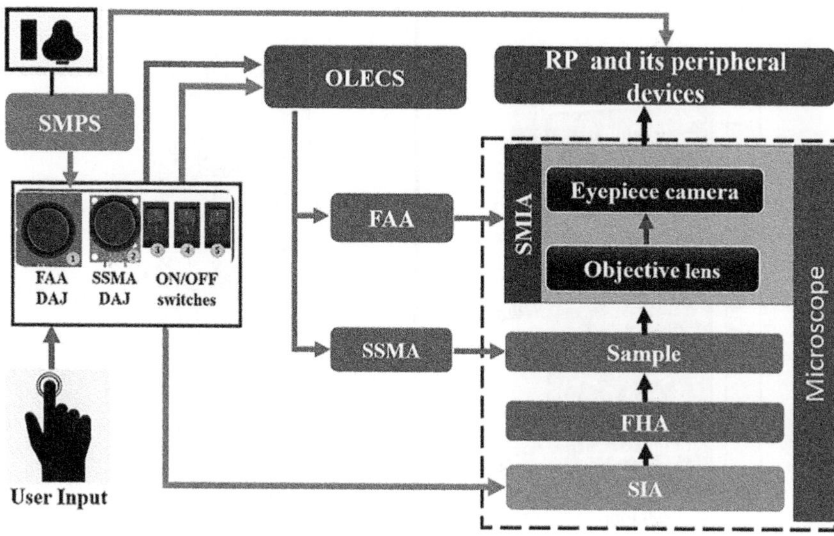

Fig. 1 Block diagram depicting the working of the proposed microscope constructed using five assemblies.

(FHA), focus adjustment assembly (FAA), and lastly, sample stage movement assembly (SSMA). All the five assemblies work in tandem with each other for the effective functioning of the microscope. Fig. 1 illustrates the block diagram depicting the working of the proposed microscope constructed using the five assemblies.

3.2.1 The sample magnification and imaging assembly (SMIA)

The SMIA of the proposed microscope comprises primarily of four elements, namely, objective lens (OL), microscope eyepiece camera (MEC), single-chip computer (Raspberry Pi; RP) with the peripheral devices, and finite-length rectangular lens housing (FLH). Fig. 2 illustrates the schematic diagrams of different parts of the SMIA. In the proposed microscope, the sample magnification is carried out using the OL (magnification: $10\times$; numerical aperture: 0.25; generic DIN semiplan achromatic; India). The magnified sample image was captured using a MEC, located at 160 mm from OL. The FLH, using 6 mm blackened plywood sheets, was used for housing the OL and the MEC in an optically aligned manner.

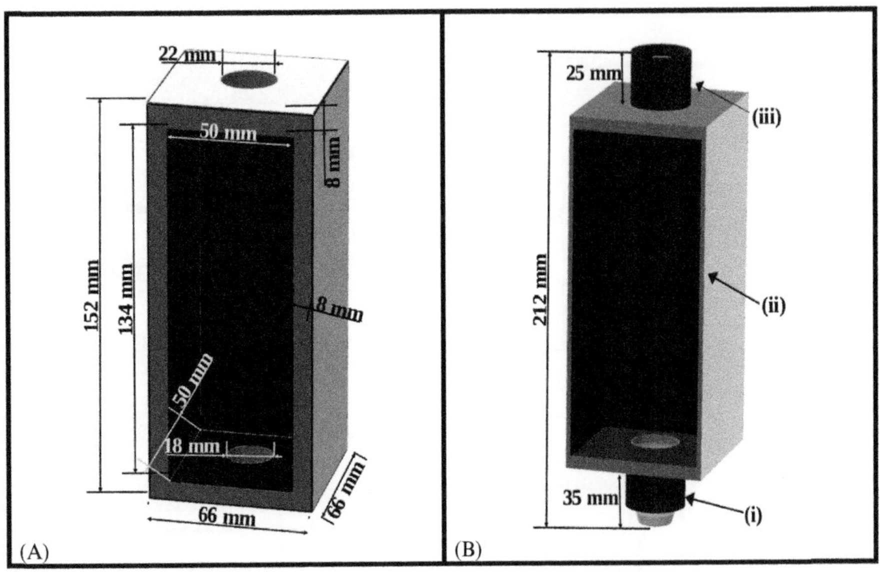

Fig. 2 Schematic diagram of different parts of the sample magnification and imaging assembly. (A) Finite-length rectangular lens housing (FLH) and (B) cross-sectional view of the magnification and imaging assembly. (i) The objective lens, (ii) FLH, and (iii) the microscope eyepiece camera (MEC).

3.2.2 The sample illuminator assembly (SIA)

The SIA of the proposed microscope encompasses a white LED (1-W; 3.3 V; 350 mA) with an aluminum heat sink in a cuboid-shaped antireflective black enclosure (Fig. 3A). The top of the SIA's enclosure was covered using a white translucent diffuser (40 mm × 30 mm × 1 mm; material: plastic sheet from a white container) to generate soft white light (Fig. 3B). The power supply circuit that was used to power the SIA is shown in Fig. 3C. A precision potentiometer was employed within the power supply unit to control the illumination intensity of the SIA.

3.2.3 The filter holder assembly (FHA)

An FHA was developed and placed over the SIA. The FHA was designed as a two-slot enclosure wherein two optical filters could be stacked to give a combined visual effect (Fig. 4A). The bottom filter slot (48 mm × 43 mm × 6 mm) was designed to house oblique illumination and polarization filters. In contrast, the upper filter slot (44 mm × 37 mm × 2 mm) was designed for either a dark field or Rheinberg illumination filter. Each filter slot consisted of a circular hole (Ø: 28 mm) at its center, which allows the light from the SIA to transmit to the light condenser (LC; Abbe condenser type;

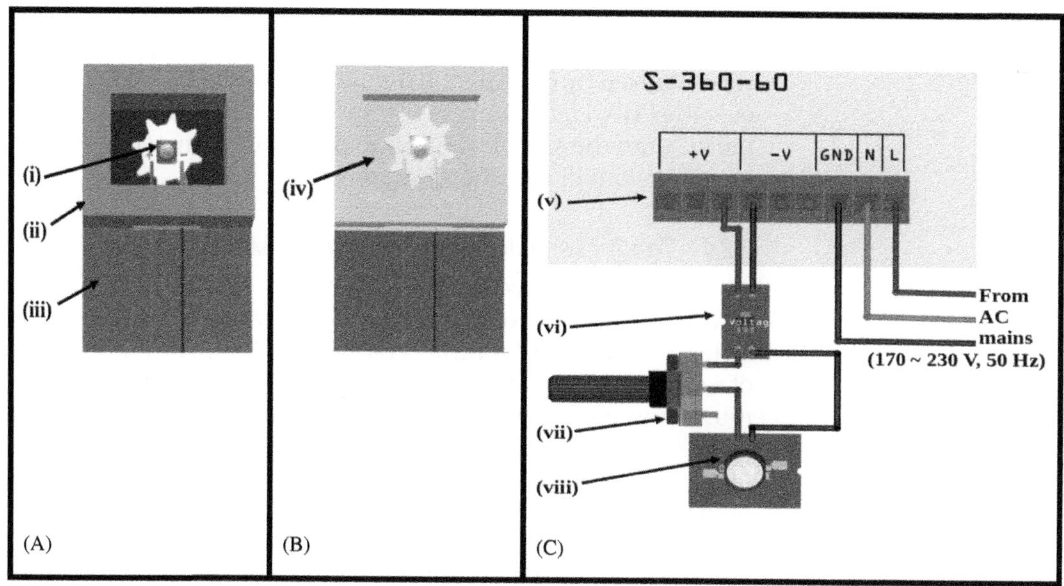

Fig. 3 Schematic diagram of different parts of the sample illuminator assembly. (A) The internal construction of sample illuminator's enclosure, (B) pictorial representation of sample illuminator with the diffuser, and (C) power supply circuit of the LED illumination system. (i) 1-W LED with aluminum heat sink, (ii) cuboid-shaped antireflective black enclosure, (iii) base plate, (iv) white translucent plastic diffuser, (v) SMPS (230 V AC to 12 V–10 A DC) supplying power to the microscope's electronic modules, (vi) CA-1235 adjustable power module supplying power to LED (3.3 V–350 mA), (vii) multiturn precision potentiometer (0–1 kΩ), and (viii) 1-W LED.

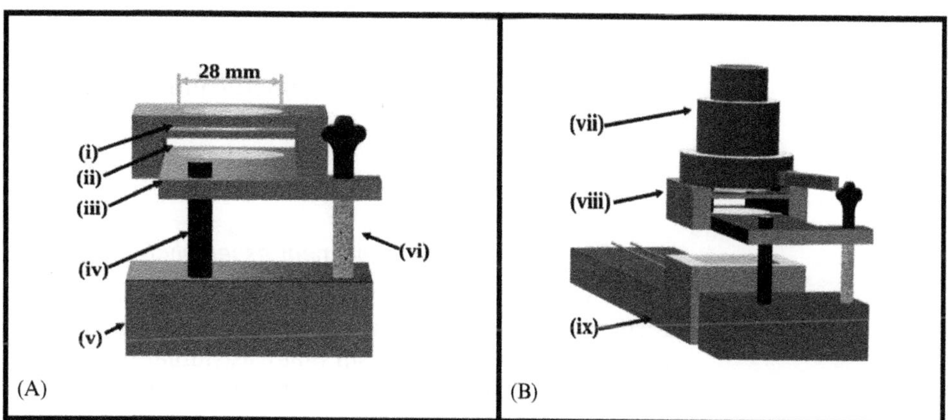

Fig. 4 Pictorial representation of FHA and its integration with SIA. (A) FHA and (B) figure depicting the integrated system formed after integrating SIA, FHA, and the LC. (i) upper filter slot for dark-field and Rheinberg filters, (ii) lower filter slot for oblique illumination and polarization filters, (iii) filter holding enclosure, (iv) stainless steel support rod (thickness: 6 mm) for filter holder assembly's height adjustment, (v) support block of filter holder assembly, (vi) stainless steel threaded rod (thickness: 6 mm) for filter holder assembly's height adjustment, (vii) the LC, (viii) the FHA, and (ix) the SIA.

numerical aperture: 1.25) of the microscope. A provision to adjust the height of the FHA was also included (Fig. 4A). This adjustment was achieved by rotating the threaded rod. The LC was then fixed over the FHA. Light from the FH was then gathered and focused by the LC onto the sample. Fig. 4B depicts the 3D image of the integrated system of the SIA, FHA, and LC.

3.2.4 The focus adjustment assembly (FAA)

An FAA was developed to carry out the focus adjustment (Z-axis movement) operation of the SMIA. Fig. 5 illustrates the schematic diagrams of various parts of the FAA. The FAA consisted of a specially designed unit named the general electromechanical movement module (GEMM). As mentioned earlier, the unit's primary function was to generate movement in a specific axis (z-axis), which is necessary for focusing the microscopic image onto the SMIA (Fig. 5A). The GEMM unit generates the movement using a mechanical movement apparatus (MMA; Fig. 5B). The SMIA was attached to MMA's holding block using screws (Fig. 5C). The upward and downward movements of SMIA were achieved by rotating the free end of the MMA's threaded rod using a stepper motor either in the clockwise or anticlockwise direction. Herein, the distance and direction of the movement were controlled using a specially designed open-loop electrical control system (OLECS; Fig. 5D). A dual-axis joystick module (DAJ) was used to acquire the user input, which was then processed using a microcontroller to control the movement of the SMIA. The microcontroller generates the control signals for initiating movements in the stepper motor through the motor driver module (DRV8825). The communication between the microcontroller, stepper motor, and motor driver module was established using the Reprap Arduino Mega Pololu Shield (RAMPS). The metrics of the movement of the SMIA have been summarized in Table 1.

3.2.5 The sample stage movement assembly (SSMA)

The SSMA was developed to move the sample in X and Y directions. The bi-directional movement of the SSMA was achieved using a movement mechanism that was similar to FAA. The SSMA was comprised of two GEMM units and a circular sample stage. Fig. 6 illustrates the schematic diagrams that represent various parts of the SSMA. The circular sample stage had a central circular window ($\emptyset = 40\,mm$). The two GEMM units of SSMA were perpendicularly stacked on each other in a horizontal orientation to the microscope's base plate. Subsequently, the circular sample stage was attached to the top GEMM unit using adhesive (Fig. 6A). In this

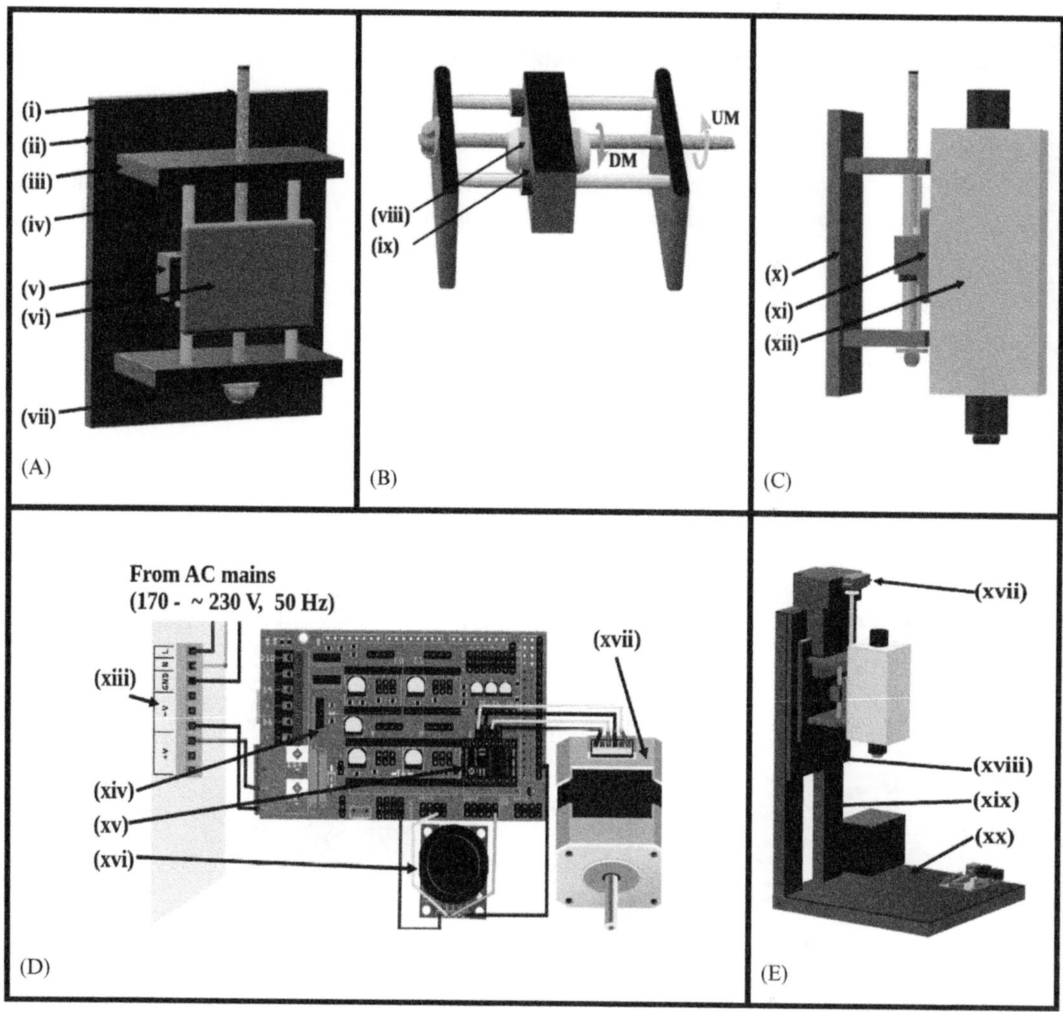

Fig. 5 Schematic diagrams of various parts employed in the FAA's construction. (A) The FAA, (B) MMA in GEMM unit of FAA, (C) side view of SMIA attachment to FAA, (D) OLECS employed for producing movements in FAA, and (E) SMIA-FAA-OLECS integrated setup. (i) Threaded stainless steel rod ($\emptyset = 6$ mm), (ii) back support plate, (iii) GEMM support plates, (iv) smooth stainless steel rods ($\emptyset = 6$ mm), (v) holding block (thickness: 22 mm) of GEMM, (vi) SMIA attachment plate, (vii) brass stopper, (viii) flanged brass nut inserts ($\emptyset = 6$ mm), (ix) linear motion ball bearings ($\emptyset = 6$ mm), (x) the FAA, (xi) SMIA attachment plate, (xii) the SMIA, (xiii) SMPS of OLECS, (xiv) RAMPS+AM unit, (xv) DRV8825 stepper motor driver, (xvi) DAJ, (xvii) stepper motor coupled to MMA's threaded rod, (xviii) back support assembly of the FAA, (xix) support beams for holding FAA, and (xx) microscope base plate.

setup, the bidirectional movement of the SSMA's sample stage was controlled using two stepper motors and the OLECS. The OLECS setup used in SMIA's movement control was modified to control the movements of the sample stage with the inclusion of additional

Table 1 The metrics of the movement of SMIA according to user input acquired from the DAJ.

DAJ movement	Movement type	Motor shaft movement direction	SMIA movement direction	Approximate distance moved per stroke (μm)
Upward	Coarse	Clockwise	Upward	125
Downward	Coarse	Anticlockwise	Downward	125
Right	Fine	Clockwise	Upward	3.125
Left	Fine	Anticlockwise	Downward	3.125

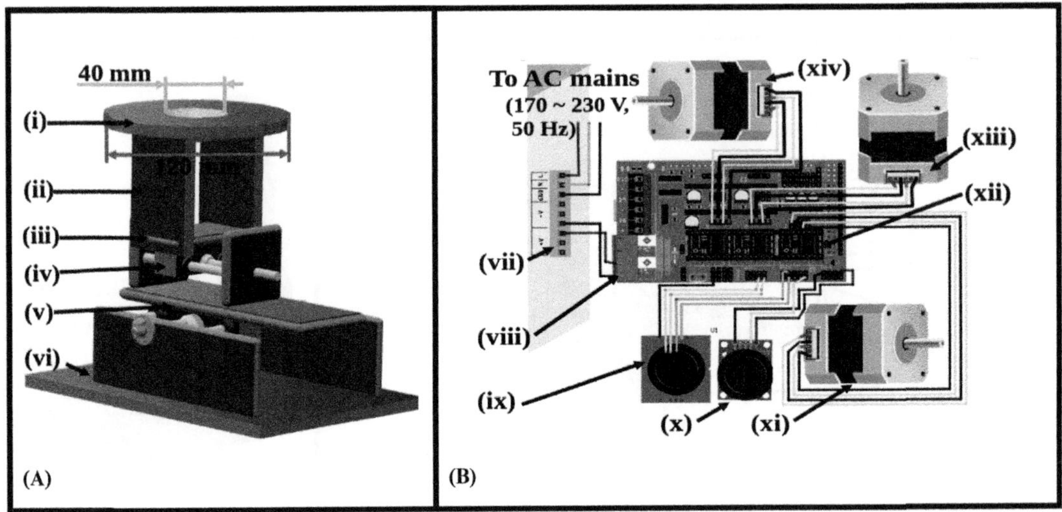

Fig. 6 Schematic diagram of various parts of SSMA. (A) The SSMA unit and (B) OLECS controlling the SSMA-FAA integrated setup. (i) Sample stage, (ii) sample stage support plates, (iii) top plate of Y-axis GEMM unit, (iv) Y-axis GEMM unit, (v) top plate of X-axis GEMM unit, (vi) SSMA base plate, (vii) SMPS supplying power to components of OLECS, (viii) AM+RAMPS control unit, (ix) DAJ of SSMA, (x) DAJ of FAA, (xi) stepper motor of the FFA, (xii) DRV8825 drivers, (xiii) stepper motor of the X-axis GEMM unit in SSMA, and (xiv) stepper motor of the Y-axis GEMM unit in SSMA.

hardware components (Fig. 6B). The components included an additional DAJ and two more DRV8825 motor drivers that helped control the sample stage's movements. The modified OLECS acquired the user input through the additional DAJ associated with SSMA movements and accordingly generates sample stage movements in positive or negative X and Y axes. The metrics of the sample stage movement have been summarized in Table 2. Fig. 7 illustrates

Table 2 The SSMA's sample stage movement metrics according to user input acquired from the DAJ.

DAJ movement	Motor shaft movement direction	Sample stage movement direction	Distance moved per stroke (μm)
Upward	Clockwise	Positive Y-axis	156.25
Downward	Anticlockwise	Negative Y-axis	156.25
Left	Anticlockwise	Negative X-axis	156.25
Right	Clockwise	Positive X-axis	156.25

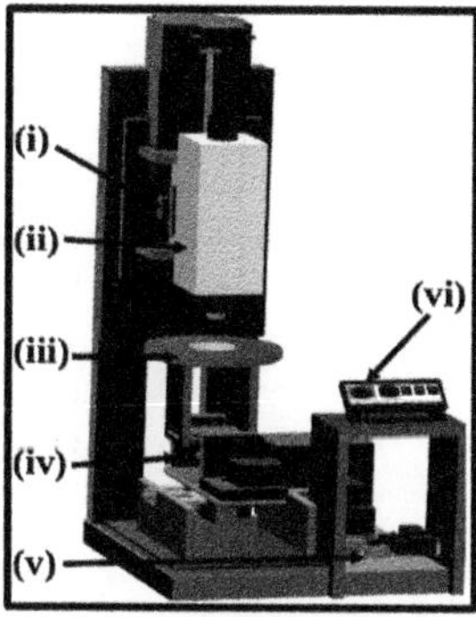

Fig. 7 Schematic representation of the setup obtained after integrating SMIA, FAA, SSMA, and the OLECS. (i) FAA, (ii) SMIA, (iii) circular sample stage, (iv) combined bi-directional movement unit of SSMA, (v) OLECS, and (vi) control panel housing the two DAJ's associated with movements in FAA and SSMA.

the schematic diagram of the setup obtained after integrating the SMIA, FAA, SSMA, and the modified OLECS.

3.3 Development of the optical filter set of the microscope

The optical filter set employed in the microscope's FHA filter slots consisted of four different filters, namely, dark field illumination filter (DF/DI), Rheinberg illumination filters (RF/RI), oblique illumination filter (OF/OI), and polarization illumination filter (PF/PI). Fig. 8 illustrates the properties of the filter set that were developed for the proposed microscope. The DF and RF were meant to be placed in the upper filter slot. Hence, the design

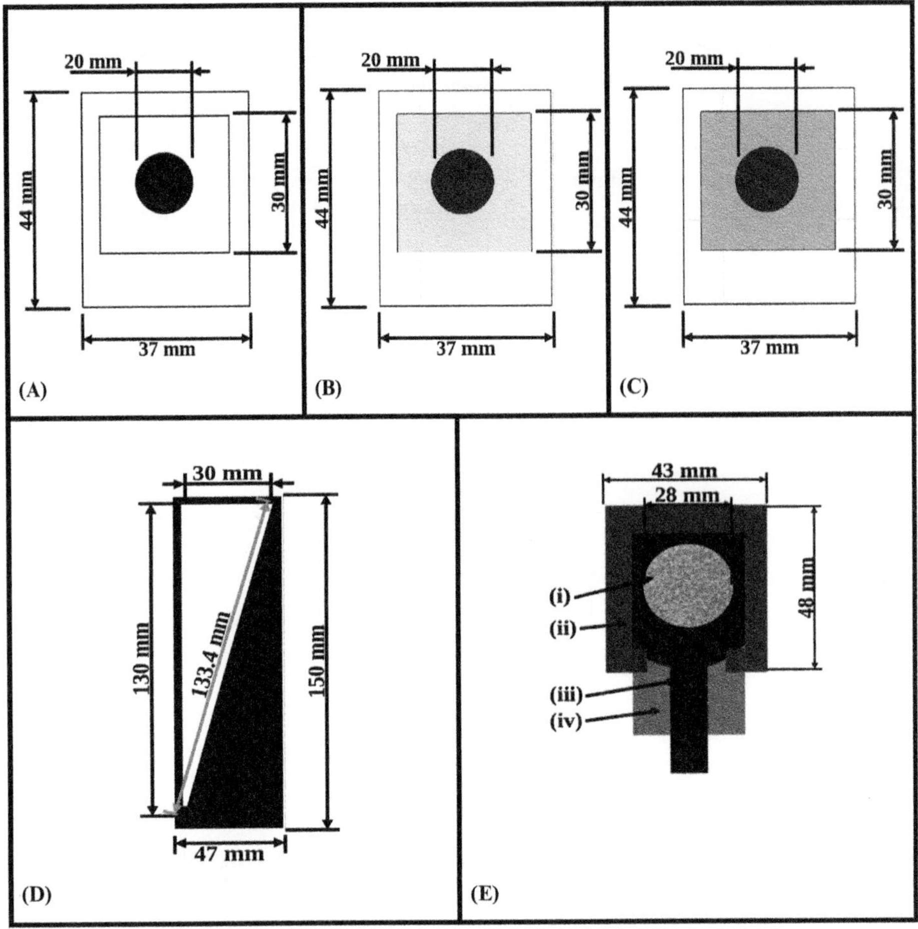

Fig. 8 Schematic representation of the filter set developed for the proposed microscope with their dimensions. (A) DF, (B) RF 1 (circle: *blue* (dark gray in the print version); square: *yellow* (gray in the print version)), (C) RF 2 (circle: *blue* (dark gray in the print version); square: *green* (gray in the print version)), (D) OF, and (E) PF. (i) Circularly cut polarization film, (ii) square-shaped sleeve black paper sleeve, (iii) rectangular arm to rotate the polarization film, and (iv) cuboidal-shaped enclosure base plate. (For interpretation of the references to color in this figure legend, the reader is referred to the web version of this article.)

and dimension of these filters were maintained according to the dimension of the upper filter slot. These two filters were designed using QCAD 2D design and drafting software (Version). The DF consisted of a black circle (Ø: 14 mm) centered within a transparent square (side: 30 mm). The RF set consisted of two filters RF1 and RF2, of the same dimensions as the DF. However, the color combinations within and outside the circular area differed (RF1: blue and green; RF2: blue and yellow). These designed files were then printed on overhead projector sheets (thickness: 0.1 mm) using an HP laser color printer (Fig. 8A–C), which were then cut out as per the required dimensions. The filters were then developed by stacking two pieces of each cut-out.

The OF and PF were meant to be placed in the bottom filter slot of FHA. The OF was constructed using a rectangle-shaped FR4 copper clad board (150 mm × 47 mm × 1.5 mm) coated with matte-black paint. A provision to pass light through OF was made using a window (side 1: 130 mm; side 2: 30 mm; hypotenuse: 133.4 mm) in the shape of a right-angled triangle on the OF (Fig. 8D). Lastly, the PF (47.5 mm × 42.5 mm × 5.5 mm) was constructed using a cuboid-shaped blackened foam sheet enclosure (thickness: 4 mm) and linear polarizer film. The PF had a central circular window (28 mm). A square-shaped black paper sleeve (side: 40 mm; thickness: 1.5) was attached on top of the cuboidal enclosure of PF to securely hold the polarizer film directly on its central circular window. Then, a circularly cut polarization film (Ø: 30 mm) attached to a rectangular arm (10 mm × 30 mm × 2 mm; material: black cardboard) was inserted into the square-shaped sleeve. The rectangular arm was meant to help the polarization film to rotate freely inside the sleeve by an angle of 55° in both clockwise and anticlockwise directions from its central position (Fig. 8E).

3.4 Development of the software

The proposed microscope uses two custom-developed software: "Hi-Conf Movement Regulator" and "Hi-Conf Microscope Visualizer v1.0." The "Hi-Conf Movement Regulator" was developed in Arduino IDE using C++ programming language, while the "Hi-Conf Microscope Visualizer v1.0" was created using the python programming language. The "Hi-Conf Movement Regulator" was designed to control the SMIA's focus adjustment and bi-directional sample movements (X- and Y-axes) in the microscope. This software acquires the user input from the dual-axis joystick modules present on the microscope's control panel. Based on the user input, the software evaluates the position to which the movement assemblies are to be moved. Further, it directs the stepper motors to turn their shafts in either clockwise or anticlockwise directions. The flowchart depicting the sequence of events that take place during the process is represented in Fig. 9.

The "Hi-Conf Microscope Visualizer v1.0" is an interactive GUI application that was developed for the visualization of the camera feed and also for image acquisition. Various tools and libraries such as "QT Designer," and "PyQt5" GUI development library

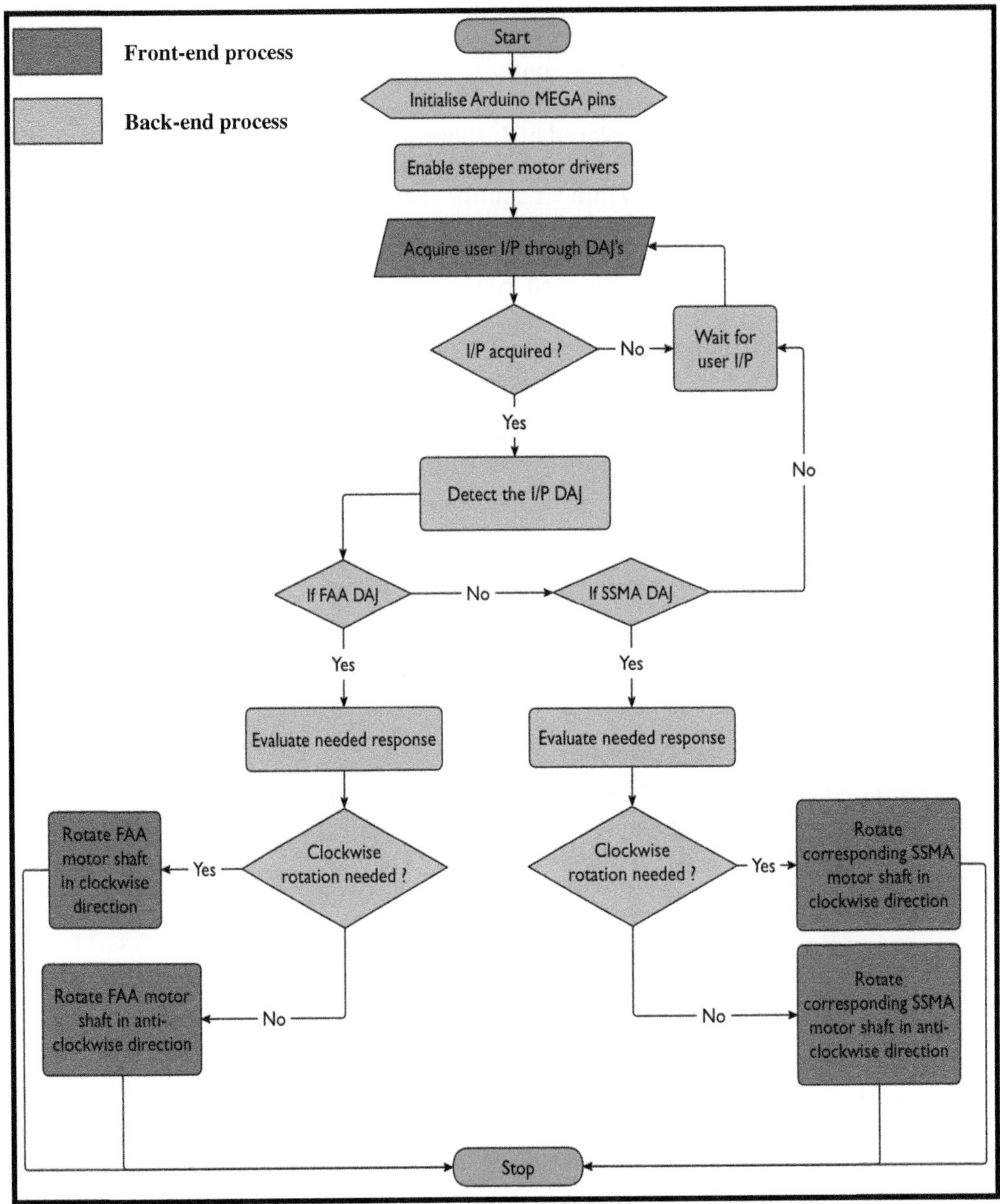

Fig. 9 Process flowchart of the "Hi-Conf Movement Regulator."

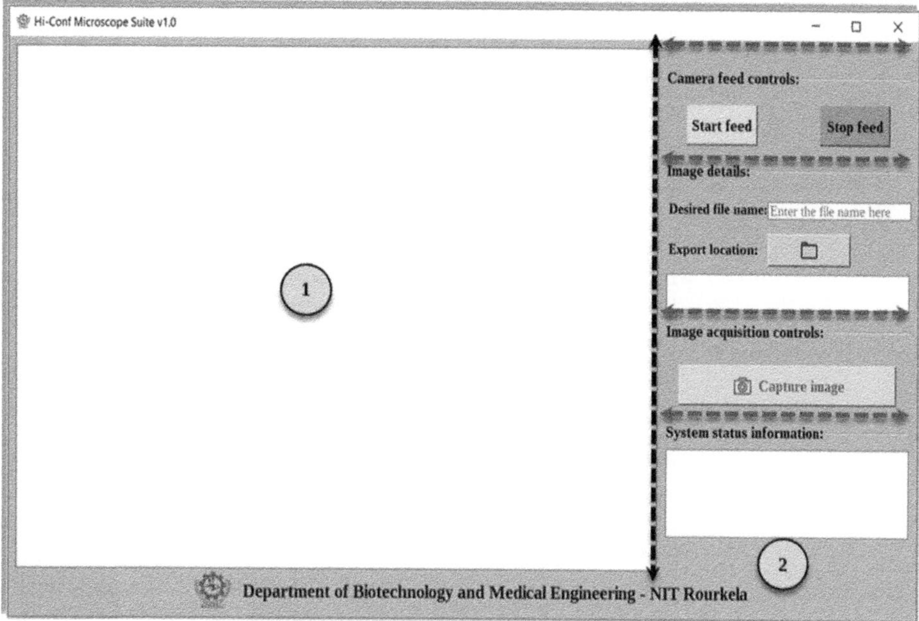

Fig. 10 Graphical user interface of the "Hi-Conf Microscope Visualizer v1.0" software and its components. (1) Camera feed visualizing panel and (2) control panel designed for performing operations like starting or stopping the camera feed and capture images.

"OpenCV" were utilized for the development of "Hi-Conf Microscope Visualizer v1.0." The software consisted of a main window divided into two vertical sections, one on the right side and the other on the left side. The left-side section embedded the camera feed visualizing panel, whereas the right-side section was further divided into four horizontal subsections, as represented in Fig. 10. Herein, each subsection is dedicated to performing a particular function. The camera feed controls section houses the "Start feed" and "Stop feed" control buttons, which activates or deactivates the camera feed visualization panel on the left side of the GUI. The image details section was designed to save the image as per the user's requirement. This section asks the user to input the desired file name and the location of the destination file where the image is to be stored. The image acquisition control section houses the "Capture image" button, which signals the RBP to capture and store the frame shown in the camera feed visualization panel at the selected location. The system status information section displays the state of the camera feed visualization panel. This section displays the camera feed starting and stopping notification based on the user input acquired from the camera feed control section. The process flowchart of the software is depicted in Fig. 11.

3.5 Testing of the developed microscope

The functionality of the proposed device was tested by analyzing a diverse range of sample specimens. These samples include microbes and milk proteins from curd, melted dairy milk chocolate, cultured wastewater microbes, and oleogel. The details of the method followed during the sample preparation for each specimen are discussed below.

3.5.1 Microbes and milk protein

The observation slide of the curd was prepared by adding a drop of diluted curd (curd: water ratio of 1:10) over the glass slide. A drop of dilute methylene blue solution was then added over the glass slide and mixed gently for 10 s. The mixture was then covered with a coverslip and was subsequently observed under the microscope.

3.5.2 Melted chocolate

The milk chocolate was melted at a constant temperature of 70 °C in the water bath. A drop of the molten milk chocolate was transferred over the glass slide with the help of a toothpick. A coverslip was then placed over the molten chocolate drop, evenly spreading the molten chocolate into a thin layer. The slide was then observed under the microscope.

3.5.3 Wastewater cultured microbes

Wastewater was collected from the drain pipe of the hostel area. The pH and temperature of the wastewater were measured before further use. An additional step for enriching ethanol-resistant bacteria was performed in the minimal salt media (MSM) using a previously discussed method [21]. The culture was maintained at 30 °C for a week at 150 rotations min^{-1}. The sample was serially diluted to 10^{-12} and spread onto the plates of MSM. The bacterial colony was gained by performing quadrant streaking. A smear of the microbial sample was dried, and heat fixation was performed to adhere the bacteria on the slide. A coverslip was placed at the heat-fixed area on the glass slide and was subsequently observed under the microscope.

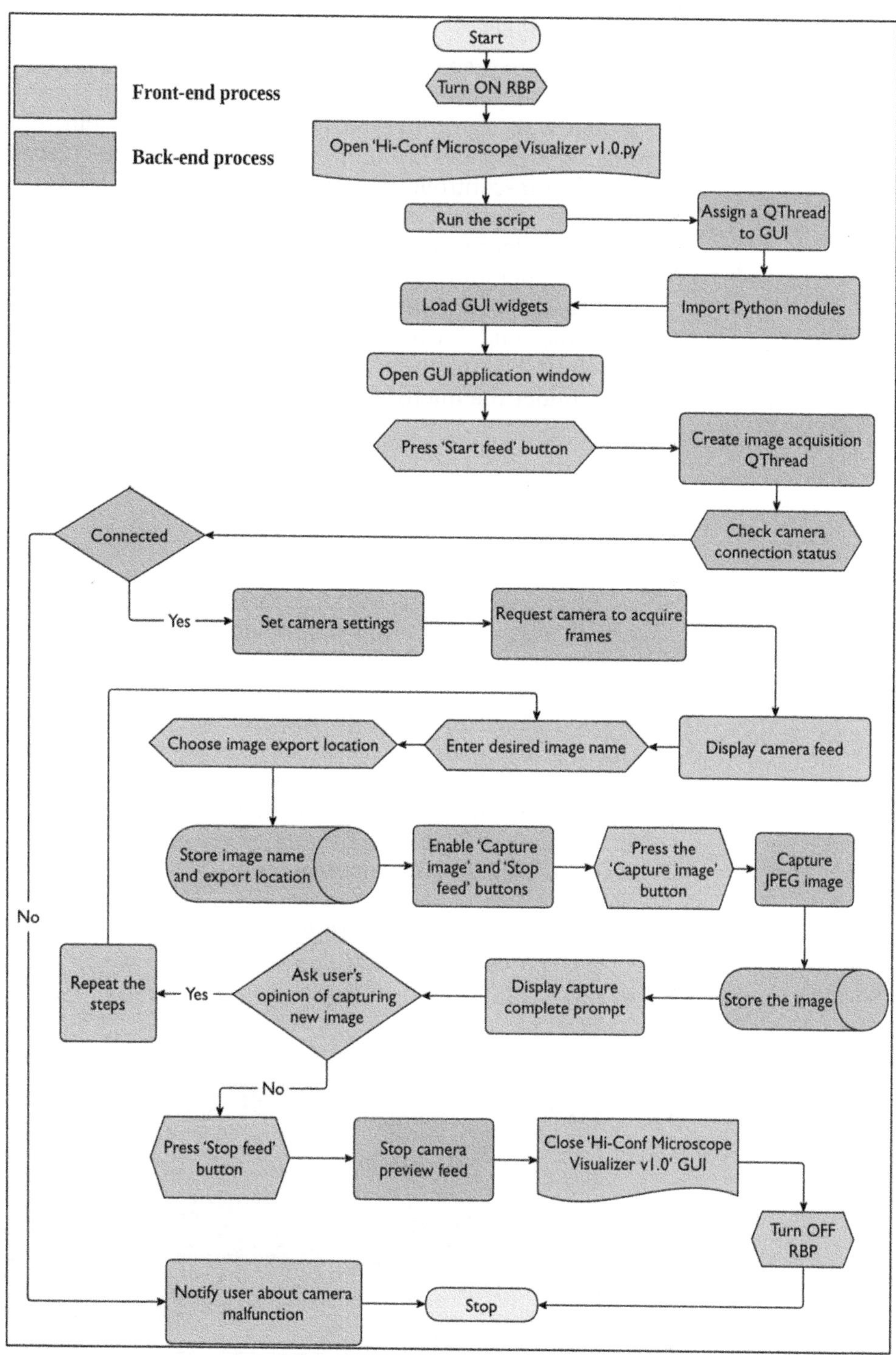

Fig. 11 Process flowchart of the "Hi-Conf Microscope Visualizer v1.0."

3.5.4 Oleogels

In order to prepare a 5% (w/w) oleogel, sunflower wax (1 g) was added to sunflower oil (14 g). Further, the mixture was supplemented with 5 g of 0.1% SPAN-80 (in sunflower oil) to achieve 5 mg of emulsifier content. This mixture was placed in a temperature-controlled water bath (80 °C) until the wax and the emulsifier dissolved in the oil to form a clear homogenous solution. This clear solution was then kept in a thermal cabinet at room temperature (25 °C) for 30 min to induce gelation. For microscopy, a small amount of molten oleogel was held on the glass side, and further, a coverslip was placed over for even spreading. The micro-arrangement in the oleogel was then visualized under the microscope.

4. Results and discussion

4.1 Development of the microscope

The proposed microscopic device is an integration of hardware and software units. The fully functional prototype of the proposed microscope after integrating all the five assemblies is depicted in Fig. 12. High-strength construction materials (e.g., marine-grade plywood sheet and high-quality adhesive) were used for constructing the prototype device to increase stability and robustness. Additionally, a matte-black sticker was adhered to the microscope structure's inner side to minimize the internal reflection of the light. The current prototype was made with plywood, which may absorb moisture from the atmosphere. Hence, a tight

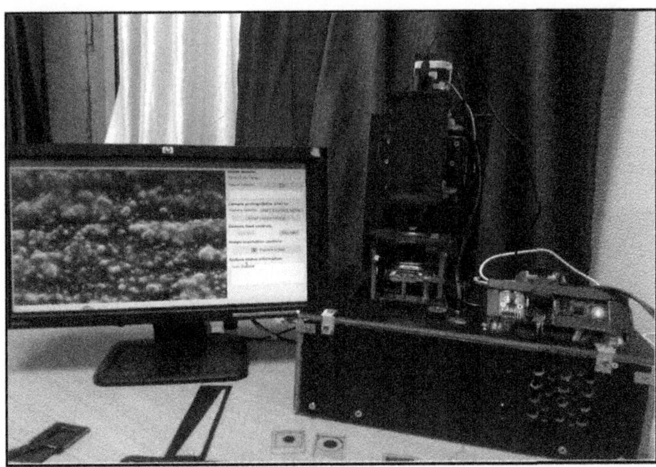

Fig. 12 The final prototype of the proposed microscope.

metallic enclosure will be considered as a replacement for plywood in our future development. The integration of OL, MEC, RBP with the peripheral devices and FLH in SMIA has resulted in a seamless optical path setup and enabled the device to perform digital microphotography.

Further, the illumination setup helped the proposed device generate controlled illumination for a wide variety of samples. The FHA unit has enabled the microscope to use multiple optical filters independently or as a combination of two per user requirements. The visual filter set developed for the prototype microscope comprises four different filters, as shown in Fig. 13. The clear transparent plastic film used in constructing the dark fields and Rheinberg illumination filters helped reduce the design cost.

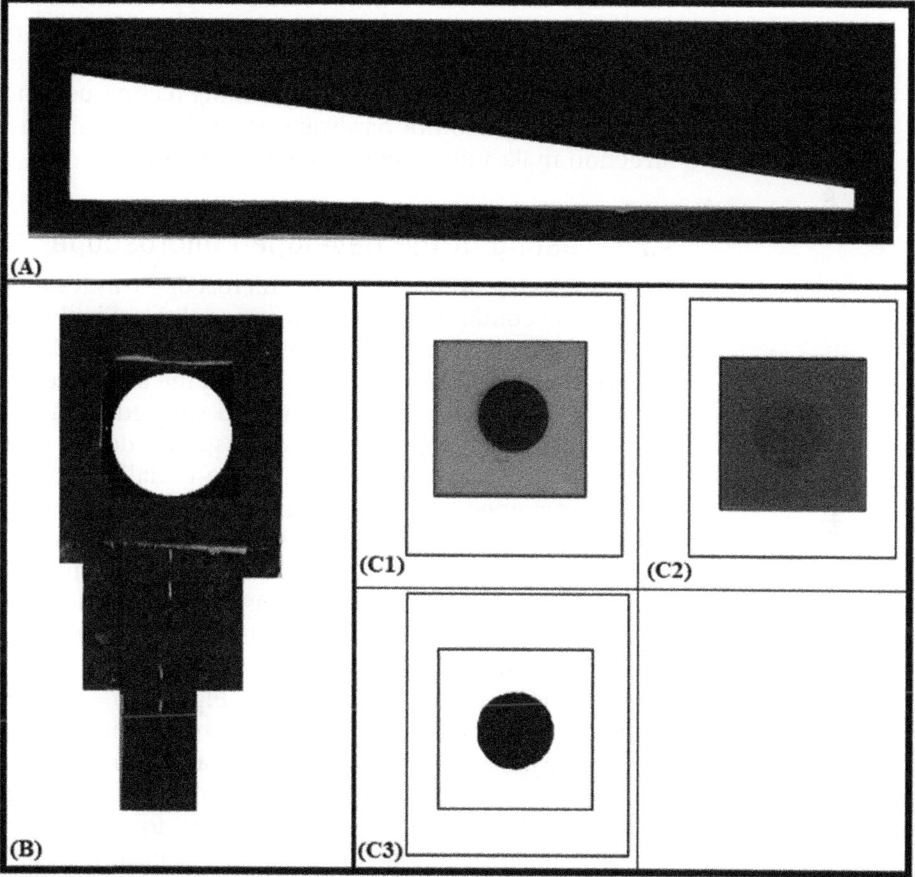

Fig. 13 The optical filter set of the proposed microscope (A) oblique illumination filter, (B) polarization filter, and (C) filter set (RF1, RF2, and DF).

Also, it ensured fast and easy replacement in case of loss or damage to the filters. The smooth working of the stepper motors, used for the movement of the stage, ensured the acquisition of blur-free digital images. Also, using a control panel (OLECS) containing two joystick modules (with separate ON/OFF switches) made the exploration of the sample microstructure an easy task. In the future, motors having lower steps per rotation will be employed to achieve better performance.

The software applications developed for the prototype device were working parallelly without any significant lag when tested. The "Hi-Conf Movement regulator" runs on the Arduino MEGA R3, whereas the "Hi-Conf Microscope Visualizer v1.0" runs on the RBP. During the working of the proposed system, no evidence of interference was noticed. Since the "Hi-Conf Microscope visualizer" is associated with a series of operations, a few seconds of lag while opening the GUI is observed compared to the time for opening the "Hi-Conf Movement Regulator." This issue can be resolved by employing suitable threading techniques. Inclusively, the tight integration of hardware and software units in the construction makes the system reliable and efficient.

4.2 Testing of the developed microscope

The working of the prototype microscope was tested in all the 12 possible combinatorial imaging modalities. Firstly, the microscope was tested using the stained dilute curd sample to observe milk proteins and bacteria. After testing the slide under different modes, the resultant images obtained showed variations in the visible structures' appearance, contrast, and depth. The BI (Fig. 14A) although was able to assist in the visualization of proteins and a few stained microbes (marked yellow); however, the image had limited contrast with poor resolution. The OI (Fig. 14B) of the same sample had better contrast and resolution along with few 3D depths. Since the illumination was not uniform, the obtained image showed variation in the contrast across the micrograph. The absence of fats in the sample did not significantly improve images' visualization through PI (Fig. 14C). DI (Fig. 14D) improved the contrast of the visible bright proteins from the background, which was dark. Though the images were of high contrast due to the oblique projection of light onto the sample, the protein structures looked more planer due to the absence of 3-dimensional depths as in OI. At the same time, the visibility of the stained microbes was also reduced in DI. The images with the DI+OI (Fig. 14E) modality were less bright and lower in contrast than the DI. The curd sample was also looked at under RI

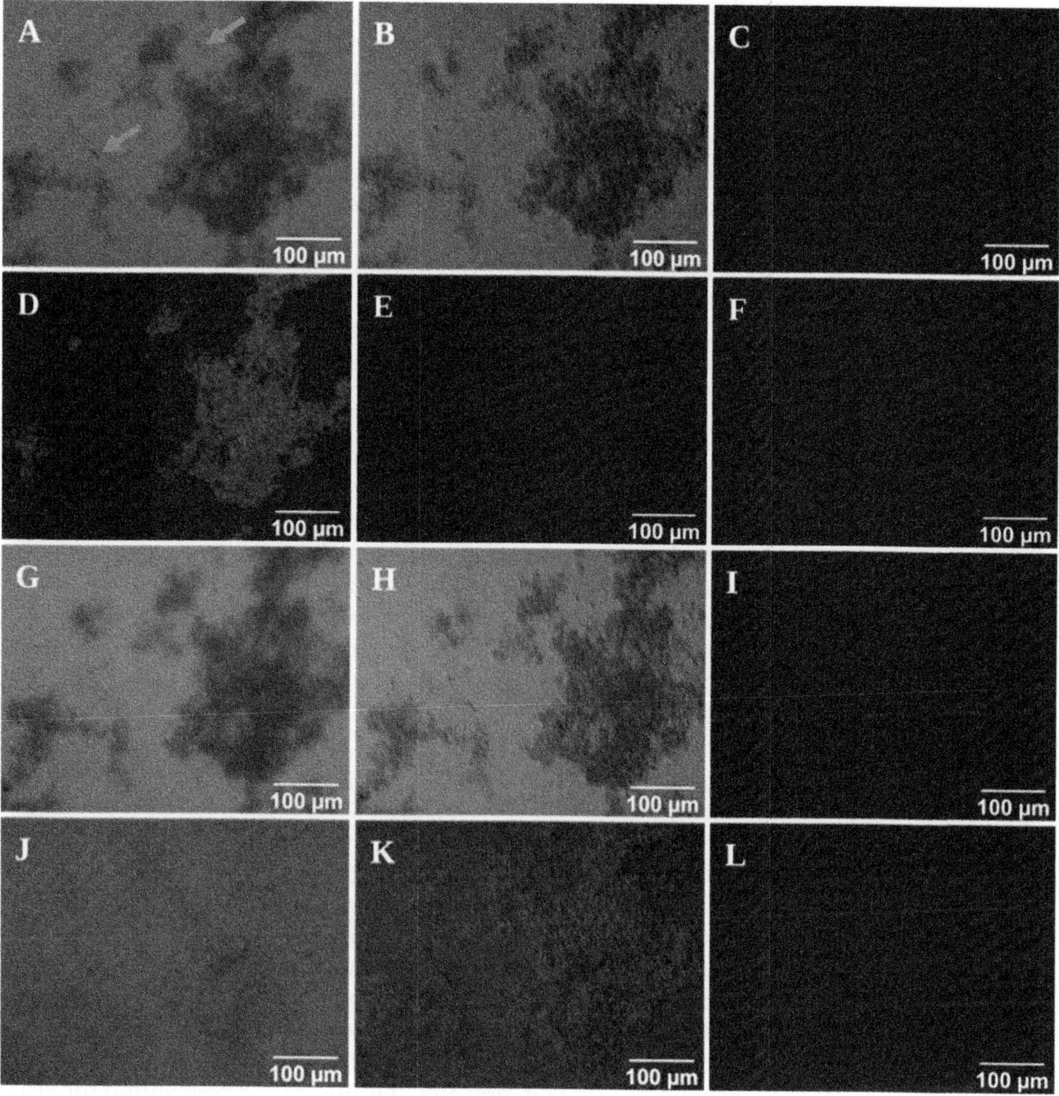

Fig. 14 Resultant magnified images of the curd sample taken by the microscope in 12 different imaging modalities. (A) BI, (B) OI, (C) PI, (D) DI, (E) DI+OI, (F) DI+PI, (G) RI1, (H) RI1+OI, (I) RI1+PI, (J) RI2, (K) RI2+OI, and (L) RI2+PI (BI: bright field illumination, OI: oblique illumination).

filters. The use of RI filters helped to assign a color to the foreground and the background. It was observed that the selection of a combination of colors for the RF is crucial to get images with better contrast, as evident from the micrographs. The individual and combinatorial modes used in RI2 (yellow annulus) showed better contrast and brightness images than RI1 (green annulus). The closeness between the green and blue RF in terms of their hue values can be the reason behind the poor contrast between the structures and the background (Fig. 14G and H). The RI2 (Fig. 14J) showed the protein structures, but the resolution was unclear. However, combining it with OI provided better clarity and contrast to the microscopic structures (Fig. 14K). The results demonstrate that DI, OI, and RI2+OI modes are best suited for visualizing the milk proteins and microbes such as lactobacillus within the curd samples.

After that, the microscope was tested with melted chocolate placed on a slide and covered with a coverslip (Fig. 15). Chocolates are regarded as suspensions that are made using varying components like sugar, cocoa particle, and cocoa butter [22]. Some chocolates may contain a certain amount of milk. The BI (Fig. 15A) displayed uniform grooves (marked in orange) like arrangements on a continuous phase. Unfortunately, the contrast was quite limited. A better resolution and depths of the grooves were visible under the OI (Fig. 15B). Interestingly, the PI (Fig. 15C) revealed the best picture of the arrangement of different constituents of the chocolate. The white sugar crystals (marked in pink) are distributed in the continuous fat phase. The dark fragments are of the cocoa particles as observed through the PI. The DI alone and in combination with OI (Fig. 15D and E) was insufficient to reveal much information from the sample. The possible reason can be the poor contrast developed between the constituents and the background. The micro-arrangement within the chocolates was better visualized with DI+PI (Fig. 15F) than other DI modalities. Regrettably, the image's brightness was significantly lower than PI. Both colored filters used in RI and an oblique projection of light (Fig. 15H and K) enhanced the overall appearance of the obtained images in terms of color and brightness compared to BI. The effect of PI in combination with RI caused a decreased brightness of fat and sugar crystals. It is imperative to conclude that the microscope's PI, RI1+OI, and RI2+OI modes are best suited for visualizing the samples containing milk proteins, fats, and crystalline substances.

The microscope was further used to test a slide prepared from the cultured wastewater microbes. The resultant images obtained after testing the slide are shown in Fig. 16. As observed, BI (Fig. 16A) failed to locate microbes. However, the OI (Fig. 16B) displayed an array of microbes with 3-dimensional depth and better resolution. Nevertheless, the contrast was found nonuniform due to variation in the illumination. The absence of fat structures showed no significant betterment in visualizing the samples

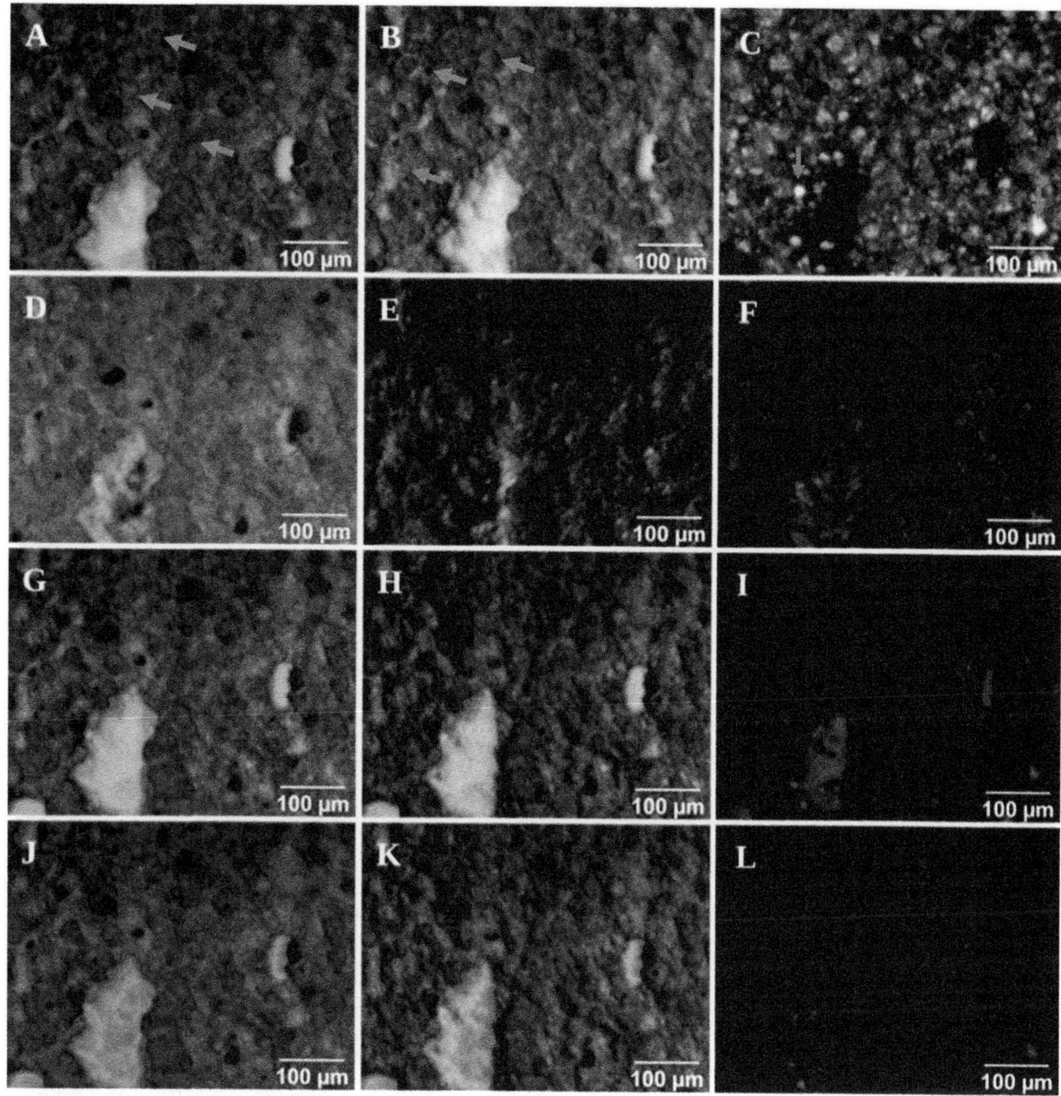

Fig. 15 Resultant magnified images of the melted dairy milk sample taken by the microscope in 12 different imaging modalities. (A) BI, (B) OI, (C) PI, (D) DI, (E) DI+OI, (F) DI+PI, (G) RI1, (H) RI1+OI, (I) RI1+PI, (J) RI2, (K) RI2+OI, and (L) RI2+PI.

through PI (Fig. 16C). The DI (Fig. 16D) showed an improved contrast of bright microbial colonies from the background, which was dark. Unlike OI, the image appeared more planar in case of DI. Combining DI with OI (Fig. 16E) reduced the image's overall brightness, thus giving microbes poor visibility.

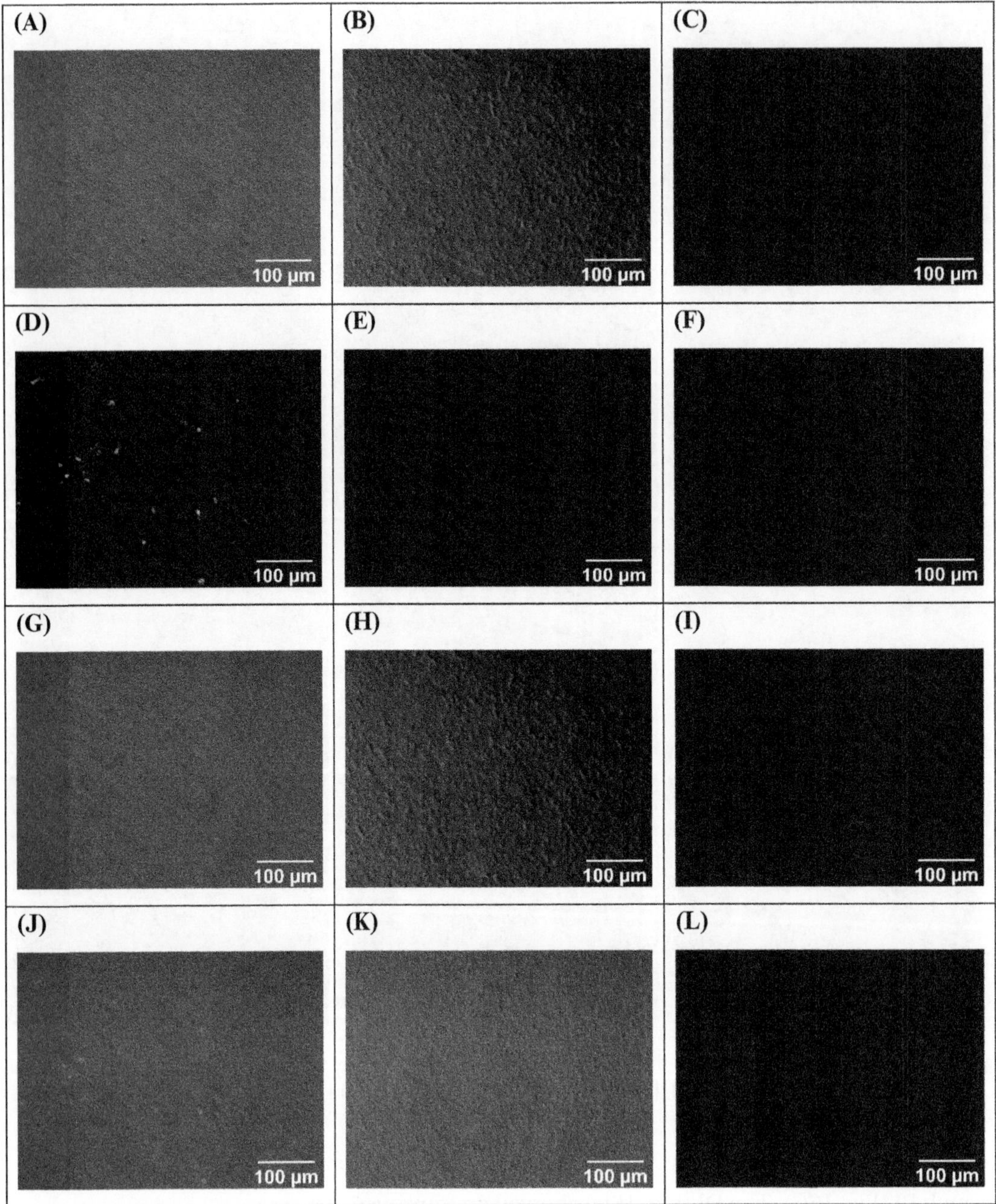

Fig. 16 Resultant magnified images of the wastewater cultured microbes sample taken by the prototype microscope in 12 different imaging modalities. (A) BI, (B) OI, (C) PI, (D) DI, (E) DI+OI, (F) DI+PI, (G) RI1, (H) RI1+OI, (I) RI1+PI, (J) RI2, (K) RI2+OI, and (L) RI2+PI.

Further, RI1 (Fig. 16G) could not create a contrast, suggesting that the combination of filters used in this case was inaccurate for visualizing microbial colonies. Looking at the slide in RI1 +OI (Fig. 16H), visualization of the microbial colony was comparable to the OI. The combination of colors for the RF in RI2 (Fig. 16J) was suitable for visualizing the microbial colonies, wherein the microbial colonies appeared as yellow (annulus color) on a blue background. The microbial colonies did not show any texture. It is to note further that some of the microbial colonies appeared brighter. This observation can be attributed to the increased microbial density of these colonies, which helped them diffract more of the yellow light. Combining it with OI revealed an image of microbial colonies having a 3-dimensional appearance. Imaging modes DI, RI2, and RI2 +OI, were found to contain high contrast differences. These images divulged maximum details about the microbial colonies. OI, DI+OI, and RI1+OI contained sufficient details, but those images' contrast differences and details were inconclusive. Using an even higher magnification objective lens (100×) might present a better picture of the nature of cultured microbes present in the sample.

Lastly, the microscope was tested using the prepared oleogel slide. The resultant images obtained after testing the slide are shown in Fig. 17. The BI (Fig. 17A) of oleogels displayed most but not all fiber-like structures present in the microstructural arrangement of the oleogel [23]. Further, the oleogel under OI (Fig. 17B) showed densely packed thick fibers associated with many thin fibers. Although the fibers tend to display 3D characteristics, the nonuniformity in the illumination is quite evident from the image. An even better microstructural arrangement was confirmed through PI (Fig. 17C) of the oleogel, which displayed needle-like planar fat structures [24]. Few of the amorphous region (marked in orange) was also seen in the image. The DI (Fig. 17D) proved to be very effective as the fibers were visible. The obtained image had a good contrast; however, the image's resolution was further improvised when combined with OI (Fig. 17E). DI+PI (Fig. 17F) reduced the image's overall brightness, making it difficult to visualize the fiber network of fats in the oleogel. Among the two combinations of RF, illumination done by the second combination gave a better idea regarding the fats' microstructural arrangement (Fig. 17J). In this case, the network formed by the gelator molecule appeared yellow over a blue background of oil. RI2+OI (Fig. 17K) was also capable of providing information regarding the network structure with an enhanced resolution.

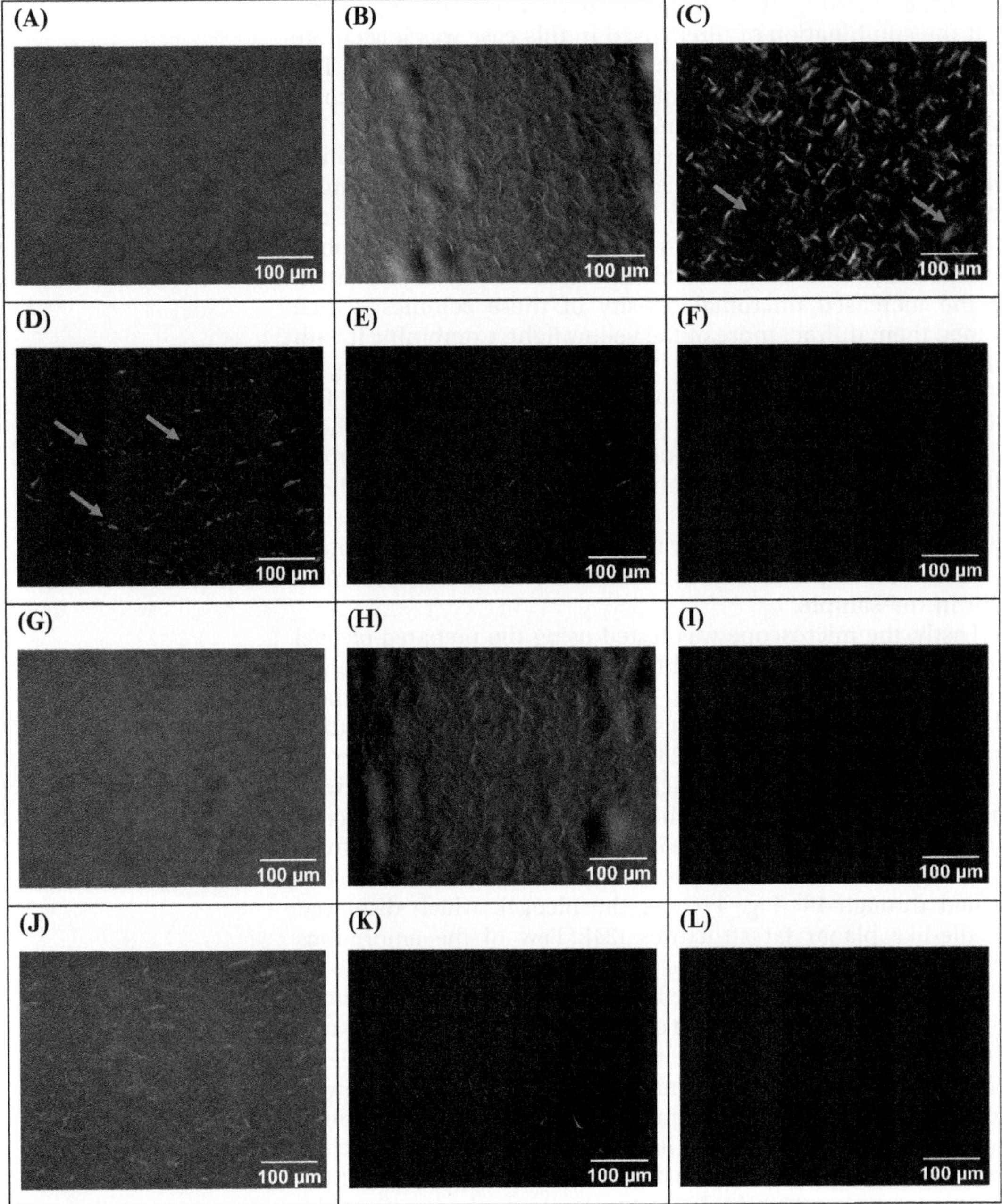

Fig. 17 Magnified images of the freshly prepared oleogel sample taken by the prototype microscope in 12 different imaging modalities. (A) BI, (B) OI, (C) PI, (D) DI, (E) DI + OI, (F) DI + PI, (G) RI1, (H) RI1 + OI, (I) RI1 + PI, (J) RI2, (K) RI2 + OI, and (L) RI2 + PI.

This clearly shows that the microscope's OI, PI, DF, and RI2+OI modes are best suited for visualizing crystal structure and fat networking in oleogel samples.

After testing the prototype microscope using six different samples, it was observed that the microscope could perform digital photomicrography in multiple imaging modalities without any noticeable issues. The overall contrast in final digital images was enhanced significantly in some imaging modalities compared to others. Also, the details present in the obtained images were highlighted quite considerably. The use of DI, RI, OI, and PI modes, either independently or concurrently, could improve the overall contrast and minute details within the microstructures of different types of samples. All these benefits make the prototype microscope an excellent alternative to high-cost laboratory microscopes.

5. Conclusion and future scope

The present study reports the construction and development of a prototype microscope capable of performing high magnification digital imaging in different imaging modalities independently or simultaneously. The developed microscope uses an AmScope microscope eyepiece camera, general-purpose ARM computer (Rasberry Pi) in conjunction with a GUI software application for sample magnification. The movements for focus and sample stage adjustments were achieved with SSMA, FAA, and OLES units. The main advantage of the proposed device is that it can perform imaging in 12 different modes. Several multimodal microscopes have been developed. However, this is the first device covering such a high range of imaging modalities cost-effectively. The use of many imaging modalities will enable the microscope to produce a larger imaging dataset for a sample, which provides the user with more discrete information about the sample. This further aid in making better inferences about the changes that occur in the samples. The acquired image showed overall contrast enhancement and highlighted details in some imaging modalities than others. The performance of the microscope was more than satisfactory. Since the components used in the proposed system are modular and user-replaceable, it provides a better possibility for upgradation than other OEM-based microscopes. In the future, the device can be integrated with the Internet of Things (IoT) technology so that multiple devices can be connected remotely and store the microscopic images centrally. Also, in the future additional imaging modalities will be incorporated to maximize the capability of the developed microscope.

Acknowledgments

The authors acknowledge the financial support obtained from the project sanctioned by the Department of Science and Technology, Government of India, vide sanction order IDP/MED/03/2017 dated: 13.10.2017. We also acknowledge the information provided in https://www.microbehunter.com/ that helped us in the successful completion of this research.

References

[1] J.C.D. Cruz, R.G. Garcia, M.I.D. Avilledo, J.C.M. Buera, R.V.S. Chan, P.G.T. Espana, Microscopic image analysis and counting of red blood cells and white blood cells in a urine sample, in: Proceedings of the 2019 9th International Conference on Biomedical Engineering and Technology, 2019, pp. 113–118.

[2] C. Aguilar-Avelar, et al., High-throughput automated microscopy of circulating tumor cells, Sci. Rep. 9 (1) (2019) 1–9.

[3] I. Bachelet, J.J. Pollak, D. Levner, Y. Bilu, N. Yorav-Raphael, Apparatus and method for automatic detection of pathogens. Google Patents, 2016.

[4] W.D. Pan, Y. Dong, D. Wu, Classification of malaria-infected cells using deep convolutional neural networks, in: Machine Learning: Advanced Techniques and Emerging Applications, vol. 159, IntechOpen, 2018.

[5] P. Ghosh, D. Bhattacharjee, M. Nasipuri, Blood smear analyzer for white blood cell counting: a hybrid microscopic image analyzing technique, Appl. Soft Comput. 46 (2016) 629–638.

[6] W. Watanabe, R. Maruyama, H. Arimoto, Y. Tamada, Low-cost multimodal microscope using Raspberry Pi, Optik 212 (2020), 164713.

[7] D. Rabha, S. Biswas, N. Chamuah, M. Mandal, P. Nath, Wide-field multimodal microscopic imaging using smartphone, Opt. Lasers Eng. 137 (2021), 106343.

[8] H.R. Kent, J.P. Bacon, Microsco-pi: a novel and inexpensive way of merging biology and IT, Sch. Sci. Rev. 98 (363) (2016) 75–82.

[9] U.A. Gurkan, et al., Miniaturized lensless imaging systems for cell and micro-organism visualization in point-of-care testing, Biotechnol. J. 6 (2) (2011) 138–149.

[10] E.O. Fernandez, et al., Microcontroller-based automated microscope for image recognition of four urine constituents, in: TENCON 2018–2018 IEEE Region 10 Conference, IEEE, 2018, pp. 1689–1694.

[11] W. Gao, et al., The design and application of an automated microscope developed based on deep learning for fungal detection in dermatology, Mycoses 64 (3) (2021) 245–251.

[12] S. Rawat, S. Komatsu, A. Markman, A. Anand, B. Javidi, Compact and field-portable 3D printed shearing digital holographic microscope for automated cell identification, Appl. Opt. 56 (9) (2017) D127–D133.

[13] G.G. Leppard, Evaluation of Electron Microscope Techniques for the Description of Aquatic Colloids, CRC Press, 2019.

[14] S. Pacheco, et al., High resolution, high speed, long working distance, large field of view confocal fluorescence microscope, Sci. Rep. 7 (1) (2017) 1–10.

[15] F. Li, X. Zhang, R. Zhang, X. Qin, Design of an adaptive regulator for an automated microscope stage, in: LIDAR Imaging Detection and Target Recognition 2017, vol. 10605, International Society for Optics and Photonics, 2017, p. 106054F.

[16] N. Sarkar, G. Lee, D. Strathearn, M. Olfat, R.R. Mansour, A multimode single-chip scanning probe microscope for simultaneous topographical and thermal metrology at the nanometer scale, in: 2016 IEEE 29th International Conference on Micro Electro Mechanical Systems (MEMS), IEEE, 2016, pp. 55–58.

[17] D.S. Mehta, S. Tayal, A. Saxena, V. Singh, V.K. Dubey, Field-portable multimodal chip-based fluorescence, bright field and quantitative phase microscopy using smartphone detecting system, in: Optics and Biophotonics in Low-Resource Settings VI, vol. 11230, International Society for Optics and Photonics, 2020, p. 112300A.

[18] B. Dong, et al., Isometric multimodal photoacoustic microscopy based on optically transparent micro-ring ultrasonic detection, Optica 2 (2) (2015) 169–176.

[19] V.Y. Shklover, et al., A complex structural study of a particle of lunar regolith by multiscale and multimodal bulk microscopy, J. Anal. Chem. 75 (10) (2020) 1358–1369.

[20] J. Li, et al., Effect of recombinant interleukin-12 on murine skin regeneration and cell dynamics using in vivo multimodal microscopy, Biomed. Optics Express 6 (11) (2015) 4277–4287.

[21] D. Sarkar, S. Prajapati, K. Poddar, A. Sarkar, Production of ethanol by Enterobacter sp. EtK3 during fruit waste biotransformation, Int. Biodeterior. Biodegradation 145 (2019), 104795.

[22] M. Torres-Moreno, E. Torrescasana, J. Salas-Salvadó, C. Blanch, Nutritional composition and fatty acids profile in cocoa beans and chocolates with different geographical origin and processing conditions, Food Chem. 166 (2015) 125–132.

[23] S. Cabrera, J. Rojas, A. Moreno, Oleogels and their contribution in the production of healthier food products: the fats of the future, J. Food Nutr. Res. 8 (2020) 172–182.

[24] A.I. Blake, E.D. Co, A.G. Marangoni, Structure and physical properties of plant wax crystal networks and their relationship to oil binding capacity, J. Am. Oil Chem. Soc. 91 (6) (2014) 885–903.

Index

Note: Page numbers followed by *f* indicate figures, *t* indicate tables and *b* indicate boxes.

CPI Antony Rowe
Eastbourne, UK
September 04, 2023